W9-ARQ-922

QUICK CONSULT® GUIDE: PRIMARY CARE AND EMERGENCY MEDICINE

YEAR 2003 UPDATE
1ST EDITION

Community-Acquired Pneumonia • Urinary Tract Infection • Bacterial Infection of the Respiratory Tract • Acute Coronary Syndromes

Project Editor-in-Chief: **Gideon Bosker, MD, FACEP,** Assistant Clinical Professor, Section of Emergency Services, Yale University School of Medicine; Associate Clinical Professor, Oregon Health Sciences University; Editor-in-Chief, *Clinical Consensus Reports.*

Associate Editor: **Gregory A. Volturo, MD, FACEP,** Vice Chairman and Associate Professor, Department of Emergency Medicine, University of Massachusetts Medical School, Worcester, Massachusetts.

© 2003 American Health Consultants®
3525 Piedmont Road, Northeast,
Six Piedmont Center, Suite 400, Atlanta, GA 30305.
(404) 262-7436 or (800) 688-2421

Editor-in-Chief: Gideon Bosker, MD, FACEP
Vice President/Sponsored Education Programs: Milo Falcon
Senior Managing Editor: Suzanne Zunic
Cover Design: Mark Gulledge, Jeff Dannels

ISBN# 1-931107-20-3

Opinions expressed are not necessarily those of this publication. Mention of products or services does not constitute endorsement. Clinical, legal, tax and other comments are offered for general guidance only; professional counsel should be sought for specific situations.

Note: The indications for and dosages of medications recommended conform to practices at the time of publication of each chapter. References to specific products are incorporated to serve only as guidelines; they are not meant to exclude a practitioner's choice of other, comparable drugs. Every attempt was made to ensure accuracy and appropriateness.

CME Accreditation

American Health Consultants is accredited by the Accreditation Council for Continuing Medical Education (ACCME) to provide continuing medical education for physicians.

American Health Consultants designates this continuing medical education activity for up to 16 hours in category 1 credit toward the AMA Physician's Recognition Award. Each physician should claim only those hours of credit that he/she actually spent in the educational activity.

This CME activity was planned and produced in accordance with the ACCME Essentials.

CME Objectives

After completing the program, physicians will be able to:

a. Understand the epidemiology, etiology, pathophysiology, and clinical features of specific conditions

b. Apply state-of-the-art therapeutic techniques (including the implications of pharmaceutical therapy discussed) to patients with specific conditions

c. Understand the differential diagnosis of entities discussed

d. Understand both likely and rare complications that may occur

Conflict of Interest Disclosure

In order to reveal potential bias in this publication, and in accordance with Accreditation Council for Continuing Education guidelines, physicians have reported the following relationships with companies related to the field of study covered by this CME program. We disclose that Dr. Bosker (project editor) is on the speaker's bureau for Pfizer and Aventis. Dr. Bosker also acknowledges that he receives royalties, commissions, and other compensation relating to the sale of symposia, textbooks, reprints of articles, and other written materials from the following pharmaceutical companies: Pfizer, Genentech, Aventis, Pharmacia, Roche, and Bayer. Dr. Volturo (associate editor) is affiliated with grants/research support for Roche Pharmaceuticals, is a consultant for Pfizer and Aventis, and receives honorarium from Roche and Pfizer.

QUICK CONSULT GUIDE

Quick Consult® Guide: Emergency and Primary Acute Care Medicine
is published by American Health Consultants,
publishers of:

Critical Care Alert®
Emergency Medicine Reports®
Emergency Medicine Alert®
Internal Medicine Alert®
Drug Utilization Review®
Primary Care Reports®
Clinical Cardiology Alert®
Clinical Consensus Reports®
Hospital Medicine Consensus Reports®
Hospital Pharmacist Consensus Reports®

Charles V. Pollack, MA, MD, FACEP
Chairman, Department of Emergency
  Medicine, Pennsylvania Hospital
Associate Professor of Emergency
  Medicine
University of Pennsylvania School of
  Medicine
Philadelphia, Pennsylvania

Robert Powers, MD, MPH, FACP, FACEP
Chief and Professor, Emergency Medicine
University of Connecticut
School of Medicine
Farmington, Connecticut

David J. Robinson, MD, MS
Research Director and Assistant Professor
Department of Emergency Medicine
The University of Texas Houston Medical Center
Director, Diagnostic Observation Center
Memorial Hermann Hospital
Houston, Texas

Steven G. Rothrock, MD, FACEP, FAAP
Associate Professor of Emergency Medicine
University of Florida College of Medicine,
Department of Emergency Medicine
Orlando Regional Medical Center
Orlando, Florida

Barry H. Rumack, MD
Director, Emeritus
Rocky Mountain Poison and Drug Center
Clinical Professor of Pediatrics
University of Colorado Health Sciences Center
Denver, Colorado

Richard Salluzzo, MD, FACEP
Chief Executive Officer and Chief
  Medical Officer
Conemaugh Health System
Johnstown, Pennsylvania

Sandra M. Schneider, MD
Professor and Chair
Department of Emergency Medicine
University of Rochester School of Medicine
Rochester, New York

John A. Schriver, MD
Chief, Section of Emergency Medicine
Yale University School of Medicine
New Haven, Connecticut

David Sklar, MD, FACEP
Professor and Chair
Department of Emergency Medicine
University of New Mexico School of Medicine
Albuquerque, New Mexico

Corey M. Slovis, MD, FACP, FACEP
Professor and Chairman
Department of Emergency Medicine
Vanderbilt University School of Medicine,
Medical Director
Metro Nashville EMS
Nashville, Tennessee

J. Stephan Stapczynski, MD
Professor and Chairman
Department of Emergency Medicine
University of Kentucky Medical Center
Lexington, Kentucky

Charles E. Stewart, MD, FACEP
Emergency Physician
Colorado Springs, Colorado

David A. Talan, MD, FACEP
Chairman and Professor of Medicine
UCLA School of Medicine
Department of Emergency Medicine
Olive View/UCLA Medical Center
Los Angeles, California

Gregory A. Volturo, MD, FACEP
Vice Chairman and Associate Professor
Department of Emergency Medicine
University of Massachusetts Medical School
Worcester, Massachusetts

Albert C. Weihl, MD
Program Director
Emergency Medicine Residency
Assistant Professor of Medicine and Surgery
Department of Surgery
Section of Emergency Medicine
Yale University School of Medicine
New Haven, Connecticut

Steven M. Winograd, MD, FACEP
Attending Physician
Department of Emergency Medicine
Jeannette District Memorial Hospital
Jeannette, Pennsylvania;
St. Clair Memorial Hospital
Pittsburgh, Pennsylvania
University of Pittsburgh Medical Center

Allan B. Wolfson, MD, FACEP, FACP
Program Director,
Affiliated Residency in Emergency Medicine
Professor of Emergency Medicine
University of Pittsburgh
Pittsburgh, Pennsylvania

TABLE OF CONTENTS

GLOSSARY OF TERMS

ABM	Acute Bacterial Meningitis
ACEIs	Angiotensin-converting Enzyme Inhibitors
ACS	Acute Coronary Syndromes
AECOPD	Acute Exacerbation of Chronic Obstructive Pulmonary Disease
AMI	Acute Myocardial Infarction
aPTT	Activated Partial Thromboplastin Time
ARB	Angiotensin Receptor Blocker
ARS	Acute Retroviral Syndrome
CAD	Coronary Artery Disease
CAP	Community-Acquired Pneumonia
CHF	Congestive Heart Failure
CSF	Cerebrospinal Fluid
DM	Diabetes Mellitus
DVT	Deep Vein Thrombosis
GCSE	Generalized Convulsive Status Epilepticus
GP	Glycoprotein
HF	Heart Failure
HIV	Human Immunodeficiency Virus
ICP	Intracranial Pressure
IDSA	Infectious Disease Society of America
INR	International Normalized Ratio
IOTT	Intensification of Treatment Trigger
LFT	Liver Function Test
LMA	Laryngeal Mask Airway
LMWH	Low Molecular Weight Heparin
LP	Lumbar Puncture
MI	Myocardial Infarction
NNRTI	Non-Nucleoside Reverse Transcriptase Inhibitor
Non-Q MI	Non-Q wave Myocardial Infarction
NRTI	Nucleoside Reverse Transcriptase Inhibitor
NSAIDs	Non-steroidal Anti-inflammatory Drugs
NSTEMI	Non-ST Elevation Myocardial Infarction
PCI	Procedural Coronary Intervention
PEP	Post-exposure Prophylaxis
PI	Protease Inhibitor
PMN	Polymorphonuclear Leukocytes
PPPD	Prescription, Parent, Patient, Drug resistance

PT	Prothrombin (time)
PTCA	Percutaneous Transluminal Coronary Angioplasty
PTT	Partial Thromboplastin Time
SE	Status Epilepticus
SERF	Severity of Exacerbation and Risk Factor
SGPT	Serum Glutamic-pyruvic Transaminase
SLE	Systemic Lupus Erythematosus
STDs	Sexually Transmitted Diseases
STSS	Streptococcal Toxic Shock-like Syndrome
TIA	Transient Ischemic Attack
t-PA	Tissue-type Plasminogen Activator
UA	Unstable Angina
UFH	Unfractionated Heparin
UTI	Urinary Tract Infection
WBC	White Blood Cell

COMMONLY USED EQUATIONS

Alveolar Gas Equation

$$PaO_2 = FIO_2 (PB - P H2O) - \frac{PaCO_2}{R}$$

PB = Barometric Pressure (760 mm at Sea Level)
$P H_2O$ = Partial pressure of water (47 mm at sea level)
R = Respiratory Quotient (0.8 = normal)

At sea level
$PaO_2 = FIO2 \times (713) - PaCO_2/ 0.8$ or
$PaO_2 = 150 - PaCO_2/ 0.8$ (on room air at Sea Level)

Alveolar - Arterial Oxygen gradient

$$PaO_2 - PAO_2$$ Normal = 13-16 if < than 30

Blood Gas pH changes

PCO_2 increase of 10 corresponds to a pH drop of 0.08
pH drop of 0.15 corresponds to a base excess decrease of 10 meq/l

Mean Arterial Pressure

$$MAP = (1/3) (SBP - DBP) + DBP$$ Normal = 70-105

Creatinine Clearance

$$(ml /min) = \frac{(140 - Age)\ (Wt\ in\ kg)}{72 \times Serum\ Creatinine\ (mg / dl)}$$

$$= \frac{Urine\ Creatinine\ (gm/ day)}{Serum\ Creatinine\ (mg/ dl)} \times 70$$

Normal > 100 ml/ min

Fractional Excretion of Sodium
FE Na = {urine Na x serum creatinine / serum Na x urine creatinine }x 100

Hyponatremia - Calculated Na deficit
Na deficit (meq) = 0.6 (wt. in Kg) (140 - Na) + (140) (volume deficit in liters)

Hypernatremia - Calculated water deficit
Water deficit = 0.6 (wt. in Kg) x ({Na / 140} - 1)

Anion gap
Anion gap = Na - (CL + HCO_3)   Normal = < 8-12

Estimated Serum Osmolality
Estimated Serum Osmolality = 2 (Na) + $\frac{glucose}{18}$ + $\frac{BUN}{2.8}$ + $\frac{ETOH}{4.6}$

Normal @ 290 mOsm/ kg H2O

Osmolal Gap
Osmolal gap = Osm (measured - (Osm calculated)

Corrected Calcium
Corrected CA++ = measured Ca++/ $\frac{(0.6 + total\ protein)}{8.5}$

Body Mass Index
BM = $\frac{W\ in\ kg}{Ht\ in\ km}$ x Height in meters

Temperature Conversion
Temperature F = Temperature C° x (1.8) + 32
Temperature C = Temperature F° -32 /1.8

CLINICAL MONOGRAPHS

Community-Acquired Pneumonia (CAP)—Antibiotic Selection and Outcome Effective Management

Year 2003 ASCAP (Antibiotic Selection for Community-Acquired Pneumonia) Panel Report

INTRODUCTION

The therapeutic landscape for managing patients with community-acquired pneumonia (CAP) continues to shift, especially as new clinical trials, surveillance studies, and epidemiological data are factored into a complex management equation that is designed to cure CAP patients today and protect the community against accelerating drug resistance tomorrow. In this regard, a number of therapy-altering advances, process-of-care changes, and triage refinements have emerged in the area of CAP management over the past year.

Among the important new developments and reports evaluated by the ASCAP (Antibiotic Selection for CAP) Clinical Consensus Panel is the growing awareness and reporting of levofloxacin-resistant respiratory isolates of *S. pneumoniae,* including documented treatment failures; the importance of the emergency department (ED) as the clinical "hot zone" for diagnosing, assessing, and treating patients with CAP; the mounting evidence favoring combination ceftriaxone/azithromycin therapy for severely ill patients with bacteremic pneumococcal pneumonia; and the association between levofloxacin use and the emergence of resistance among both gram-negative organisms and methicillin-resistant *Staphylococcus aureus* (MRSA). *(See Table 1).*

In addition, increasing emphasis has been placed on prompt administration (i.e., within 4 hours of presentation) of antibiotics in patients in whom the diagnosis of CAP is strongly suspected or confirmed, and on the potential in-hospital drug administration delays and compliance-compromising errors associated with antibiotics requiring multiple daily doses. Resistance-induction studies and sensitivity surveillance data have highlighted the potential advantages of moxifloxacin as compared to levofloxacin for initial CAP therapy in patients in whom advanced generation fluoroquinolones are indicated. It also has been recognized that effecting positive outcomes with potent, excessively broad-spectrum agents must be balanced against the pitfalls of inducing resistance to agents, especially fluoroquinolones, that are currently effective but have a propensity for developing resistance at a disproportionately accelerated rate in respiratory pathogens. Finally, the need to prophylax against development of DVT in hospitalized patients with CAP has become a quality-of-care measure.

The importance of the ED as a clinical zone where process-of-care measures for patients with CAP should be instituted is supported by a recent study linking quality of care and resource utilization.[1] This has been confirmed in an analysis of quality-of-care variables observed in randomly selected cases of CAP.[1] In this study, three quality-of-care measures for CAP were analyzed: 1) site of initial antibiotic treatment (ED vs floor); 2) door-to-needle time; and 3) appropriateness of antibiotic selection. A regression analysis revealed that all three quality-of-care measures were associated with prolonged length of stay (LOS). The implication is that implementation of process-of-care measures in the ED environment can have a positive effect on patient outcome, and in particular length of stay.

The landscape shift in CAP management and antibiotic selection has spawned the concept of curing patients today, while protecting the community tomorrow; that is, identifying pharmacotherapeutic strategies which not only optimize short-term, in-hospital clinical outcomes for CAP—in which curing patients is the preeminent goal—but also achieve this end point while reducing the likelihood of developing drug resistance. Additional resource utilization goals, including reducing length of stay (LOS), eliminating nursing time for drug administration, and minimizing treatment failures and pharmacological reservicing, must be factored into the drug selection equation. The mandate to both cure patients acutely and preserve long-term antimicrobial efficacy represents one of the most important challenges that emergency physicians, hospitalists, other clinicians, pharmacists, formulary managers, and health policy planners face when developing protocols and pathways for in-hospital management of such life-threatening infectious conditions as CAP.

A common cause for admission to the hospital, CAP continues to be a serious, growing health problem in the United States. It has an incidence estimated at 5.6 million cases annually.[2,3] Approximately 1.7 million hospitalizations for CAP are reported each year at an annual cost of about $23 billion.[2,4] The elderly consume the majority of these expenses, account for the majority of CAP-related hospitalizations, and have longer LOS. Mortality rates among the most seriously affected patients with CAP (the majority of whom are in the geriatric age group) approaches 40%, and causative pathogens are identified in fewer than 50% of patients.[5] Accordingly, empiric antibiotic regimens frequently are chosen in hospitalized patients with CAP on the basis of results of clinical trials and expert panel recommendations.

S. pneumoniae is the leading cause of both CAP and bacteremia, which can lead to meningitis. According to the Centers for Disease Control and Prevention (CDC), *S. pneumoniae* infections cause 100,000-135,000 pneumonia-related hospitalizations and more than 60,000 cases of invasive disease each year, including 3300 cases of meningitis. Bacteria resistant to any one antibiotic drug, regardless of class, cause up to 40% of these infections; 15% are due to a bacterial strain that is resistant to three or more drugs.[20]

Despite a general consensus that empiric treatment of CAP requires, at the least, mandatory coverage of such organisms as *Streptococcus pneumoniae, Haemophilus influenzae,* and *Moraxella catarrhalis,* as well as atypical organisms (*Mycoplasma pneumoniae, Chlamydia pneumoniae,* and *Legionella pneumophila),* antibiotic selection strategies for achieving this spectrum of coverage vary widely. To provide physicians and pharmacists current, evidence-supported standards for antimicrobial therapy in CAP, new treatment guidelines have been issued by a number of national panels and/or associations, including the American Thoracic Society Guidelines (2001), Infectious Disease Society of America (IDSA), the ASCAP (Antibiotic Selection for Community-Acquired Pneumonia) Consensus Panel, and the Centers for Disease Control and Prevention's Drug-Resistant *Streptococcus pneumoniae* Therapeutic Working Group (CDC-DRSPWG).

As might be expected, although there are consistencies among expert-endorsed recommendations, there also are variations, with some panels prioritizing one treatment strategy over another. In some cases, panel recommendations lag behind the emergence of new data that would force a reevaluation of current practices. For example, beginning in January 2002, the National Committee on Clinical Laboratory Standards (NCCLS) officially adopted new breakpoint minimum inhibitory concentrations (MICs) for two third generation cephalosporins for non-meningeal sources of *S. pneumoniae*. Stemming from discrepancies between microbiologic failure and clinical cure, the NCCLS reviewed and accepted revised breakpoint MICs for ceftriaxone and cefotaxime. Based on the new microbiologic standards, a drug-resistant *Streptococcus pneumoniae* (DRSP) of non-meningeal sources is defined with a breakpoint MIC of ≥ 4 mcg/mL to cefotaxime or ceftri-axone. The only treatment guidelines that recognized the new NCCLS breakpoints for cefotaxime and ceftriaxone are those published by the CDC-DRSPWG. Nevertheless, the clinical implications of the revised breakpoints already have become widespread, as subsequent treatment guidelines are reevaluating the role of third generation cephalosporins for initial therapy of all inpatients with CAP.

Deciphering the strengths, subtleties, and weaknesses of recommendations issued by different authoritative sources can be problematic and confusing. Because patient disposition practices and treatment pathways vary among insti-tutions and from region to region, management guidelines for CAP patient must be "customized" for the local practice environment. Unfortunately, no single set of guidelines is applicable to every patient or practice setting; therefore, clinical judgment must prevail. This means taking into account local antibiotic resistance patterns, epidemiological and infection incidence data, and patient demographic features.

It also is becoming clear that outcomes in patients with CAP can be maxi-mized by using risk-stratification criteria that predict mortality in various patient subgroups. Associated clinical findings such as hypotension, tachypnea, impaired oxygen saturation, multi-lobar involvement, elevated blood urea nitrogen, and altered level of consciousness are predictive of more serious disease, as are age and acquisition of CAP in a nursing home environment. These factors may assist clinicians in initial selection of intravenous antibiotic therapy for hospitalized patients.

With these considerations in clear focus, this landmark review presents a comprehensive, state-of-the-art assessment of diagnostic strategies and antimicrobial guidelines for management of patients with CAP. Special emphasis has been given to both epidemiological data demonstrating the importance of correct spectrum coverage with specific cephalosporins (ceftriaxone, Rocephin®) in combination with a macrolide (azithromycin, Zithromax®) or monotherapy with a fluoroquinolone, as well as the selection of initial intravenous antibiotics for in-hospital management of CAP. In addition to antibiotic therapy, comprehensive management of the patient with CAP includes not only supportive respiratory and hemodynamic measures, but also risk-stratifying patients according to the Fine Pneumonia Severity Index (PSI). The ASCAP Consensus Panel has addressed the need to provide prophylaxis against venous thromboembolism (VTE) with enoxaparin in hospitalized patients with pneumonia with or without such comorbid conditions as congestive heart failure (CHF) and/or respiratory failure.

A detailed analysis and comparison of two-drug (ceftriaxone plus a macrolide) approaches vs. monotherapeutic options (azithromycin or advanced generation fluoroquinolones [moxifloxacin, levofloxacin, gatifloxacin]) are provided. In this regard, although one national association (2001 American Thoracic Society Guidelines) has proposed the option of intravenous monotherapy with a macrolide for inpatient management of CAP in selected, younger patients without co-morbidity, most experts and national panels agree that monotherapy with IV azithromycin is not advisable for inpatients with CAP. Hospitalized patients are at sufficiently high risk for CAP-related morbidity, complications, and mortality to require combination therapy that includes a cephalosporin (i.e., ceftriaxone, cefotaxime, etc.) with significant activity against *S. pneumoniae, H. influenzae,* and *M. catarrhalis,* along with a macrolide to provide activity against atypical organisms. One recent study suggests that CAP patient outcomes in those with bacteremic, pneumococcal pneumonia may be improved with two-drug, combination regimens as compared to monotherapeutic approaches using fluoroquinolones or other agents.[21] Additionally, increasing rates of macrolide-resistant *S. pneumoniae* may warrant avoiding monotherapy in the inpatient setting with this class of antibiotics. Detailed discussions of this important controversy and practical antibiotic selection implications of the year 2002 NCCLS breakpoints are presented to

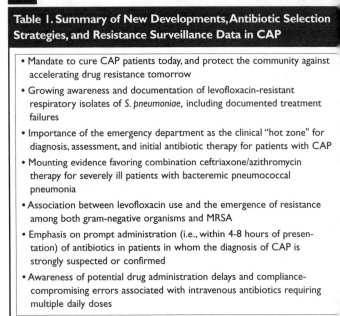

Table 1. Summary of New Developments, Antibiotic Selection Strategies, and Resistance Surveillance Data in CAP

- Mandate to cure CAP patients today, and protect the community against accelerating drug resistance tomorrow

- Growing awareness and documentation of levofloxacin-resistant respiratory isolates of *S. pneumoniae,* including documented treatment failures

- Importance of the emergency department as the clinical "hot zone" for diagnosis, assessment, and initial antibiotic therapy for patients with CAP

- Mounting evidence favoring combination ceftriaxone/azithromycin therapy for severely ill patients with bacteremic pneumococcal pneumonia

- Association between levofloxacin use and the emergence of resistance among both gram-negative organisms and MRSA

- Emphasis on prompt administration (i.e., within 4-8 hours of presentation) of antibiotics in patients in whom the diagnosis of CAP is strongly suspected or confirmed

- Awareness of potential drug administration delays and compliance-compromising errors associated with intravenous antibiotics requiring multiple daily doses

provide evidence-based guidance in the area of empiric drug selection for CAP.

Finally, to ensure that clinicians are current with and can apply the latest evidence-based strategies for CAP treatment to their patient populations, detailed antibiotic selection guidelines (see Table 2) issued by the ASCAP Consensus Panel are provided. Drawing upon clinical trials, epidemiological data, and other association guidelines, these antimicrobial protocols are linked to risk-stratification criteria and specific clinical profiles of patients presenting to the hospital or acute ambulatory setting with CAP.

INTRODUCTION: THE ASCAP (ANTIBIOTIC SELECTION FOR CAP) 2003 CONSENSUS PANEL AND SCIENTIFIC ROUNDTABLE

To address the complex issues surrounding antibiotic selection and care of

- Resistance-induction studies and sensitivity surveillance data favoring ceftriaxone as cephalosporin of choice
- The need to prophylax against the development of deep venous thrombosis and the efficacy of enoxaparin for this patient subgroup
- The importance of the emergency department as a clinical zone where process-of-care measures for patients with CAP should be instituted
- Differentiating among advanced generation fluoroquinolones and identifying moxifloxacin as preferred agent within this class
- Emphasis on achieving resource utilization goals, including decrease in length of stay (LOS), reducing unnecesary nursing time for drug administration, and minimizing treatment failures
- Endorsement of the mandate to both cure patients acutely and preserve long-term antimicrobial efficacy
- Use of expert-endorsed CAP guidelines to ensure outcome-effective, best practice strategies

the hospitalized patient with pneumonia, the ASCAP Year 2003 Consensus Panel and Scientific Roundtable was convened. Its mission statement was to review, analyze, and interpret published, evidence-based trials assessing the safety and efficacy of antibiotic therapy for CAP. In addition, the ASCAP Consensus Panel was charged with both developing strategies that would ensure appropriate use of antibiotics in this population and making recommendations for how patients with respiratory infections should be evaluated and managed in the inpatient setting.

Treatment guidelines generated by the ASCAP 2003 Consensus Panel are reported in this consensus statement. They are based on evidence presented in well-designed clinical trials, and focus on hospital management delivered by the emergency physician, hospitalist, internist, critical care specialist, and/or infectious disease specialist. Detailed review and analyses of national consensus guidelines issued by the American Thoracic Society (ATS), Infectious Disease Society of

America (IDSA), CDC Drug-Resistant *Streptococcus pneumoniae* Working Group
(CDC-DRSPWG), and the Year 2002 Antibiotic Selection in Community-Acquired
Pneumonia (ASCAP) Consensus Panel also were evaluated and included in the
decision-making process. *(See Tables 3 and 4.)*

With these objectives in clear focus, the purpose of this comprehensive
review, which includes the ASCAP 2003 Consensus Panel report on assessment
strategies and treatment recommendations, is to provide an evidence-based, state-
of-the-art clinical resource outlining, in precise and practical detail, clinical protocols for the acute management of CAP. To achieve this goal, all of the critical
aspects entering into the equation for maximizing patient outcomes, while minimizing costs—including systematic patient evaluation, disposition decision trees,
and outcome-effective antibiotic therapy—will be discussed in detail. In addition, because appropriate disposition of patients with CAP has become essential
for cost-effective patient management, this review includes critical pathways and
treatment tables that incorporate risk stratification tools that can be used to identify and distinguish those patient subgroups that are appropriately managed in the
outpatient setting from those more appropriately admitted to the hospital for
more intensive care.

COMMUNITY-ACQUIRED PNEUMONIA: EPIDEMIOLOGY, DIAGNOSIS, AND EVALUATION

CAP affects 5.6 million adults annually in the United States, with 1.7 million
patients requiring hospitalization.[22] It is the sixth leading cause of death overall
and the most common cause of death from infection,[22,23] with an overall case-
fatality rate of about 5%. Mortality is substantially greater (about 13.6%) among
hospitalized patients.[24] Expert committees have published treatment guidelines
intended to improve the care of pneumonia patients, but the guidelines have not
been prospectively validated.[6,25] Prior studies of pneumonia guidelines have
reported decreased lengths of stay, admission rates, and costs, but no change in
clinical outcomes.[7,26,27] Expert endorsed guidelines are difficult to implement,
and traditional continuing medical education has an incomplete effect on physician practice.[28-33] However, studies by Dean and others[115] indicate that adoption
of institutional pathways for CAP management have an effect on mortality and

outcome (see below: Treatment Guidelines for CAP Outcomes, Value, and Institutional Implementation).

The introduction of antibiotic agents dramatically reduced mortality from pneumococcal pneumonia. However, the mortality rate from bacteremic pneumococcal CAP has shown little improvement in the past three decades, remaining between 19% and 28% depending on the population and institution studied. The aging population, increased prevalence of comorbid illnesses, human immunodeficiency virus, and increasing microbial resistance probably all have contributed to maintaining the high mortality rate despite advances in medical care. However, even allowing that some patients are seen too late to benefit from the antibiotic therapy, the continued high mortality rate, despite apparently appropriate antibiotic therapy, is a cause for concern.

The annual incidence of pneumonia in patients older than age 65 is about 1%.[8] The typical presentation of pneumococcal pneumonia with fever, rigors, shortness of breath, chest pain, sputum production, and abnormal lung sounds is easy to recognize. Unfortunately, the changing epidemiology of pneumonia presents a greater diagnostic challenge, especially in the aging patient. Atypical agents or opportunistic infections in immunocompromised individuals have a much more subtle presentation. In particular, pneumonia in older patients frequently has an insidious presentation and fewer characteristic features of pneumonia, which may be confused with CHF or respiratory compromise associated with chronic lung disease.

The definitive, etiologic diagnosis of pneumonia is verified by the recovery of a pathogenic organism(s) from either the blood, sputum, or pleural fluid in the setting of a patient with a radiographic abnormality suggestive of pneumonia. In the case of atypical organisms, the diagnosis usually is made by the comparison of acute and convalescent sera demonstrating a rise in appropriate titers, or by other sophisticated techniques such as direct florescent antibody testing. A gram stain is occasionally helpful with establishing the diagnosis, but requires practitioners or technicians who are highly skilled in this diagnostic methodology. An adequate gram stain must have fewer than 25 epithelial cells per low-powered field. The finding of more than 10 gram-positive, lancet-shaped diplococci in a high-powered field is a sensitive and specific predictor of pneumococcal pneu-

Table 2. Year 2003 ASCAP (Antibiotic Selection for Community-Acquired Pneumonia) Guidelines

PATIENT PROFILE/ETIOLOGIC AGENTS

Otherwise Healthy
< 60 years of age (Patients deemed to be
suitable for outpatient/oral therapy, i.e., no
systemic toxicity, high likelihood of compliance,
and supportive home environment)*

Otherwise Healthy
> 60 years of age (Patients deemed to be
suitable for outpatient/oral therapy, i.e., no
systemic toxicity, high likelihood of compliance,
and supportive home environment)*

In-Hospital (not in intensive care unit)
underlying risk factors or comorbid conditions:
In-Hospital management (COPD,
history of pneumonia, diabetes, etc.)

CAP acquired in the nursing home environment
(increased likelihood of gram-negative, *E. coli,
Klebsiella pneumoniae*)

CAP in the elderly individual with chronic alcoholism
(Increased likelihood of *Klebsiella pneumonige* infection)

Severe bacteremic CAP with documented
***S. pneumoniae* species showing high-level**
resistance to macrolides and/or penicillin, but
maintaining high sensitivity to extended
spectrum quinolones and cephalosporins

Severe CAP complicated by structural disease
of the lung (bronchiectasis): Increased
likelihood of *Pseudomonas* and polymicrobial
infection

FIRST-LINE ANTIBIOTIC THERAPY[†]	ALTERNATIVE FIRST-LINE ANTIBIOTIC THERAPY
Azithromycin PO	Moxifloxacin PO (preferred) *OR* Levofloxacin PO *OR* Clarithromycin *OR* Gatifloxacin PO
Azithromycin PO *OR* Moxifloxacin PO	Levofloxacin PO *OR* Clarithromycin *OR* Gatifloxacin PO
Ceftriaxone IV[D] plus azithromycin IV[†††]	Moxifloxacin (preferred) *OR* Levofloxacin IV *OR* Gatifloxacin IV
Ceftriaxone IV plus azithromycin IV	Moxifloxacin (preferred) *OR* Levofloxacin IV *OR* Gatifloxacin IV
Ceftriaxone IV plus azithromycin IV	Levofloxacin IV *OR* Cefepime IV plus azithromycin IV
Ceftriaxone IV plus moxifloxacin	Vancomycin[¶] plus azithromycin IV *OR* Ceftriaxone IV plus levofloxacin IV
Cefepime IV plus levofloxacin IV plus/minus aminoglycoside *OR* Ciprofloxacin IV plus amino-glycoside IV plus azithromycin IV	Ciprofloxacin IV plus cefepime IV plus azithromycin IV *OR* Carbapenem IV plus azithromycin IV plus aminoglycoside

Table continued on next page

Table 2. Year 2003 ASCAP (Antibiotic Selection for Community-Acquired Pneumonia) Guidelines *(continued)*

CAP in a patient with suspected aspiration
(increases the likelihood of gram-negative
and anaerobic infection**)

Severe CAP in a compromised host with a
previous hospitalization for, or who resides in
a community or facility with a high reported
incidence of methicillin-resistant *S. aureus* (MRSA)***

**CAP patient with severe pneumonia
requiring ICU hospitalization***

* Oral therapy/outpatient treatment recommendations are appropriate
only for those otherwise healthy patients with CAP of mild enough severity
that they are judged to be suitable candidates for outpatient management
with oral antibiotics.

§ Quinolones are restricted for use in patients > 18 years of age.

¶ If *S. pneumoniae* demonstrates complete resistance to extended spectrum
quinolones (very rare), third-generation cephalosporins, and macrolides,
then vancomycin may be required as part of initial therapy, although this
would be necessary only in rare circumstances.

† First-line therapy recommendations take into consideration cost of the
drug (which may vary from one institution to another), convenience of dosing, daily dose frequency, spectrum of coverage, side effects, and risk of
drug-drug interactions.

††† Some institutions may use oral macrolide therapy for patients with mild-
to-moderate CAP.

** When anaerobic organisms are suspected as one of the possible etiolog-
ic pathogens in a patient with CAP, clindamycin or a β-lactam/β-lactamase
inhibitor (ampicillin/sulbactam, tricarcillin/clavulanate, or pipercillin/tazobac-
tam) is recommended.

Ceftriaxone IV plus azithromycin IV plus clindamycin IV	Levofloxacin IV plus clindamycin IV OR Levofloxacin IV plus metronidazole IV OR Gatifloxacin IV plus clindamycin IV
Moxifloxacin IV plus vancomycin IV	Levofloxacin IV plus vancomycin IV
Ceftriaxone IV plus levofloxacin IV plus/minus aminoglycoside (Pseudomonas strongly suspected) OR Ceftriaxone IV plus moxifloxacin IV plus/minus anti-pseudomonal agent	Ceftriaxone IV plus azithromycin IV plus/minus anti-pseudomonal agent OR Cefepime IV plus aminoglycoside IV plus moxifloxacin IV OR Carbepenem IV plus aminoglycoside IV plus azithromycin IV

[D]Cefotaxime may be used as an alternative to ceftriaxone, although it should be noted that Year 2002 NCCLS breakpoints for cefotaxime apply ONLY when this antibiotic is dosed on a q 8 hr basis and considerations regarding in-hospital medication administration/compliance must be considered when making such a substitution. In addition, consistently greater susceptibilities by one tube or more have been observed for ceftriaxone vs. cefotaxime in the ARM (Antibiotic Resistance Management) database, which support use of ceftriaxone as the agent of choice for co-therapy with a macrolide for CAP, although comparative clinical outcome data is still lacking.

*** High community prevalence of, previous history of hospitalization, or increasing local incidence of methicillin-resistant S. aureus (MRSA) in a patient with a clinical presentation consistent with S. aureus pneumonia; vancomycin should be considered as component for initial therapy.

‡ Adapted from references 3,4, 6-19

§§ Cefotaxime may be substituted for ceftriaxone, although ceftriaxone is preferred because of its once-daily dosing.

Table 3. IDSA — Year 2000 Guidelines. Empirical Selection of Antimicrobial Agents for Treating Patients with CAP

Outpatients

- Generally preferred are (not in any particular order): doxycycline, a macrolide, or a fluoroquinolone
- Selection considerations
- These agents have activity against the most likely pathogens in this setting, which include *Streptococcus pneumoniae*, *Mycoplasma pneumoniae*, and *Chlamydia pneumoniae*
- Selection should be influenced by regional antibiotic susceptibility patterns for *S. pneumoniae* and the presence of other risk factors for drug-resistant *S. pneumoniae*
- Penicillin-resistant pneumococci may be resistant to macrolides and/or doxycycline
- For older patients or those with underlying disease, a fluoroquinolone may be a preferred choice; some authorities prefer to reserve fluoroquinolones for such patients

Hospitalized Patients

- General medical ward
- Generally preferred are: an extended-spectrum cephalosporin combined with a macrolide or a β-lactam/β-lactamase inhibitor combined with a macrolide or a fluoroquinolone (alone)

monia. Unfortunately, gram stain rarely is helpful with determining other causes of pneumonia. The IDSA Guidelines recommend gram stain, whereas the ATS considers gram stain optional.

Transtracheal aspiration or bronchial washings are a more accurate means of obtaining specimens for gram stain and culture, although this procedure rarely is indicated in the outpatient setting. Overall, fewer than 50% of patients with CAP will be able to produce sputum. Of these, one-half of the sputum specimens obtained will be inadequate. When an adequate gram stain is obtained, however, it has a negative predictive value of 80% when compared to a sputum culture. The blood culture is helpful in about 15% of patients, while serology will establish the diagnosis in 25% of patients.[6,8] About 40% of sputum cultures will identify a patho-

Intensive Care Unit

- Generally preferred are: an extended-spectrum cephalosporin or β-lactam/β-lactamase inhibitor plus either a fluoroquinolone or macrolide
- Alternatives or modifying factors
- Structural lung disease: antipseudomonal agents (piperacillin, piperacillin-tazobactam, carbapenem, or cefepime) plus a fluoroquinolone (including high-dose ciprofloxacin)
- β-lactam allergy: fluoroquinolone ± clindamycin
- Suspected aspiration: fluoroquinolone with or without clindamycin, metronidazole, or a β-lactam/β-lactamase inhibitor

Note: β-lactam/β-lactamase inhibitor: ampicillin-sulbactam or piperacillin-tazobactam. Extended-spectrum cephalosporin: cefotaxime or ceftriaxone. Fluoroquinolone: gatifloxacin, levofloxacin, moxifloxacin, or other fluoro-quinolone with enhanced activity against *S. pneumoniae* (for aspiration pneumonia, some fluoroquinolones show in vitro activity against anaero-bic pulmonary pathogens, although there are no clinical studies to verify in vivo). Macrolide: azithromycin, clarithromycin, or erythromycin ± with or without.

logic organism. Bronchoscopy and thoracentesis occasionally may be necessary, but these procedures generally are reserved for seriously ill patients, particularly those who require management in the intensive care unit (ICU).[4,6,9] While the above statistics note the occasional times that a gram stain or blood culture are use-ful, in most cases patients may be adequately managed without these studies. The treatment of CAP is almost always empiric.

Differential Diagnosis. Especially in the elderly patient, the signs and symp-toms of pneumonia may be mimicked by many disorders, including pulmonary embolism (PE), CHF, lung cancer, hypersensitivity pneumonitis, tuberculosis, chronic obstructive pulmonary disease (COPD), granulomatosis disease, and fungal infections. A variety of drugs also can induce pulmonary disease.

Table 4. Recommended Year 2000 CDC DRSP-WG Empiric Regimens for Treating Community-Acquired Pneumonia*

Empiric treatment**	Penicillin ≤ 0.06	Penicillin 0.12-1
Outpatients		
Macrolide (erythromycin, clarithromycin, or azithromycin)	+++	+
Doxycycline (or tetracycline)	+++	++
Oral β-lactam (cefuroxime axetil, amoxicillin, or amoxicillin-clavulanate potassium)	+++	++
Fluoroquinolones (levofloxacin, moxifloxacin, or gatifloxacin)†	+++	+++
Hospitalized (Nonintensive		
Parenteral β-lactam (cefuroxime, cefotaxime sodium, ceftriaxone sodium, or ampicillin sodium-sulbactam sodium) plus macrolide (erythromycin, clarithromycin, or azithromycin)	+++	+++
Fluoroquinolones (e.g., moxifloxacin, levofloxacin, gatifloxacin, or trovafloxacin)†	+++	+++
Intubated or		
Intravenous β-lactam (ceftriaxone or cefotaxime) plus intravenous macrolide (erythromycin or azithromycin)	+++	+++
Intravenous β-lactam (ceftriaxone or cefotaxime) plus fluoroquinolone (e.g., gatifloxacin, levofloxacin, moxifloxacin, or trovafloxacin)†	+++	+++
Fluoroquinolones (e.g., moxifloxacin, levofloxacin, gatifloxacin, or trovafloxacin)†	++	++

MIC mcg/mL			
2	**4**	**≥ 8**	**Comments**
±	-	-	Covers atypical pathogens (*Mycoplasma* spp, *Chlamydia* spp, and *Legionella* spp)
+	-	-	Covers atypical pathogens; not FDA-approved for children younger than 8 years
+	-	-	Does not cover atypical pathogens, alternatively cefpodoxime or cefprozil may be used
+++	++	++	Not first-line treatment because of concerns about emerging resistance; not FDA-approved for use in children; covers atypical pathogens
Care Unit) Patients			
++	±	-	Ceftriaxone and cefotaxime have superior activity against resistant pneumococci in comparison with ampicillin-sulbactam and with cefuroxime.
+++	++	++	See previous comments about fluoroquinolones.
Intensive Care Unit Patients‡			
++	±	-	Ceftriaxone or cefotaxime are preferred over other β-lactams because of their superior activity against resistant pneumococci; clarithromycin has no intravenous formulation.
++	++	++	Ceftriaxone or cefotaxime are preferred over other β-lactams; see previous comments about fluoroquinolones.
++	++	++	See previous comments about fluoroquinolones; efficacy of monotherapy for critically ill persons with pneumococcal pneumonia has not been established.

Table continued on next page

Table 4. Recommended Year 2000 CDC DRSP-WG Empiric Regimens for Treating CAP* (continued)

Key:

† The relative antipneumococcal activity of these agents differs slightly, with that of trovafloxacin equal or superior to that of grepafloxacin, which equals that of sparfloxacin, which is superior to that of levofloxacin. Because of new data showing an association with serious liver damage, the FDA issued a public health advisory recommending that trovafloxacin be used only for patients with serious and life- or limb-threatening infections who receive initial treatment in an inpatient health care facility and for whom physicians believe that the benefit of the agent outweighs its potential risk.

** Adaptations made to reflect introduction of new agents since report was published.

Cytotoxic agents; non-steroidal anti-inflammatory drugs (NSAIDs); and some antibiotics, including sulfonamides and certain antiarrhythmics (e.g., amiodarone or tocainide), can mimic pulmonary infection. In addition, common analgesics, including salicylates, propoxyphene, and methadone, also may precipitate acute respiratory symptoms. Such collagen vascular diseases as systemic lupus erythematosus, polymyositis, and polyarteritis nodosa may cause fever, cough, dyspnea, and pulmonary infiltrates, thereby mimicking symptoms of pneumonia. Rheumatoid arthritis can cause an interstitial lung disease, although it usually does not cause fever or alveolar infiltrates.

Initial Stabilization and Adjunctive Measures. Prompt, aggressive, and adequate supportive care must be provided to patients who present to the hospital with pneumonia. As is the case with other serious conditions, supportive care frequently must be performed in conjunction with the history, physical examination, and diagnostic testing. Among initial stabilization measures, managing the airway and ensuring adequate breathing, oxygenation, ventilation, and perfusion are of paramount importance.

Upon arrival to the hospital, oxygenation status should be assessed immediately using pulse-oximetry. Patients with an arterial oxygen saturation of less than

* FDA indicates Food and Drug Administration. Ratings estimate clinical efficacy and in vitro susceptibility among persons with pneumococcal pneumonia. In-depth information on empiric treatment of pneumonia is given by the Infectious Disease Society of America and the American Thoracic Society guidelines.

‡ Vancomycin hydrochloride may be indicated for the treatment of selected critically ill children with community-acquired pneumonia for whom coverage of drug-resistant Streptococcus pneumoniae must be ensured.

90% should receive supplemental oxygen, and should be considered candidates for admission, prompt evaluation, and treatment if the diagnosis is confirmed. Arterial blood gases are especially helpful in patients suspected of hypercarbia and respiratory failure. This laboratory modality may be useful in patients with COPD, decreased mental status, and fatigue. Patients with hypoxia who do not respond to supplemental oxygen, as well as those with hypercarbia accompanied by respiratory acidosis, may be candidates for mechanical ventilation. This patient population also has a poorer prognosis. Support may be accomplished with either intubation and mechanical ventilation or non-invasive ventilation (bilevel positive pressure ventilation [BiPAP]). Recent studies have shown BiPAP to be successful for treatment of patients with respiratory failure due to pneumonia.[25] When this technique is available, it may avert the need for endotracheal intubation and its potential complications. Finally, patients with evidence of bronchospasm on physical examination, as well as those with a history of obstructive airway disease (asthma or COPD) may benefit from inhaled bronchodilator therapy.

Evidence of inadequate perfusion may range from mild dehydration with tachycardia to life-threatening hypotension due to septic shock. Patients with septic shock usually will show evidence of decreased tissue perfusion, such as confusion and oliguria in association with a hyperdynamic circulation. In either case, initial therapy consists of intravenous fluids (normal saline or lactated Ringer's solution) administered through a large bore IV. In elderly patients, fluid overload is a potential complication, and it is prudent to administer IV fluids with frequent assessment of clinical response.

RISK STRATIFICATION AND PATIENT DISPOSITION: OUTPATIENT VS. INPATIENT MANAGEMENT

Determining whether to admit or discharge patients suspected of having CAP is one of the most important decisions an emergency physician, pulmonologist, or internist can make. For this reason, there have been increasing efforts to identify patients with CAP who can appropriately (i.e., safely) be treated as outpatients.[7,26,27,34] The disposition decision for patients with pneumonia should take into account the severity of the pneumonia, as well as other medical and psychosocial factors that may affect the treatment plan and clinical outcome.[35-37]

Patient Disposition. In the absence of respiratory distress or other complicating factors, many young adults can be adequately treated with appropriate oral antibiotic therapy. In fact, guidelines issued by the IDSA and ATS support oral antibiotic therapy in patients deemed to be at low risk for complications and/or mortality associated with CAP. This option is utilized less frequently in the case of elderly patients with CAP because comorbid conditions and other risk factors that may complicate the course of the illness frequently are present. Even following appropriate treatment and disposition, patients may have symptoms, including cough, fatigue, dyspnea, sputum production, and chest pain that can last for several months. To address the issue of patient disposition and treatment setting, a variety of investigators have proposed risk-stratification criteria to identify patients requiring hospitalization.

Among the factors most physicians use to make admission decisions for pneumonia are the presence of hypoxemia, overall clinical status, the ability to maintain oral intake, hemodynamic status, and the patient's home environment. Such factors as hypotension, tachypnea, multi-lobar involvement, elevated BUN, and confusion have been linked to inferior outcomes in patients with CAP. Using clinical judgment, however, physicians tend to overestimate the likelihood of death from pneumonia.[35] These findings have led some investigators to employ more stringent prediction rules. For example, the chest radiograph may help identify patients who are at high risk for mortality. The presence of bilateral effusions, moderate-size pleural effusions, multi-lobar involvement, and bilateral infiltrates are associated with poorer outcomes.

A landmark study (outlined below) presented a prediction rule (Pneumonia Severity Index [PSI]) to identify low-risk patients with CAP.[7] Using such objective criteria as patient age, coexisting medical conditions, and vital signs, patients are assigned either to a low-risk class, which has a mortality rate of about 0.1% in outpatients, or to higher risk categories. Patients with any risk factors are then evaluated with a second scoring system that assigns individuals to one of three higher risk categories, which have mortality rates ranging from 0.7% to 31%.[53] In addition to the factors noted in this prediction rule, patients who are immunocompromised as a result of AIDS or chronic alcohol use frequently require hospitalization.

Once the clinician has determined hospitalization is required, the need for ICU admission also must be evaluated. A variety of factors are associated with an increased risk for mortality, including increasing age (> 65 years), alcoholism, chronic lung disease, immunodeficiency, and specific laboratory abnormalities, including azotemia and hypoxemia. These patients may require admission to the ICU.

Prognostic Scoring. There have been many efforts to assess severity and risk of death in patients with pneumonia.[36,38,39] The study by Fine and colleagues has received considerable attention and is used as a benchmark by many clinicians.[35] This study developed a prediction rule, the PSI, to assess 30-day mortality in patients with CAP. The rule was derived and validated with data from more than 52,000 inpatients, and then validated with a second cohort of 2287 inpatients and outpatients as part of the Pneumonia PORT (Pneumonia Patient Outcomes Research Team Cohort) study. Subsequent evaluation and validation has been performed with other cohorts, including geriatric patients and nursing home residents.[40,41]

In this risk-stratification model, patients are assigned to one of five risk classes (1 is lowest risk, 5 is highest risk) based upon a point system that considers age, co-existing disease, abnormal physical findings, and abnormal laboratory findings. Elderly patients cannot be assigned to Class 1, as a requirement is age younger than 50 years. In older patients, age contributes the most points to the overall score. For example, it should be noted that males ages older than 70 years and females ages older than 80 years would be assigned to Class 3 on the basis of age alone, without any other risk factor. In the Fine study, patients assigned to Classes 1 and 2 were typically younger (median age, 35-59 years) and patients in Classes 3-5 were older (median age, 72-75 years).

Outpatient management is recommended for Classes 1 and 2, brief inpatient observation for Class 3, and traditional hospitalization for Classes 4 and 5.[36] For a geriatric patient to qualify for outpatient treatment based on these recommendations, he or she would have to be younger than age 70 if male or younger than age 80 if female, and have no additional risk factors. Inpatient observation or traditional hospitalization would be recommended for all other patients based on this rule. Other studies have suggested outpatient management for Class 3 patients, but most authorities consider Class 3 patients to be appropriate candidates for hospital admission or for management in an observation unit or skilled nursing facility.[7,42]

As a rule, patients considered eligible for management as outpatients must be able to take oral fluids and antibiotics, comply with outpatient care, and carry out activities of daily living (ADLs) or have adequate home support to assist with ADLs. Other factors cited in previous studies but not included in the PSI also have been found to increase the risk of morbidity or mortality from pneumonia. These include: other comorbid illnesses (diabetes mellitus, COPD, post-splenectomy state), altered mental status, suspicion of aspiration, chronic alcohol abuse or malnutrition, and evidence of extrapulmonary disease.[6] Additional laboratory studies that may suggest increased severity of illness include white blood cell count less than 4000 or greater than 30,000; absolute neutrophil count less than 1000; elevated protime or partial thromboplastin time; decreased platelet count; or radiographic evidence of multilobar involvement, cavitation, and rapid spreading.[6]

Severe pneumonia may require ICU admission. In the Fine study, 6% of patients in Class 3, 11% of patients in Class 4, and 17% of patients in Class 5 required ICU admission.[35] The ATS guidelines define severe pneumonia as the presence of at least one of the following: respiratory rate greater than 30, severe respiratory failure ($PaO_2/FIO_2 < 250$), mechanical ventilation, bilateral infiltrates or multilobar infiltrates, shock, vasopressor requirement, or oliguria (urine output < 20 cc per hour). The presence of at least one of these is highly sensitive (98%), but provides low specificity (32%) for the need to manage the patient in the ICU.[43] It is emphasized that the above guidelines for admission should not supercede clinical judgment when assessing the need to hospitalize patients.[6,35,36,44]

ANTIBIOTIC MANAGEMENT FOR HOSPITALIZED CAP PATIENTS: AN OVERVIEW OF CURRENT CONTROVERSIES, ISSUES, AND GUIDELINES

Timing of Antibiotic Administration. Antibiotic therapy is the mainstay of management for patients with CAP. It should be stated at the outset that antibiotic therapy should be initiated promptly, as soon as the diagnosis is strongly suspected or confirmed, and after appropriate microbiological studies or samples have been obtained. However, antibiotic administration should not be delayed for microbiologic sampling. More and more, institutional guidelines are mandating administration of antibiotics within 4-8 hours of patient presentation to the hospital, since mortality rates rise when antibiotic administration is delayed beyond eight hours.[45] The Joint Commission on Accreditation of Healthcare Organizations' (JCAHO) guidelines currently mandate that for hospitalized patients with CAP, antibiotics must be administered no later than eight hours after patient presentation. The Healthcare Financing Administration (HCFA) recommends IV antibiotic administration within four hours in Medicare patients with CAP.

Previous studies evaluating the effect of changing process of care, including administration of antibiotics within four hours of hospital admission for patients with CAP, have demonstrated a relationship between early antibiotic administration and lower three-day mortality rate.[46,47] More recently, data from the Medicare Quality Indicator System pneumonia module revealed a 15% lower odds ratio of 30-day mortality when antibiotics were administered within eight hours of hospital arrival.[48]

Based on a review of medical evidence, the 6th Scope of Work National

Pneumonia project has issued revised performance measures for CAP. One of these modifications is the shortening of the time from initial hospital arrival to the first dose of antibiotics from eight hours to four hours. The ASCAP Consensus Panel noted that the eight-hour target is based on published guidelines. However, recent data from the 6th Scope of Work project indicate that several thousand deaths could be prevented every year among hospitalized Medicare patients with pneumonia if the initial dose of antibiotic were administered *within four hours of arrival*. In recognition of improved outcomes linked to early antibiotic administration, the Medicare Quality Improvement Organization will revise the published guidelines downward. Specifically, in the 7th Scope of Work project, the Quality Improvement Organization will attempt to positively impact patient outcomes by decreasing door-to-drug time to a four-hour threshold instead of the current eight-hour threshold.

The link between quality of care and resource utilization also has been confirmed in an analysis of quality-of-care variables observed in randomly selected cases of CAP.[1] In this study, three quality-of-care measures for CAP were analyzed: 1) site of initial antibiotic treatment (ED vs floor); 2) door-to-needle time; and 3) appropriateness of antibiotic selection. A regression analysis revealed that all three quality-of-care measures were associated with prolonged length of stay (LOS). Further analysis revealed that, on average, patients who received their initial antibiotic treatments in the ED had a door-to-treatment time of 3.5 ± 1.4 hours, while patients who had their initial antibiotic treatments on the inpatient floor had a door-to-needle time of 9.5 ± 3 hours ($p < 0.001$).[1] Based on these data, and in anticipation of new federal guidelines, the ASCAP Consensus Panel recommends that initial antibiotic therapy be administered in the ED, and that whenever possible such administration occur within a four-hour door-to-needle time frame.

Antibiotic Administration Errors: Compliance Issues in the Hospital and Emergency Department. The importance of ensuring medication compliance in the outpatient setting has had a measurable effect on physician prescribing practices, which now emphasize the use of once-daily formulations whenever possible. Recently, however, it has become clear that in-hospital medication errors have become a national concern, and that daily dose frequency may play a role in ensuring adequate drug intake for hospitalized patients, and perhaps may even influence clinical outcomes.[49,50]

To identify the prevalence of medication errors, a prospective cohort study was conducted in hospitals accredited by JCAHO,[49] nonaccredited hospitals, and skilled nursing facilities in Georgia and Colorado. The study evaluated medication doses given (or omitted) during at least one medication pass during a one- to four-day period by nurses in high medication volume nursing units. The target sample was 50-day shift doses per nursing unit or until all doses for that medication pass were administered.

In the 36 institutions, 19% of the doses (605 of 3216) were in error. The most frequent errors by category were wrong time (43%), omission (30%), wrong dose (17%), and unauthorized drug (4%). The authors concluded that medication errors were extremely common (nearly 1 of every 5 doses in the typical hospital and skilled nursing facility). The percentage of errors rated potentially harmful was 7%, or more than 40 per day in a typical 300-patient facility.[49]

Further confirmation of this problem, and its potential effect on antibiotic administration, was reported in an abstract (No. 127) at the American College of Emergency Physicians (ACEP) Scientific Assembly (2002).[50] The investigators evaluated antibiotic compliance in patients with CAP, the majority of whom received their initial dose in the ED, and the second dose in the inpatient unit, or occasionally, in an observation unit. Delays of the first antibiotic dose have been documented and targeted for quality improvement (see above). Delays in the second dose have not been studied, but are likely to be important if the delay results in serum-antibiotic concentrations of less than therapeutic levels.[50]

Investigators from the University of Rochester School of Medicine and Dentistry and the University of Chicago Hospitals attempted to characterize the epidemiology of delayed antibiotics after transfer to an inpatient unit in patients with CAP, and to compare differences in delays among antibiotics dosed every six hours (q6) and every 24 hours (q24). The study was conducted by performing a retrospective chart review of patients with CAP admitted to the medicine service between July 1997 and June 1999. In all, 359 patients were identified. The mean age was 61 years; 62% were female. Of those, 185 (34%) were ordered q6 and 332 (62%) were ordered q24. Twenty-four percent of those receiving a q6 antibiotic received their second dose within six hours, whereas 80% of patients receiving a q24 antibiotic received their second dose within 24 hours (p < 0.001). The authors concluded that patients with CAP who are prescribed antibiotics that require frequent dosing are more likely to receive a delayed second antibiotic dose, and that physicians should consider using long-acting, once-daily antibiotics when possible.[50]

In light of the importance of process-of-care issues related to optimizing outcomes in patients with CAP, the ASCAP Consensus Panel recommends the preferential use of ceftriaxone over cefotaxime as the cephalosporin of choice for patients with CAP. Although both agents underwent NCCLS breakpoint revisions in 2002, the NCCLS noted that the breakpoint for cefotaxime applied specifically to a dose of at least 1 g q8 hours. Given the potential problems associated with delayed antibiotic administration, the increased nursing time and resource costs required for more frequent administration, and additional data from the Antimicrobial Resistance Management (ARM) surveillance network suggesting greater *in vitro* efficacy of ceftriaxone as compared to cefotaxime for *S. pneumoniae* respiratory isolates, the panel identified ceftriaxone as the cephalosporin of choice for initial empiric use in hospitalized patients with CAP.

Consensus Panel Recommendations. It should be stressed that there is no absolute or consistent consensus about precisely which drug, or combination of drugs, constitutes the most outcome-effective choice for pneumonia in patients with CAP. However, a recent study suggests improved mortality rates with regimens using two-drug combinations rather than monotherapy in patients with bacteremic pneumococcal pneumonia.[21] Most panels and guideline documents agree that antimicrobial coverage must include sufficient activity against the principal bacterial pathogens *S. pneumoniae, H. influenzae,* and *M. catarrhalis,* as well as against the atypical pathogens *Mycoplasma, Legionella,* and *C. pneumoniae.* In about 5% of cases, antimicrobial activity against *S. aureus* also is required. Therefore, such regimens as ceftriaxone/cefotaxime plus azithromycin or monotherapy with an advanced generation fluoroquinolone such as moxifloxacin—given some qualifications regarding outcomes and resistance issues to be discussed later—have emerged as preferred options for treatment of inpatients with CAP.

Beyond this non-negotiable caveat mandating coverage for the six aforementioned pathogens, there are important differences among recommendations and expert panels for empiric treatment of pneumonia. Variations among the guidelines usually depend upon: 1) their emphasis or focus on the need to empirically cover drug-resistant *Streptococcus pneumoniae* (DRSP) as part of the initial antimicrobial regimen; 2) their concern about using antimicrobials (fluoroquinolones, i.e., levofloxacin) with an over-extended (too broad) spectrum of coverage; 3) their concern about the potential of growing resistance to a class (fluoroquinolones) which has agents that currently are active against DRSP; 4) their preference for monotherapeutic vs. combination therapy; 5) when the guidelines were released (recent vs several years old); and 6) their emphasis on drug costs (see Table 5), patient convenience, and options for step-down (IV to oral) therapeutic approaches. Clearly, these factors and the relative emphasis placed on each of them will influence antimicrobial selection for the patient with pneumonia.

With these issues and drug selection factors in mind, the most recent guidelines issued by the CDC-DRSPWG and American Thoracic Society attempt to both risk-stratify and "drug-stratify" patients according to their eligibility for receiving agents as initial empiric therapy that have activity against DRSP. Before presenting a detailed discussion of the current treatment landscape for CAP, the following points from the ASCAP expert's panel should be emphasized. First, the relative importance of *S. pneumoniae* as a cause of *outpatient* CAP is difficult to determine. Nevertheless, a review of the literature suggests that *S. pneumoniae* accounts for 2-27% of all cases of CAP treated on an outpatient basis.[8,51] In addition, surveillance studies have suggested that about 7% of invasive *S. pneumoniae* species in the United States show a significant degree of penicillin resistance.[52] This group estimates that only 0.14% (7% of 2%) to 1.9% (7% of 27%) of outpatients with bacterial pneumonia have pneumococcal infections with levels of resistance high enough to warrant consideration of alternative treatment.

This analysis has prompted the CDC panel to conclude that because CAP in patients who are appropriately triaged and risk-stratified is generally not immediately life-threatening and because *S. pneumoniae* isolates with penicillin MICs of no less than 4 mcg/mL are uncommon, antibiotics with predictable activity against highly penicillin-resistant pneumococci are not necessary as part of the initial regimen. From a practical, drug-selection perspective, the working group, therefore, suggests that oral fluoroquinolones are not first-line treatment in outpatients with CAP because of concerns about emerging resistance. Consequently, oral macrolide or beta-lactam monotherapy is recommended by the CDC-DRSPWG as initial therapy in patients with pneumonia considered to be amenable to outpatient management. Because atypical pathogens are an important cause of outpatient CAP, the ASCAP Consensus Panel recommends macrolides over beta-lactam monotherapy for outpatients. If a fluoroquinolone is used for outpatients with CAP, moxifloxacin is the preferred agent.

It should be noted, however, that even for hospitalized (non-ICU) patients, this panel, while noting the effectiveness of monotherapy with selected fluoro-quinolones, recommends the combination of a parenteral beta-lactam (ceftriax-one, cefotaxime, etc.) plus a macrolide (azithromycin, erythromycin, etc.) for ini-tial therapy.[3] Regardless of the panel or critical pathway, one of the important, consistent changes among recent recommendations for initial, empiric manage-ment of patients with CAP is mandatory inclusion of a macrolide (which covers atypical pathogens) when a cephalosporin (which has poor activity against atypi-cal pathogens) is selected as part of the regimen. For critically ill patients, first-line therapy should include an intravenous beta-lactam such as ceftriaxone plus an intravenous macrolide such as azithromycin or, alternatively, a respiratory fluoro-quinolone such as moxifloxacin (see discussion below).

The option of using a combination of a parenteral beta-lactam (ceftriaxone, etc.) plus a fluoroquinolone with improved activity against DRSP also is pre-sented. Once again, however, the committee issues clarifying, and sometimes cautionary, statements about the role of fluoroquinolone monotherapy in the crit-ically ill patient, stating that care should be exercised because the efficacy of the new fluoroquinolones as monotherapy for critically ill patients has not been determined.[3] Based on this cautionary statement, it is recommended that a par-enteral beta-lactam such as ceftriaxone be used in combination with a fluoro-quinolone in ICU patients with serious CAP.

Clearly, however, fluoroquinolones are an important part of the antimicrobial arsenal in the elderly, and the CDC-DRSPWG has issued specific guidelines gov-erning their use in the setting of outpatient and inpatient CAP. In general, this panel has recommended that fluoroquinolones be reserved for selected patients

Table 5. Daily Drug Cost (WAC)*

Drug and Dosage	Cost/Day
Azithromycin IV 500 mg	$18.96
Ceftriaxone 1 g IV qd	36.06
Levofloxacin 500 mg IV qd	33.00
Erythromycin 500 mg IV qid	5.20
Ciprofloxacin 400 mg IV bid	48.00
Cefotaxime 1 g IV tid	25.00
Tricarcillin-clavulanate 3.1 g qid	48.32
Moxifloxacin IV	30.00

*WAC = Wholesale acquisition cost

Hospital formulary pricing guide, August 1999. WAC may not necessarily reflect actual pharmacy costs or costs associated with drug administration cost and comparisons.

with CAP, and these experts have identified specific patient subgroups that are eligible for initial treatment with extended-spectrum fluoroquinolones. For hospitalized patients, these include adults for whom one of the first-line regimens (e.g., ceftriaxone plus a macrolide) has failed, those who are allergic to the first-line agents, or those who have a documented infection with highly drug-resistant pneumococci (i.e., penicillin MIC > 4 mcg/mL).[3] The rationale for this approach is discussed in subsequent sections.

EMERGENCE OF FLUOROQUINOLONE RESISTANCE AMONG *Streptococcus pneumoniae*

The only treatment guideline that recognizes the potential effect of widespread fluoroquinolone resistance also is the only treatment guideline that recommends fluoroquinolones be reserved for selected patients with CAP (CDC-DRSPWG). With revised breakpoint MICs for cefotaxime and ceftriaxone, the percent of resistant *S. pneumoniae* to these third generation cephalosporins is below 3-5% nationally. This has required clinicians to reexamine the published treatment guidelines that recommend fluoroquinolones as initial therapy for CAP.

Widespread, indiscriminate use of fluoroquinolones may be associated with rising resistance rates to selected gram-positive and gram-negative organisms. Previous assumptions that fluoroquinolones will be more clinically effective vs. DRSP than ceftriaxone or cefotaxime must be reevaluated. Based on the 2002 NCCLS guidelines, both ceftriaxone and cefotaxime are expected to provide comparable microbiologic end points and clinical cures in patients with non-meningeal *S. pneumoniae* infections as compared to the anti-pneumococcal fluoroquinolones. The clinician will be asked to incorporate geographic specific resistance rates and the ecology of microorganisms into his/her decision about how to empirically treat the patient with CAP.

When first introduced in 1987, ciprofloxacin was promoted for the treatment of respiratory tract infections, including those due to *S. pneumoniae*. Early trials demonstrated clinical success for patients with respiratory infections.[53,54] However, subsequent studies found that the use of ciprofloxacin against *S. pneumoniae* was associated with poor eradication rates both in acute exacerbations of chronic bronchitis (AECB) and pneumonia.[55-57] Reports of the development of resistance soon appeared.[58-62] Knowing the pharmacodynamic parameters of ciprofloxacin and *S. pneumoniae*, this was not unexpected. The AUC24/MIC generally accepted to be most predictive of bacterial eradication and clinical success is greater than 35.[63-66] The C_{max}/MIC ratio generally accepted to be most predictive for prevention of resistance selection is greater than 4.[67,68] Following a 750 mg oral dose of ciprofloxacin, the C_{max} is only 3 mg/L and the AUC24 is 31 mg/h/L.[69] The MIC_{90} of *S. pneumoniae* is 1 mg/L giving a C_{max}/MIC of 3 and an AUC/MIC of 31.[63]

Although ciprofloxacin was not promoted or widely used for the treatment of CAP, it was used for the treatment of AECB at a dose of 500 mg twice daily. Eradication rates of *S. pneumoniae* in AECB varied from 63% to 90%.[71,72] This failure to eradicate was associated with the development of resistance during therapy in some patients.[71,72] This may, in part, explain the emergence of pneumococci with reduced susceptibility to the fluoroquinolones and, in particular, to ciprofloxacin.

Emergence of resistance in *S. pneumoniae* to the fluoroquinolones has been described in Canada, Spain, Hong Kong, and Northern Ireland. In Canada, Chen et al found that the prevalence of ciprofloxacin-resistant pneumococci (MIC ≥ 4 mcg/mL) increased from 0% in 1993 to 1.7% in 1997-1998 (p = 0.01).[73] In adults, the prevalence increased from 0% in 1993 to 3.7% in 1998. This was associated with an increase in the consumption of fluoroquinolones. Overall, the number of fluoroquinolone prescriptions increased from 0.8 to 5.5 per 100 persons per year between 1988 and 1997.[73] In addition to the increase in prevalence of pneumococci with reduced susceptibility to fluoroquinolones, the degree of resistance also increased. From 1994 to 1998, there was a statistically significant increase in the proportion of isolates with a MIC for ciprofloxacin of 32 mcg/mL or greater (p = 0.04).

Linares et al found an increase of ciprofloxacin-resistant pneumococci in Spain from 0.9% in 1991-1992 to 3% in 1997-1998.[74] Ho and colleagues documented a marked increase in the overall prevalence of non-susceptibility to the fluoroquinolones when comparing results of surveillance carried out in Hong Kong in 1998 and 2000.[6,75,76] Over a two-year period, the prevalence of levofloxacin non-susceptibility increased from 5.5% to 13.3% among all isolates and from 9.2% to 28.4% among the penicillin-resistant strains. In Northern Ireland, ciprofloxacin resistance was linked to penicillin resistance. Eighteen (42.9%) of 42 penicillin-resistant pneumococci were resistant to ciprofloxacin.[77] Current rates of resistance in the United States are low.[78-79] Doern et al reported ciprofloxacin resistance rates of 1.4%.[79] The CDC Active Bacterial Core Surveillance (ABCs) program carried out during 1995-1999 reported levofloxacin resistance rates of 0.2%.[78] They have not included ciprofloxacin as one of the agents they test.

One study group reviewed 181 S. pneumoniae isolates in Hong Kong in 1998. Hong Kong is an environment with uniquely high rates of resistance, which may provide a vision of what can occur when fluoroquinolone resistance is observed with S. pneumoniae.[75] Within three years, the resistance of S. pneumoniae to fluoroquinolones has increased from less than 0.5% for ofloxacin, to 5.5% for levofloxacin. In addition, 4% of penicillin resistance isolates also were resistant to trovafloxacin, an agent that was only approved for use in October 1998; this demonstrates the cross resistance to newer quinolones. Resistance to levofloxacin and trovafloxacin was found only in isolates that also were penicillin resistant.

A recent study has documented that the increased use of fluoroquinolones has resulted in an increase in pseudomonas and gram-negative resistance to these drugs, particularly ciprofloxacin; although levofloxacin resistance is not mentioned in this particular report, similar reports have identified development of gram resistance for this agent as well. Furthermore, the development of resistance to fluoroquinolones also has accompanied an increased incidence of resistance to other potent antibiotics. This study provides further argument for limiting the use of fluoroquinolones, especially levofloxacin and gatifloxacin, according to the CDC recommendations.[191]

One abstract detailed changes in *S. pneumoniae* resistance among different drug classes. Unfortunately, although no MICs or breakpoints are given, *S. pneumoniae* resistance for levofloxacin grew from 0.1% to 0.6%, a growth rate over the period of about 600%. While *S. pneumoniae* grew in several antibiotic classes and among various agents, including macrolides, trimethoprim-sulfamethoxazole (TMP-SMX), and cefuroxime, the greatest growth in resistance was seen with levofloxacin.[82] In another study evaluating emergent resistance,[83] it was found that compared to cephalosporins and combination therapy, fluoroquinolones were associated with the greatest risk for acquiring emergent resistance during therapy, had the highest treatment failure due to emergent resistance, the largest increase in treatment duration due to resistance, and the largest decrease in clinical response due to emergent resistance.[83]

Recent Trends in *S. pneumoniae* Resistance to Levofloxacin. The increasing use of broad-spectrum fluoroquinolones for the treatment of respiratory tract infections has led to concerns regarding the potential for emergence and spread of resistance to these agents, particularly among *S. pneumoniae*. Recently, there has been evidence suggesting an increasing prevalence of fluoroquinolone resistance among *S. pneumoniae* isolated in the United States during the winter of 2000-2001.[84] As part of a longitudinal surveillance study (PROTEKT US), 10,103 isolates of *S. pneumoniae* were collected during the 2000-2001 winter from outpatients with respiratory tract infections in 154 cities/metropolitan areas in 44 states across the United States. MICs and susceptibilities to 13 antimicrobials were determined centrally using NCCLS broth microdilution method breakpoints.

Overall, the fluoroquinolone mode MIC and MIC_{90} (levofloxacin) were both

1 mcg/L, MIC range 0.12-16 mcg/L. Fluoroquinolone resistance (levofloxacin MIC > 8 mcg/L) was found in 81 (0.8%) isolates, and intermediate resistance (levofloxacin MIC 4 mcg/L) in eight (0.08%) isolates. States with high fluoroquinolone resistance prevalence were: Massachusetts (4.8%) and Colorado (4.6%); cities with high fluoroquinolone resistance prevalence were: Salem (21.8%), Stamford (11.8%), Abington (7.7%), Dayton (5.9%), and Denver (5.6%). The ASCAP Consensus Panel concurred that, considering levofloxacin frequently is used to manage hospitalized, high-risk, Fine Category 3-5 patients, this agent should be avoided as an initial, empiric agent in communities demonstrating fluoroquinolone resistance exceeding 5-10% in surveillance studies. Although the precise relationship between documented resistance rates of this magnitude in particular states and clinical outcomes in CAP was not addressed by the study, the likelihood of treatment failures with levofloxacin in such communities may be increased. Accordingly, a more prudent approach would suggest the use of combination therapy with ceftriaxone and azithromycin, or alternatively, the use of a respiratory fluoroquinolone (i.e., moxifloxacin) with documented lower MICs against *S. pneumoniae.*

Levofloxacin resistance among *S. pneumoniae* may play an especially important role in older patients. With higher mortality rates from CAP in the elderly, the initial choice of antibiotic is crucial and surveillance data confirming antibiotic activity becomes more important. To address this question, the Canadian Bacterial Surveillance Network, in 1988 and from 1993-2001, tested 2187 *S. pneumoniae* isolates from patients ages 65 or older for antibiotic susceptibility as per NCCLS guidelines. Respiratory samples included sputums, bronchial washings, and endotracheal tube aspirates. Results indicate that since 1988, rates of *S. pneumoniae* resistance have increased substantially for penicillin, erythromycin, and the fluoroquinolones in this age group. Most alarming was the rapid rise of levofloxacin resistance over the past three years. The authors concluded that with increasing fluoroquinolone resistance in *S. pneumoniae* isolates from the elderly population, hospitals and microbiology laboratories will need to more vigilantly look for clinical resistance to fluoroquinolones. As the prevalence of resistance in these Canadian isolates is 4.3% and first-step mutants are 7.2%, they conclude it may not be prudent to use a fluoroquinolone as empiric therapy in this group of patients.[85]

In aggregate, what these studies make clear is that with the rising prevalence of levofloxacin-resistant *S. pneumoniae,* it is prudent for hospitals to test those agents they use (i.e., fluoroquinolones) to document clinically effective sensitivities and MICs, and conversely to use only those agents that have been tested and that demonstrate MICs predictive of bacterial eradication and positive clinical outcomes.

Clinical Implications. Although treatment failures due to beta-lactams, macrolides, and TMP-SMX resistance in pneumococci have been reported with meningitis and otitis media, the relationship between drug resistance and treatment failures among patients with pneumococcal pneumonia is less clear.[86,87] However, fluoroquinolone resistance in pneumococci causing pneumonia in association with clinical failures, although anecdotal, has been well described.[55-58,88,89]

Reports of the development of resistance and clinical failures appeared shortly after the introduction of ciprofloxacin in 1987.[58-62] Weiss and colleagues described a nosocomial outbreak of fluoroquinolone-resistant pneumococci.[89] Over the course of a 20-month period, in a hospital respiratory ward where ciprofloxacin often was used as empirical antimicrobial therapy for lower respiratory tract infections, 16 patients with chronic bronchitis developed lower respiratory tract infections caused by a strain of penicillin- and ciprofloxacin-resistant *S. pneumoniae* (serotype 23 F). The MIC of ciprofloxacin for all isolates was 4 mcg/mL or greater. All five patients with AECB due to the resistant strain who were treated with ciprofloxacin failed therapy. Davidson et al report four cases of pneumococcal pneumonia, treated empirically with oral levofloxacin, that failed therapy.[88] All cases were associated with the isolation of an organism that was either resistant to levofloxacin prior to therapy or had acquired resistance during therapy. Two of the four patients had been or were on fluoroquinolones prior to initiating levofloxacin.

From these and other studies, a number of risk factors may identify the patients who are likely to be colonized or infected with a fluoroquinolone-resistant pneumococci: patients who are older than age 64, have a history of chronic obstructive lung disease, and/or a prior fluoroquinolone exposure.[73,76,78,81,90] None of the CAP position papers published since the introduction of the fluoroquinolones for the treatment of pneumococcal pneumonia has suggested that a history of previous fluoroquinolone use should be a reason for caution when using one of these antimicrobials. However, the aforementioned study by Davidson suggests recent (i.e., < 3 months) fluoroquinolone use may predispose patients to developing resistance to this class, and that other options should be considered.

One recent review[91] has noted a significant correlation between increased levofloxacin use and declining fluoroquinolone susceptibilities among ICU isolates of *K. pneumoniae* (96% to 79% [p < 0.008]) and *P. aeruginosa* (82% to 67% [p < 0.01]). Similarly, another group[92] reported that after levofloxacin was added to the formulary, levofloxacin use as a proportion of total fluoroquinolone use increased from less than 2% to greater than 22% over a six-month period (from 3rd quarter 1999 to 1st quarter 2000). During the period of first quarter 1998 to second quarter 2000, the susceptibility of *P. aeruginosa* to ciprofloxacin decreased by 11% (82% to 71%).

Because the ICU has been a focal point of antimicrobial resistance, the CDC initiated Project ICARE in 1996.[93] Specific data regarding fluoroquinolone use and fluoroquinolone susceptibility among *P. aeruginosa* isolates were presented for the period 1996-1999 by Hill et al.[94] No correlation was found between prevalence of quinolone resistance and total use of ciprofloxacin/ ofloxacin. However, significant associations were found between fluoroquinolone resistance and the combined use of ciprofloxacin, ofloxacin, and levofloxacin (p < 0.019); and by use of levofloxacin alone (p < 0.006).[94]

Likewise, recent studies suggest that using a less potent fluoroquinolone against *S. pneumoniae* for treating community and hospital respiratory tract infections may be affecting the sensitivity to the drug class and may be associated with an increase in treatment failures. Inappropriate use of antimicrobial agents has been associated with adverse consequences, including therapeutic failure, development of resistance, and increased healthcare costs. One example of a mismatch between pharmacodynamics and clinical infection was in the use of ciprofloxacin for CAP. The pharmacodynamics of the dose typically prescribed in these cases (ciprofloxacin 250 mg bid) are inappropriate for treating pneumococcal pneumonia, especially in seriously ill patients. By 1994, approximately 15 cases of *S. pneumoniae* infections that did not respond to ciprofloxacin had been reported, primarily in seriously ill patients.[68] These events prompted the U.S. Food and Drug Administration to modify the package insert to warn against empiric use of ciprofloxacin for respiratory infections in which *S. pneumoniae* would be a primary pathogen.

By contrast, greater than 50% of levofloxacin use has been for the treatment of respiratory infections. Since 1999, at least 20 case reports of pulmonary infections that did not respond to levofloxacin therapy have been published.[95-104] Three of the patients died due to fulminant pneumococcal infections that were unresponsive to levofloxacin therapy at approved dosage. Very few of these cases were in immunosuppressed patients. Reports of pneumococcal failures on the standard dosage of levofloxacin, 500 mg every 24 h, also have been described in two clinical trials, one in a patient with acute exacerbation of chronic bronchitis and the other in a patient with CAP.[95-100] In some of the 21 case reports, the treatment failed and the pathogen developed levofloxacin resistance during therapy, as was previously mentioned in the series by Davidson et al.

Both Weiss et al[105] and Ho et al[106] demonstrated clear risk factors associated with the development of fluoroquinolone resistance, including prior exposure of the patient to first- or second-generation fluoroquinolones (i.e., ciprofloxacin, levofloxacin, and ofloxacin), and history of COPD.

YEAR 2002 NCCLS BREAKPOINTS: EVIDENCE-BASED SUPPORT FOR ADOPTION OF NEW STANDARDS

Prior to revising the NCCLS MIC breakpoints for *S. pneumoniae*, the clinical significance of the original S, I, and R breakpoints (originally published in NCCLS document M100-S9) of the parenteral aminothiazolyl cephalosporins ceftriaxone/cefotaxime in systemic non-meningeal pneumococcal infections was not fully elucidated.

To evaluate clinical outcomes in patients managed with ceftriaxone/cefotaxime, one group, during the period January 1994 through October 2000, studied 522 episodes (in 499 adult patients) of non-meningeal pneumococcal infections (448 of severe pneumonia [clinical and x-ray findings together with positive blood or invasive lower respiratory tract cultures] and 74 of bacteremia from other origin). Of the 522, 74% had serious underlying diseases, 14% nosocomial infections, and 7% polymicrobial infections.[107] The 30-day mortality rate was 21%. Ceftriaxone/cefotaxime MICs according to NCCLS were determined by microdilution methods and Mueller-Hinton broth with lysed horse blood. The frequency distribution in terms of ceftriaxone/cefotaxime MICs of strains was S <= 0.5 mcg/mL 413 (79%), I = 1 mcg/mL 79 (15%), and R = 2 mcg/mL 30 (6%); no strain with a ceftriaxone/cefotaxime MIC of greater than 2 mcg/mL was found.

In ceftriaxone/cefotaxime-resistant strains, the most commonly encountered serotypes were 14, 9, 23, and 6. In the 429 episodes of community-acquired pneumococcal infection (polymicrobial and nosocomial cases were excluded), the ceftriaxone/cefotaxime MICs and antibiotic therapy (prescribed according to the attending physician's criteria) were correlated with the 30-day mortality rate. In 185 episodes treated with 1 g/d of ceftriaxone (n = 171) or 1.5-2 g/8 h of cefotaxime (n = 14), the mortality rates for patients with S, I, and R strains were 18% (26/148), 13% (3/24), and 15% (2/13), respectively (p = 0.81). In the 244 patients treated with other antibiotics, the mortality rates for patients with S, I, and R strains were 18% (36/200), 12% (4/33), and 9% (1/11), respectively (p = 0.55).[107]

Patients infected with pneumococci with ceftriaxone/cefotaxime MIC of 1 or 2 mcg/mL categorized as I or R by NCCLS did not show an increased mortality rate compared to S strains in non-meningeal pneumococcal infections when treated with ceftriaxone (1 g/d) or cefotaxime (1.5-2 g/8 h). These data support the higher breakpoints for ceftriaxone/cefotaxime by the NCCLS that went into effect in January 2002 for non-meningeal pneumococcal infections. This study demonstrates that parenteral aminothiazolyl cephalosporins such as ceftriaxone (1 g/day) or cefotaxime (1.5-2 g/8 h) work well in adult patients with systemic non-meningeal pneumococcal infections caused by strains with ceftriaxone/cefotaxime MIC up to 1 mcg/mL. Based on their limited experience, they concluded it also is probable that this observation is true for strains with ceftriaxone/cefotaxime MICs of 2 mcg/mL.

The available data in children[108] and adults suggest the NCCLS interpretive breakpoints were appropriately modified for systemic non-meningeal pneumococcal infections, and considered susceptible up to a ceftriaxone/cefotaxime MIC of 1 mcg/mL (NCCLS publication M100-S12 which went into effect January

2002). Until further experience with isolates with ceftriaxone/cefotaxime MIC of 2 mcg/mL accumulates, the investigators strongly recommend continued monitoring of the MIC of aminothiazolyl cephalosporins in all invasive pneumococcal isolates, and assessment of clinical and bacteriological outcomes.[108]

ANTIMICROBIAL THERAPY

With these considerations in focus, the purpose of this antimicrobial treatment section is to review the various recommendations, consensus panel statements, clinical trials, and published guidelines. A rational analysis of this information also will be performed to generate a set of evidence-based guidelines and protocols for specific populations with CAP.

Antibiotic Overview. A brief overview of agents that have been used for treatment of CAP will help set the stage for outcome-effective drug selection. *(See Table 2.)* The first generation cephalosporins have significant coverage against gram-positive organisms. By comparison, third generation cephalosporins have equal gram-positive coverage and increased coverage against aerobic gram-negative rods.[109] Ceftazidime has coverage against *Pseudomonas*, while cefoperazone has a somewhat higher MIC. Some of the second generation cephalosporins, such as cefoxitin, cefotetan, and cefmetazole, provide coverage against *Bacteroides* species. Imipenem has broad coverage against aerobic and anaerobic organisms. Aztreonam provides significant coverage for gram-negative bacilli such as *Pseudomonas*.

Among the beta-lactams, the CDC-DRSPWG identifies cefuroxime axetil, cefotaxime sodium, ceftriaxone sodium, or ampicillin-sulbactam as recommended empiric agents. The group notes, however, that among these agents, ceftriaxone and cefotaxime have superior activity against resistant pneumococci when compared with cefuroxime and ampicillin-sulbactam.[3] Because it is recommended that cefotaxime be administered in a dose of at least 1 g q8h for treatment of CAP,[3,110] and because the efficacy and safety of once-daily ceftriaxone for inpatient CAP is well established, ceftriaxone is recommended by most experts and the ASCAP Consensus Panel as the cephalosporin of choice for management of CAP.[110]

The aminoglycosides are active against gram-negative aerobic organisms.

These agents generally are used for elderly patients when severe CAP infection is suspected. As a rule, the aminoglycosides are combined with a third generation antipseudomonal or an extended spectrum quinolone antibiotic, monobactam, or an extended spectrum penicillin when used in these circumstances.[111]

The tetracyclines are active against *S. pneumoniae, H. influenza, Mycoplasma, Chlamydia*, and *Legionella*. There is, however, a growing incidence of *S. pneumoniae* resistance to tetracyclines.[112] These agents are alternatives to the macrolide antibiotics for empiric therapy for CAP in young, healthy adults.[113] Convenience and coverage advantages of the new macrolides, however, have thrust the tetracyclines into a secondary role for managing CAP. Clindamycin has activity against anaerobes, such as *B. fragilis*.[112,114] Its anaerobic coverage makes it a consideration for the treatment of pneumonia in nursing home patients suspected of aspiration. Metronidazole also has activity against anaerobic bacteria such as *B. fragilis.* It is used in combination with other antibiotics for the treatment of lung abscesses, aspiration pneumonia, or anaerobic infections.

Appropriate and Adequate Intensity of Antimicrobial Coverage. Because macrolides and extended spectrum quinolones have indications for monotherapeutic treatment of CAP, they frequently get equal billing as initial agents of choice. However, the macrolides and extended spectrum quinolones have clinically significant differences that should be considered in the antibiotic treatment equation for CAP. Accordingly, a careful analysis of the benefits and potential pitfalls of these agents should include a full accounting of the relevant similarities and differences. It will help emergency physicians, hospitalists, infectious disease specialists, and intensivists develop criteria that suggest the appropriateness and suitability that each of these classes may have in specific patient subgroups.

Although the previously cited six organisms (*S. pneumoniae, H. influenzae,* and *M. catarrhalis;* and atypical pathogens *Mycoplasma, Legionella,* and *C. pneumoniae*) are the most commonly implicated pathogens in patients with CAP, the elderly patient population also is susceptible to infection with gram-negative enteric organisms such as *Klebsiella, Escherichia coli,* and *Pseudomonas.* In other cases, the likelihood of infection with DRSP is high. When infection with these pathogens is likely, intensification of empiric coverage should include antibiotics with activity against these gram-negative species.[4,8,9] From a practical, antibiotic selection perspective, this requires that macrolides be used in combination with a cephalosporin such as ceftriaxone as initial, empiric therapy, or alternatively, an advanced generation fluoroquinolone.

Clinical features or risk factors that may suggest the need for intensification and expansion of bacterial and/or atypical pathogen coverage include the following: 1) increasing fragility (> 85 years of age, comorbid conditions, previous infection, etc.) of the patient; 2) acquisition of the pneumonia in a skilled nursing facility; 3) the presence of an aspiration pneumonia, suggesting involvement with gram-negative or anaerobic organisms; 4) chronic alcoholism, increasing the likelihood of infection with *Klebsiella pneumoniae*; 5) pneumococcal pneumonia in an underlying disease-compromised individual who has not been vaccinated with pneumococcal polysaccharide antigen (Pneumovax); 6) history of infection with gram-negative, anaerobic, or resistant species of *S. pneumoniae;* 7) history of treatment failure; 8) previous hospitalizations for pneumonia; 9) current or previous ICU hospitalization for pneumonia; 10) acquisition of pneumonia in a community with high and increasing resistance among *S. pneumoniae* species; and 11) immunodeficiency and/or severe underlying disease. Many of the aforementioned risk groups also can be treated with the combination of a third-generation cephalosporin plus a macrolide, in combination with an aminoglycoside when indicated.

As emphasized earlier in this report, most consensus panels, infectious disease experts, textbooks, and peer-reviewed antimicrobial prescribing guides recommend, as the initial or preferred choice, those antibiotics that, within the framework of monotherapy or combination therapy, address current etiologic and mortality trends in CAP. As a general rule, for empiric initial therapy in patients without modifying host factors that predispose to enteric gram-negative or pseudomonal infection, they recommend those antibiotics that provide coverage against the bacterial pathogens *S. pneumoniae, H. influenzae,* and *M. catarrhalis,* as well as against atypical pathogens *Mycoplasma, Legionella,* and *C. pneumoniae.*[38]

TREATMENT GUIDELINES FOR CAP: OUTCOMES, VALUE, AND INSTITUTIONAL IMPLEMENTATION

Based on a review of the available literature and personal communications

among the panel members, the ASCAP Consensus Panel recommends implementation of institution-wide guidelines for patients with CAP. A strong case can
be made for adopting such a strategy, especially when educational, process of
care, and quality review/improvement measures are put into place.

In one study reviewed,[115] a pneumonia guideline developed at Intermountain
Health Care included admission decision support and recommendations for
antibiotic timing and selection, based on the 1993 ATS guideline.[115] The study
included all immunocompetent patients older than age 65 with CAP from 1993
through 1997 in Utah; nursing home patients were excluded. The investigators
compared 30-day mortality rates among patients before and after the guideline
was implemented, as well as among patients treated by physicians who did not
participate in the guideline program.

Overall, the research group observed 28,661 cases of pneumonia, including
7719 (27%) that resulted in hospital admission. Thirty-day mortality was 13.4%
(1037 of 7719) among admitted patients and 6.3% (1801 of 28,661) overall.
Mortality rates (both overall and among admitted patients) were similar for both
patients of physicians affiliated and not affiliated with Intermountain Health Care
before the guideline was implemented. For episodes that resulted in hospital
admission after guideline implementation, 30-day mortality was 11.0% among
patients treated by Intermountain Health Care-affiliated physicians compared
with 14.2% for other Utah physicians. The guideline used ceftriaxone without or
without a macrolide such as azithromycin or clarithromycin.

An analysis that adjusted by logistic regression for age, sex, rural vs. urban res-
idences, and year confirmed that 30-day mortality was lower among admitted
patients who were treated by Intermountain Health Care-affiliated physicians (odds
ratio [OR]: 0.69; 95% confidence interval [CI]: 0.49 to 0.97; p = 0.04) and was
somewhat lower among all pneumonia patients (OR: 0.81; 95% CI: 0.63 to 1.03; p
= 0.08). The investigators concluded that implementation of a pneumonia practice
guideline in the Intermountain Health Care system was associated with a reduction
in 30-day mortality among elderly patients with pneumonia.

Explanations offered by the investigators for the decreased mortality after
guideline implementation include selection of more appropriate antibiotics, timing of initial antibiotic administration, and use of heparin prophylaxis against

thromboembolic disease. For example, one study[116] reported that mortality was about 25% lower among inpatients when the initial, empiric antibiotic regimen combined a third-generation cephalosporin with a macrolide compared with cephalosporins alone; whereas another investigation[43] showed a 15% reduction in mortality when antibiotics were administered within eight hours of hospitalization. The guideline that was evaluated by Intermountain Health Care recommended that antibiotics should be administered before a patient with pneumonia leaves the outpatient site of diagnosis. In addition, admission orders included prophylactic heparin.

Another group conducted a comprehensive review of the medical literature to determine whether guideline implementation for CAP reduces mortality and resource costs.[117] These investigators noted that studies have shown significant changes in the processes of care after implementation of guideline recommendations for treatment of patients with CAP.[118-120] The most extensive of these studies consisted of a randomized trial that was conducted in 19 hospitals and which included 1743 patients.[7] This study design provided reasonable internal validity (i.e., it is likely that the differences in the process of care between the nine intervention hospitals and the 10 control hospitals were due to the implementation of the critical pathway). The motivation for the trial was a desire to find means of cost-containment, inasmuch as the primary hypothesis was that the critical pathway would reduce the use of institutional resources without compromising the safety and efficacy of therapy.[7]

Two other studies have demonstrated an improvement in outcome after implementation of guidelines: improvement of patient response to antibacterial treatment in one[121] and lower mortality rates in the other.[122] Both studies used an uncontrolled, before-and-after design, but in one of the studies, the changes in the mortality rate in the intervention hospital were compared with data from 23 other hospitals.[122] In both of these studies, the improvement in outcome was accompanied by a reduction in the cost of care. A third study used an uncontrolled, before-and-after design to show that a quality improvement program reduced time to initiation of antibacterial treatment of patients with CAP, which is likely to improve patient outcome. However, there was no direct measurement of outcome. The reviewers conclude that the best-quality evidence about the effects of guideline implementation shows that they can be used to reduce unnecessary use of resources without compromising the quality of care or patient outcomes.[42,121]

CORRECT SPECTRUM COVERAGE: OUTCOME-OPTIMIZING REGIMENS FOR CAP

Because beta-lactams, advanced generation macrolides, and extended spectrum quinolones constitute the principal oral and intravenous treatment options for CAP, the following sections will discuss indications, clinical trials, side effects, and strategies for their use in CAP. The discussion will focus on antibiotics that: 1) provide, as combination therapy or monotherapy, appropriate coverage of bacterial and atypical organisms causing CAP; 2) are available for both outpatient (oral) and in-hospital (IV) management; and 3) are supported by national consensus panels or association guidelines.

Beta-Lactams: Ceftriaxone for Combination Therapy in CAP. The safety and efficacy of ceftriaxone for managing hospitalized patients with CAP has been well-established in numerous clinical trials, including recent investigations confirming its equal efficacy as compared to new generation fluoroquinolones. In this regard, one recent study attempted to determine the comparative efficacy and total resource costs of sequential IV to oral gatifloxacin therapy vs. IV ceftriaxone with or without IV erythromycin to oral clarithromycin therapy for treatment of CAP patients requiring hospitalization.[123]

Two hundred eighty-three patients were enrolled in a randomized, double-blind, clinical trial; data collected included patient demographics, clinical and microbiological outcomes, length of stay (LOS), and antibiotic-related LOS (LOSAR). Overall, 203 patients were clinically and economically evaluable (98 receiving gatifloxacin and 105 receiving ceftriaxone). It should be noted that IV erythromycin was administered to only 35 patients in the ceftriaxone-treated group, thereby putting a significant percentage (about 62%) of the ceftriaxone cohort at a "spectrum of coverage" disadvantage because of the failure to include an agent with coverage against atypical organisms. Despite this, oral conversion was achieved in 98% of patients in each group, and the investigators concluded that clinical cure and microbiological eradication rates did not differ statistically between ceftriaxone (92% and 92%) and gatifloxacin (98% and 97%).[123]

Given the concern about DRSP in hospitalized CAP patients, there has been robust debate about the effectiveness of ceftriaxone in pulmonary infections caused by DRSP. Attempting to shed light on this issue, an important study evaluating actual clinical outcomes in patients treated with beta-lactams for systemic infection outside of the central nervous system (CNS) that was caused by isolates of *S. pneumoniae* considered nonsusceptible to ceftriaxone (MIC ≥ 1.0 mcg/mL) by pre-2002 NCCLS breakpoints has recently been published by the Pediatric Infectious Diseases Section, Baylor College of Medicine.[124]

The objective of the study was to determine the actual clinical outcomes of patients treated primarily with beta-lactam antibiotics for a systemic infection outside of the CNS caused by isolates of *S. pneumoniae* nonsusceptible to ceftriaxone (MIC ≥ 1.0 mcg/mL). A retrospective review was performed of the medical records of children identified prospectively with invasive infections outside of the CNS caused by isolates of *S. pneumoniae* that were not susceptible to ceftriaxone between September 1993 and August 1999. A subset of this group treated primarily with beta-lactam antibiotics was analyzed for outcome. Among 2100 patients with invasive infections outside the CNS that were caused by *S. pneumoniae*, 166 had isolates not susceptible to ceftriaxone.

One hundred patients treated primarily with beta-lactam antibiotics were identified. From this group, 71 and 14 children had bacteremia alone or with pneumonia, respectively, caused by strains with an MIC of 1.0 mcg/mL. Bacteremia or pneumonia caused by isolates with a ceftriaxone MIC of 2.0 mcg/mL or greater occurred in six and five children, respectively. Three children with septic arthritis and one with cellulitis had infections caused by strains with an MIC to ceftriaxone of 1.0 mcg/mL. Most were treated with parenteral ceftriaxone, cefotaxime, or cefuroxime for one or more doses followed by an oral antibiotic. All but one child were successfully treated. The failure occurred in a child with severe combined immune deficiency and bacteremia (MIC = 1.0 mcg/mL) who remained febrile after a single dose of ceftriaxone followed by 12 days of cefprozil. The investigators concluded that ceftriaxone, cefotaxime, or cefuroxime are adequate to treat invasive infections outside the CNS caused by pneumococcal isolates with MICs up to 2.0 mcg/mL. Accordingly, the NCCLS breakpoints, as of January 2002, for the beta-lactam ceftriaxone and cefotaxime were modified and up-calibrated so that currently about 95% of all *S. pneumoniae* species are considered sensitive to ceftriaxone, as well as cefotaxime.[25]

OBSERVATIONAL TRENDS FROM THE ARM DATABASE: CEFTRIAXONE VS. CEFOTAXIME FOR *Streptococcus pneumoniae*

The Antimicrobial Resistance Management (ARM) program was established to help individual institutions define their antimicrobial resistance problems and establish cause-effect relationships that could lead to strategic interventions. To date, the ARM program has entered more than 121 community and teaching hospitals into a web-centered database. This observational database currently has susceptibility data on up to 19 different organisms and up to 46 different antibiotics. As of February 2003, the ARM program had collected data on more than 15 million total isolates, and sensitivity data on more than 60,000 separate isolates of *S. pneumoniae*.[125]

In a presentation made at the American College of Clinical Pharmacy (Albuquerque, New Mexico, Oct. 21, 2002, John Gums, PharmD), data from the ARM program demonstrated higher rates of resistance for cefotaxime as compared to ceftriaxone for *S. pneumoniae* isolates. In this study, University of Florida researchers analyzed data from the ARM Program in 1995-2001. National and regional susceptibility data from 143 hospitals in five U.S. regions (North Central, Northeast, South Central, Southeast, and Southwest) were examined. Sensitivity reports for pneumococcal isolates were reviewed for susceptibility to cefotaxime and ceftriaxone and compared across years and U.S. regions using a web-based analysis tool.

The results of the study showed that *S. pneumoniae* bacteria were more susceptible overall to ceftriaxone compared to cefotaxime (80.9% vs 71.7%). National susceptibility rates for cefotaxime were lower than the rates for ceftriaxone in each of the years studied, beginning at 54.7% in 1995 and progressing to 73.6% in 2001. Over the same time period, national susceptibility rates for ceftriaxone were higher, beginning at 75.2% in 1995 and increasing to 82.3% in 2001. For the most part, these national susceptibility trends also were consistent regionally, with one exception. In the Northeast, susceptibility rates were comparable for cefotaxime and ceftriaxone in each year except for 2001, when susceptibility rates for the two drugs were 70.2% and 80.7%, respectively.

Since the ARM program was originally designed as an observational database to use antibiogram trending to identify resistance patterns for individual hospitals, it is not capable of isolating the specific reason why national sensitivity differences exist between ceftriaxone and cefotaxime. Additionally, for similar reasons, the ARM program is not designed to identify why certain geographic sections of the United States demonstrate the discrepancies in sensitivities and others do not. However, subanalysis of the data suggests that the discrepancy between the third-generation cephalosporins did not exist through the whole database. The difference in sensitivity percentages appeared to emerge during the last half of the 1990-2000 decade. This coincides with the push to use cefotaxime on a twice a day basis vs. a more traditional three times daily dosing regimen.[125]

Since cefotaxime exerts its antimicrobial activity as a function of its time above the MIC of *S. pneumoniae*, a drop in dosing frequency from TID to BID will increase the percent of time that the organism is exposed to subinhibitory concentrations.[126] Without any significant post-antibiotic effect, the sensitivities of cefotaxime to *S. pneumoniae* may fall. More specific MIC analysis is required to determine if the reduced dosing frequency is causally related to the emergence of a sensitivity discrepancy between cefotaxime and ceftriaxone. The clinical implications, in terms of patient outcomes, have not been established.

Cephalosporins Vs. Fluoroquinolones: Comparing Propensity for Development of Drug Resistance.[127] Current guidelines from the Infectious Disease Society of America recommend a third generation cephalosporin such as ceftriaxone (along with a macrolide) and quinolones such as levofloxacin, gatifloxacin, and moxifloxacin (as single agents) for treatment of patients with CAP requiring hospitalization.[128] The respiratory advanced generation fluoroquinolones have a broad spectrum of activity against *S. pneumoniae, H. influenzae, Moraxella catarrhalis, Mycoplasma pneumoniae,* and *Legionella pneumophila* and are currently one of the treatments of choice for penicillin-resistant *S. pneumoniae.* However, overuse of this class of antimicrobial agents could lead to emergence of resistant mutants. A 1999/2000 National Antimicrobial

Resistance Surveillance Study showed a greater than 1% resistance to quinolones and analysis of recent SENTRY studies show a 0.9% resistance to levofloxacin.[129-31] In Canada, the prevalence of pneumococci with reduced susceptibility to fluoroquinolones in adults, increased from 0% in 1993 to 1.7% in 1997 and 1998.[132]

The prevalence of pneumococci with raised ciprofloxacin MIC ciprofloxacin MIC 4 mcg/L) also increased from 0.9% in 1991-1992 to 3.0% in 1997-1998 in Spain.[133] A recent study from Hong Kong showed an overall prevalence of quinolone resistance of 13.3%, with 27.3% quinolone resistance among penicillin-resistant isolates.[134] It is of concern that these resistant clones may spread to other parts of the world. The primary targets of fluoroquinolones are topoisomerase II (DNA gyrase) and topoisomerase IV, which alter DNA topology through transient double-stranded selected mutants, and did not have alteration in the QRDR of proteins GyrA, GyrB, ParC, and ParE.

Selecting Resistant Mutants. In one study,[127] attempts were made to select resistant pneumococcal mutants by sequential subculturing of 12 clinically isolated pneumococci (4 were penicillin sensitive [MIC 0.03-0.06 mcg/L], 4 penicillin intermediate [MIC 0.25-0.5 mcg/L], and 4 penicillin resistant [MIC 2-4 mcg/L]) in subinhibitory concentrations of ceftriaxone, levofloxacin, gatifloxacin, and moxifloxacin. Subculturing in gatifloxacin, levofloxacin, moxifloxacin, and ceftriaxone selected 12 mutants (12/12), 10 mutants (10/12), 10 mutants (10/12), and three mutants (3/12), respectively. DNA sequencing of the quinolone-resistant mutants showed that most strains had mutations in GyrA at E85 or S81. This *in vitro* mutation study demonstrated a clear distinction between the low frequency of development of resistance with ceftriaxone exposure as opposed to the high frequency with quinolone exposure.

Initial MICs of parent strains and resistant mutants resulting from serial daily subculturing in subinhibitory concentrations of antimicrobials were evaluated. The lowest mutant selection rate was obtained by ceftriaxone. Three mutants were selected by ceftriaxone with at least an eight-fold increase in their MICs for ceftriaxone. The three mutants had initial MICs of 0.125, 1, and 1 mcg/L (1 ceftriaxone sensitive and the other 2 ceftriaxone intermediate). These ceftriaxone mutants were selected in 14, 32, and 42 days. Among the quinolones tested, levofloxacin, moxifloxacin, and gatifloxacin selected 10, 10, and 12 resistant mutants, respectively. All selected mutants had the same pulsed-field electrophoresis pattern as their parent strains. The average time necessary for mutant selection was 22.7 days for levofloxacin, 24 days for moxifloxacin, and 24.3 days for gatifloxacin. All of the parent strains were sensitive to levofloxacin, gatifloxacin, and moxifloxacin. The majority of the parent strains were of intermediate resistance to ceftriaxone. After subculturing in selected antibiotics, ceftriaxone showed resistance in all of the three mutant strains, two of three had initial MICs in the ceftriaxone intermediate range, and one of three was in the ceftriaxone sensitive range.

Of 12 parent strains used for mutant selection, 10 already had substitution of I at position 460 of ParC protein by V compared with reference strains. Selection by levofloxacin, gatifloxacin, and moxifloxacin caused alterations of GyrA in eight, eight, and seven mutants selected by these antibiotics, respectively. The second most affected protein was parC for mutants produced by levofloxacin and gatifloxacin exposure. GyrB was the second most affected protein for mutants produced by moxifloxacin exposure. Among 32 mutants selected by quinolones, 25 had alterations in GyrA, 12 in ParC, nine in ParE, and eight in GyrB. The changes in GyrA were mostly at positions 81 (S81/A,F,L,Y) and 85 (E85/K,A,G). In two mutant strains selected by levofloxacin, exposure changes in two amino acids, S81Y and V101I in GyrA, were associated with the increase in the quinolone MICs. One mutant selected by levofloxacin had substitution of D by G at position 80 in GyrA. Alterations in GyrB were detected in eight mutants selected by moxifloxacin, gatifloxacin, and levofloxacin exposure. In two mutants GyrB was altered by insertion of two amino acids. The mutant selected by moxifloxacin exposure from parent 3 had insertion of I and S after position 398, and the mutant selected by levofloxacin exposure from parent 11 had insertion of E and I after.

In this study, the parenteral beta-lactam antibiotic, ceftriaxone, and three quinolone antibiotics, levofloxacin, gatifloxacin, and moxifloxacin were tested for their ability to select resistant mutants. The lowest mutation rates occurred with ceftriaxone in multi-step resistance selection experiments. No obvious differences in ability to select resistant mutants were observed among the three quinolones tested. Alterations in GyrA, GyrB, ParC, and ParE were detected among resistant mutants selected by quinolone exposure. Seventy-eight percent of resistant mutants had modifications in GyrA, showing the importance of this protein in the action of these quinolones. Mutations in ParC were found in 37% of these mutants. However, moxifloxacin exposure, in addition to selecting mutants with GyrA changes, also selected mutants with GyrB changes. GyrB is, therefore, likely to be an important target for moxifloxacin. Overall, ceftriaxone had lower rates of resistance selection compared with the respiratory quinolones. This is a similar finding to previous studies when ceftriaxone was compared with macrolides.[135] When resistant clones were selected by ceftriaxone, on average it took more subcultures for the development of resistance compared with the quinolones. Therefore, the investigators concluded, ceftriaxone may not pose an important selective pressure for resistance development compared with the fluoroquinolones and the macrolides, and may be used confidently in the treatment of CAP requiring hospitalization.[127]

Advanced Generation Macrolides. The established new generation macrolide antibiotics include the erythromycin analogues azithromycin and clarithromycin.[136,137] Compared to erythromycin, which is the least expensive macrolide, the major advantages of these newer antibiotics are significantly decreased gastrointestinal side effects, which produce enhanced tolerance, improved bioavailability, higher tissue levels, and pharmacokinetic features that permit less frequent dosing and better compliance, as well as enhanced activity against *H. influenzae*.[138,139] In particular, the long tissue half-life of azithromycin allows this antibiotic to be prescribed for a shorter duration (5 days) than comparable antibiotics given for the same indications. Given the cost differences between azithromycin and clarithromycin, as well as the improved compliance patterns associated with short-duration therapy, any rational approach to distinguishing between these agents must consider prescription, patient, and drug resistance barriers.

At the outset, it is fair to say that these macrolides—especially azithromycin—to a great degree, have supplanted the use of erythromycin in community-acquired infections of the lower respiratory tract. In addition, from the perspective of providing definitive, cost-effective, and compliance-promoting therapy, the newer macrolide antibiotics, which includes intravenous azithromycin for hospital-based management, have recently emerged as some of the drugs of choice—along with the new, extended spectrum quinolones—for outpatient management of CAP.[140] When used as oral agents, they play a central role in the management of pneumonia in otherwise healthy individuals who do not require hospitalization.

From an emergency medicine and in-hospital management perspective, the value and desirability of macrolide therapy has been significantly enhanced by the availability of the intravenous formulation of azithromycin as a cotherapeutic agent for hospitalized patients with CAP. Unlike penicillins, cephalosporins, and sulfa-based agents, azithromycin has the advantage of showing in vitro activity against both atypical and bacterial offenders implicated in CAP.[13,14]

The macrolides also have the advantage of a simplified dosing schedule, especially azithromycin, which for outpatients is given once daily for only five days (500 mg po on day 1 and 250 mg po qd on days 2-5). For oral, step-down therapy of hospitalized patients with CAP, the dose of azithromycin is 500 mg po qd for a total treatment course of 10 days. Clarithromycin requires a longer course of therapy and is more expensive. Clarithromycin costs approximately $68-72 for a complete, 10-day course of therapy vs. $42-44 for a complete course of therapy with azithromycin.

Clarithromycin, however, is an alternative among macrolides for outpatient treatment of CAP. It is now available in once-daily formulation (1000 mg/d for 10 days) for oral use, but an intravenous preparation is not currently available. In general, the decision to use a macrolide such as azithromycin rather than erythromycin is based on weighing the increased cost of a course of therapy with azithromycin against its real-world advantages, which include a more convenient dosing schedule; its broader spectrum of coverage; its favorable drug interaction profile; no pain on injection or venous thrombosis issues; and its decreased incidence of gastrointestinal side effects, which occur in 3-5% of patients taking an oral, five-day, multiple-dose regimen.[141]

Azithromycin—Coagent (i.e., with Ceftriaxone) For Combination Therapy in Hospitalized CAP. Intravenous azithromycin can be used for the management of hospitalized patients with moderate or severe CAP.[15,16,142] Currently, azithromycin is the only advanced generation macrolide indicated for parenteral therapy in hospitalized patients with CAP due to *C. pneumoniae, H. influenzae, L. pneumophila, M. catarrhalis, M. pneumoniae, S. pneumoniae,* or *Staphylococcus aureus.*[13,14,142,143] This would be considered correct spectrum coverage for empiric therapy of CAP in most patients. However, for hospitalized patients, who tend to have co-morbid conditions, including underlying cardiorespiratory disease, the addition of a beta-lactam (ceftriaxone/cefotaxime) to azithromycin is considered *mandatory* by the ASCAP Consensus Panel.

Azithromycin dosing and administration schedules for hospitalized patients are different than for the five-day course used exclusively for outpatient management, and these differences should be noted. When this advanced generation macrolide is used for hospitalized patients with CAP, 2-5 days of therapy with azithromycin IV (500 mg once daily) followed by oral azithromycin (500 mg once daily to complete a total of 7-10 days of therapy) is clinically and bacteriologically effective. For patients requiring hospitalization, the initial 500 mg intravenous dose of azithromycin should be given in the ED.

Like the oral formulation, IV azithromycin appears to be well-tolerated, with a low incidence of gastrointestinal adverse events (4.3% diarrhea, 3.9% nausea, 2.7% abdominal pain, 1.4% vomiting), minimal injection-site reactions (less than 12% combined injection-site pain and/or inflammation or infection), and a low incidence of discontinuation (1.2% discontinuation of IV therapy) due to drug-related adverse patient events or laboratory abnormalities.[144]

One recent study[145] has investigated the value of adding a macrolide to an initial beta-lactam-based antibiotic regimen in patients with bacteremic pneumococcal pneumonia. The objective was to assess the influence of including a macrolide into a beta-lactam-based empiric antibiotic regimen on bacteremic pneumococcal pneumonia mortality. This observational, 10-year study of patients with bacteremic pneumococcal pneumonia receiving a beta-lactam as initial antibiotic therapy attempted to assess the independent predictors of mortality; the available set of prognostic factors were subjected to a step-wise logistic regression procedure taking in-hospital death as the outcome variable. Among the 409 patients who were included in the study, 238 (58%) received a beta-lactam plus a macrolide with or without other antibiotics and 171 (42%) a beta-lactam with or without other antibiotics different from a macrolide. Patients not receiving a macrolide were more likely to have comorbidity (p = 0.0002); an ultimately/rapidly fatal underlying disease (p < 0.0001); neutropenia (p = 0.002); a nosocomial origin of the infection (p < 0.0001); a microorganism resistant to penicillin (p = 0.02); and an increased exposure to corticosteroids, cancer chemotherapy, and prior antibiotics. However, they were less likely to be in shock at presentation (p < 0.0001) and require ICU admission (p < 0.0001). Overall, 35 patients (9%) died. Four variables were independently associated with death: shock (p < 0.0001), age 65 or older (p = 0.02), resistance to both penicillin and erythromycin (p = 0.04), and no inclusion of a macrolide in the initial antibiotic regimen (p = 0.03). The investigators concluded that not adding a macrolide to a beta-lactam-based initial antibiotic regimen for bacteremic pneumococcal pneumonia is an independent predictor of in-hospital mortality.[145]

COMMUNITY-ACQUIRED PNEUMONIA (CAP): ASCAP CONSENSUS PANEL RECOMMENDATIONS FOR OUTPATIENT MANAGEMENT

Despite a general consensus that empiric, outpatient treatment of CAP requires, at the least, mandatory coverage of such organisms as *S. pneumoniae, H. influenzae*, and *M. catarrhalis,* as well as atypical organisms (*M. pneumoniae, C. pneumoniae*, and *L. pneumophila*), antibiotic selection strategies for achieving this spectrum of coverage vary widely. New treatment guidelines for CAP have been issued by such national associations as the IDSA (2000), the ATS (2001), and the CDC (CDC-DRSPWG, 2000).

Deciphering the strengths, subtleties, and differences among recommendations issued by different authoritative sources can be problematic and confusing. Because patient disposition practices and treatment pathways vary among institutions and from region to region, management guidelines for CAP must be "customized" for the local practice environment. Unfortunately, no single set of guidelines is applicable to every patient or practice environment; therefore, clinical judgment must prevail. This means taking into account local antibiotic resistance patterns, epidemiological and infection incidence data, and patient demographic features.

Patient Management Recommendations. The ASCAP 2003 Consensus Panel concurred that appropriate use of antibiotics requires radiographic confirmation of the diagnosis of CAP. In this regard, physicians should use clinical judgement when ordering chest x-rays, with the understanding that the diagnostic yield of this radiographic modality in CAP is increased in patients with fever greater than 38.5°C; presence of new cough; and abnormal pulmonary findings suggestive of consolidation, localized bronchoconstriction, or pleural effusion.

Accordingly, a chest x-ray is recommended and encouraged by the ASCAP Consensus Panel, as well as by such national associations as the IDSA, ATS, and American College of Emergency Physicians (ACEP), to confirm the diagnosis of outpatient CAP; however, the panel acknowledges that, on occasion, logistical issues may prevent radiographic confirmation at the time of diagnosis and treatment.

The approach to antibiotic therapy usually will be empiric, and must account for a number of clinical, epidemiological, and unpredictable factors related to antibiotic resistance patterns and respiratory tract pathogens. As a general rule, appropriate antibiotic choice for the patient with CAP requires consideration of strategies that will yield clinical cure in the patient "today," combined with antibiotic selection strategies that prevent accelerated emergence of drug-resistant organisms that will infect the community "tomorrow."

Based on the most current clinical studies, the principal six respiratory tract pathogens that must be covered on an empiric basis in individuals with outpatient CAP include: *S. pneumoniae, H. influenzae, M. catarrhalis, C. pneumoniae, M. pneumoniae*, and *L. pneumophila*. In addition, the ASCAP Consensus Panel emphasized that there may be a "disconnect" (i.e., an incompletely understood and not entirely predictable relationship between an antibiotic's MIC level and its association with positive clinical outcomes in CAP). This "disconnect" may be explained by the unique qualities of an antimicrobial, such as tissue penetration and/or pharmacokinetics, patient medication compliance, and other factors.

Double-blinded, prospective clinical trials comparing new generation macrolides vs. new generation fluoroquinolones demonstrate similar outcomes in terms of clinical cure and bacteriologic eradication rates in outpatients with CAP.[124] However, emergence of resistance among *S. pneumoniae* species to new generation fluoroquinolones has been reported in a number of geographic regions, including the United States, Hong Kong, and Canada, and this may have implications for treatment.

The frequency of DRSP causing outpatient CAP, as estimated by the CDC, is very low (i.e., in the range of 0.14-1.9%). The CDC-DRSPWG cautions against overuse of new generation fluoroquinolones in outpatient CAP, and recommends their use as alternative agents when: 1) first-line therapy with advanced generation macrolides such as azithromycin fails; 2) patients are allergic to first-line agents; or 3) the case is a documented infection with DRSP.[146]

Given concerns about antibiotic overuse, the potential for emerging resistance among DRSP to fluoroquinolones, and the increasing recognition of atypical pathogens as causative agents in patients with outpatient CAP, the panel concurs with the CDC-DRSPWG recommendation advocating macrolides as initial agents of choice in outpatient CAP. The ASCAP Consensus Panel also noted that the Canadian Consensus Guidelines for CAP Management and the 2001 ATS Consensus Guideline Recommendations also include advanced generation macrolides as initial therapy for outpatient CAP.

In this regard, two safe and effective advanced generation macrolides, azithromycin and clarithromycin, currently are available for outpatient, oral-based treatment of CAP. Based on outcome-sensitive criteria such as cost, daily dose frequency, duration of therapy, side effects, and drug interactions, the ASCAP Consensus Panel recommends as first-line, preferred initial therapy in CAP, azithromycin, with clarithromycin or doxycycline as alternative agents; and as alternative first-line therapy, moxifloxacin, gatifloxacin, or levofloxacin when appropriate, according to CDC guidelines and other association-based protocols. Among the advanced generation fluoroquinolones, moxifloxacin is preferred by the ASCAP Consensus Panel as the initial fluoroquinolone of choice because it has the most favorable MICs against *S. pneumoniae*, and a more focused spectrum of coverage against gram-positive organisms than levofloxacin or gatifloxacin. For older individuals or "higher risk" patients managed in the outpatient setting, moxifloxacin or azithromycin are the initial agents of choice.

Physicians are urged to prescribe antibiotics in CAP at the time of diagnosis and to encourage patients to fill and begin taking their prescriptions for CAP on the day of diagnosis. Ideally, patients should initiate their first course of oral therapy within eight hours of diagnosis, a time frame that appears reasonable based on studies in hospitalized patients indicating improved survival in patients who received their first IV dose within eight hours of diagnosis. Primary care practitioners also are urged to instruct patients in medication compliance. In the case of short (5-day) courses of therapy, patients should be educated that although they are only consuming medications for a five-day period, the antibiotic remains at the tissue site of infection for about 7-10 days and continues to deliver therapeutic effects during that period.

Either verbal or on-site, reevaluation of patients is recommended within a three-day period following diagnosis and initiation of antibiotic therapy. Follow-up in the office or clinic within three days is recommended in certain risk-stratified patients, especially the elderly, those with co-morbid illness, and those in whom medication compliance may be compromised. More urgent follow-up may be required in patients with increasing symptoms, including dyspnea, fever, and other systemic signs or symptoms. Follow-up chest x-rays generally are not recommended in patients with outpatient CAP, except in certain high-risk groups, such as those with right middle lobe syndrome, and in individuals in whom the diagnosis may have been uncertain.

IN-HOSPITAL MANAGEMENT OF CAP: MONOTHERAPY VS. COMBINATION THERAPY. OUTCOMES ANALYSIS AND ASCAP TREATMENT GUIDELINES

Although antibiotic recommendations based on risk-stratification criteria, historical features, sites where the infection was acquired, and other modifying factors play a role, institutional protocols, hospital-based critical pathways, resistance features, and other factors also will influence antibiotic selection. Despite variations in hospital or departmental protocols, certain requirements regarding drug selection for CAP are relatively consistent. For example, from an empiric antibiotic selection perspective, providing mandatory antimicrobial coverage against *S. pneumoniae, H. influenzae, M. catarrhalis, Legionella, M. pneumoniae,* and *C. pneumoniae* appears to be non-negotiable for managing the majority of patients with CAP. Selected populations also may be at risk for infection with *S. aureus* or gram-negative organisms, a factor that will modify antibiotic selection. As mentioned earlier, consensus reports and national guidelines support this strategy (see section on Consensus Guidelines for Antibiotic Therapy, below).

When combination cephalosporin/macrolide therapy is the accepted hospital protocol, among the beta-lactams available, IV ceftriaxone is recommended by the ASCAP 2003 Consensus Panel because of its evidence-based efficacy in moderate-to severe CAP, once-daily administration, and spectrum of coverage; and because it is supported by all major guideline panels.

One study evaluated antibiotic resistance data using data derived from community-based medical practices. Data were gathered from July 1999 to April 2000. Four of the most common isolates were: *Moraxella catarrhalis* (27%), *Haemophilus influenzae* (25%), *Staphylococcus aureus* (14%), and *Streptococcus pneumoniae* (12%); atypical organisms were not assessed.

Among *S. pneumoniae* isolates, levofloxacin exhibited a 4.8% level of resistance; for ceftriaxone, the resistance rate was only 5.8% (based on pre-2002 NCCLS MIC breakpoint). For *S. aureus*, both ceftriaxone and levofloxacin inhibited all isolates. And for *M. catarrhalis* and *H. influenzae,* no resistance was observed for either levofloxacin or ceftriaxone. The investigators concluded that levofloxacin and ceftriaxone exhibited equivalent susceptibility/resistance patterns to organisms encountered in CAP.[147]

Although ceftriaxone was introduced to the market in 1985, and despite 18 years of use, its susceptibility to multiple gram-positive and gram-negative isolates has not changed significantly. In this regard, ceftriaxone has retained potent activity against the most commonly encountered enteric species (i.e., *E. coli, K. pneumoniae, K. oxytocia,* and *P. mirabilis*), at a level of 93-99%.[147]

Azithromycin is recommended as the co-therapeutic macrolide agent (i.e., in combination with ceftriaxone) in patients with CAP for the following reasons: 1) it can be administered on a once-daily basis, thereby minimizing human resource costs associated with drug administration; 2) it is the only macrolide indicated for in-hospital, intravenous-to-oral step-down, monotherapeutic management of CAP caused by *S. pneumoniae, H. influenzae, M. catarrhalis, L. pneumophila, M. pneumoniae, C. pneumoniae,* or *S. aureus*—an important efficacy and spectrum of coverage benchmark; 3) at $19-22 per day for the intravenous dose of 500 mg azithromycin, its cost is reasonable; 4) the intravenous-to-oral step-down dose of 500 mg has been established as effective in clinical trials evaluating hospitalized patients with CAP; and 5) azithromycin has excellent activity against *L. pneumophila*, a pathogen commonly implicated in the geriatric patient with CAP. Decisions about use will be determined by intrainstitutional pathways and protocols, based on consensus recommendations and association guidelines as presented in this article.

Critical Pathways and Protocols. When patients with CAP are hospitalized in the ICU or there is a significant likelihood of gram-negative infection (i.e., *Klebsiella, E. coli,* or *P. aeruginosa*), monotherapy with a macrolide is not appropriate, and the CDC group's recent consensus report stresses the importance of using an IV macrolide in combination with other agents, and in particular third-generation cephalosporins such as ceftriaxone.[3] In these patients, a macrolide should be used in combination with a cephalosporin (i.e., ceftriaxone); when anti-pseudomonal coverage is necessary, an anti-pseudomonal cephalosporin and/or an aminoglycoside also may be required. Or alternatively, for the ICU patient with CAP, an extended spectrum fluoroquinolone such as moxifloxacin should be considered, along with a cephalosporin such as ceftriaxone.[3] When anaerobic organisms are suspected, clindamycin or a beta-lactam/beta-lactamase inhibitor is appropriate.

Accordingly, a number of critical pathways for pneumonia therapy recommend use of two-drug therapy for CAP. The therapy typically is the combination of an IV cephalosporin such as ceftriaxone plus a macrolide, which usually is initially administered by the intravenous route when the patient's condition so warrants. Perhaps the important change in CAP treatment since publication of the ATS guidelines in 1993 is the current general consensus, including guidelines presented at the 2001 ATS Scientific Conference, that atypical organisms such as *L. pneumophila, C. pneumoniae,* and *M. pneumoniae* must be covered empirically as part of the initial antibiotic regimen. Whereas previous consensus guidelines indicated that macrolides could be added to a cephalosporin on a "plus or minus" basis for initial CAP treatment, it is now emphasized that coverage of the atypical spectrum, along with coverage of *S. pneumoniae, H. influenzae*, and *M. catarrhalis,* is mandatory.[3] New guidelines from the IDSA, ATS, ASCAP, and CDC now reflect this strategy.

Although virtually all protocols using combination cephalosporin/ macrolide therapy specify intravenous administration of the cephalosporin, guidelines specifying whether initial macrolide therapy should occur via the intravenous or oral route are less concrete. Recent CDC-DRSPWG guidelines recommend an intravenous macrolide therapy for patients hospitalized in the ICU, while oral therapy is permissible in conjunction with an IV cephalosporin in the medical ward patient.[2] Because atypical infections such as *L. pneumophila* are associated with high mortality rates, especially in the elderly, and because hospitalized patients with CAP, by definition, represent a sicker cohort, it is prudent and, therefore, advisable that initial macrolide therapy in the hospital be administered by the intravenous route. The ASCAP Consensus Panel, therefore, recommends IV azithromycin therapy as the preferred initial, empiric agent in combination with ceftriaxone. The Panel acknowledges, however, that some institutions will use intravenous ceftriaxone in combination with an oral macrolide in non-ICU patients, an approach supported by a number of national panels. In patients on combination cephalosporin/macrolide therapy, step-down to oral therapy with azithromycin can be accomplished when the patient's clinical status so dictates, or when culture results suggest this is appropriate.

Monotherapy Vs. Combination Therapy. It should be pointed out that while some consensus panels (ATS Guidelines, 2001) support the use of IV azithromycin in very carefully selected hospitalized CAP patients (mild disease) as monothera-py, *or* as the macrolide component of *combination therapy,* other panels, such as CDC-DRSPWG and the IDSA 2000 Guidelines, support its use specifically as the macrolide component of *combination therapy* (i.e., to be used in combination with such agents as ceftriaxone). The ASCAP Panel supports the use of IV azithromycin as part of a combination cephalosporin/macrolide regimen for CAP.

As emphasized, advanced generation fluoroquinolones also provide a monotherapeutic option for management of CAP, and advocates of this approach argue that these agents, on an empiric basis, provide an adequate spectrum of coverage against expected respiratory pathogens at lower drug acquisition costs. Other experts make the case that although monotherapy for pneumococcal pneu-monia is standard practice in many institutions, and is identified as a treatment option in many national association guidelines, there may be a survival benefit from using a combination beta-lactam and macrolide therapy.[21] To address this issue, a group of investigators evaluated a patient database to determine whether initial empirical therapy with a combination of effective antibiotic agents would have a better outcome than a single effective antibiotic agent in patients with bac-teremic pneumococcal pneumonia.

The investigators conducted a review of adult bacteremic pneumococcal pneumonia managed in the Methodist Healthcare System, Memphis, Tennessee, between Jan. 1, 1996, and July 31, 2000. Empirical therapy was defined as all antibiotic agents received in the first 24 hours after presentation. On the basis of culture results, empirical therapy was classified as single effective therapy (SET), dual effective therapy (DET), or more than DET (MET). Acute Physiology and Chronic Health Evaluation II (APACHE II)-based predicted mortality and PSI scores were calculated.[21]

Two hundred twenty-five subjects met the inclusion criteria for analysis. An additional seven cases of CAP with pneumococcal bacteremia were identified but were excluded from the study because the isolate was resistant to the empirical therapy the patient received. Investigators noted that the subjects who received MET were significantly sicker than the subjects who received SET or DET, as measured by the PSI ($p = 0.04$) and APACHE II-based predicted mortality ($p = 0.03$). Of special significance was that there was no statistically significant difference between the prevalence of chronic disease states between the SET and DET groups.

Levofloxacin was the most commonly chosen fluoroquinolone (70.4%), with only four subjects treated with ciprofloxacin (1 in the SET group, 2 in the DET group, and 1 in the MET group, all with no fatalities). Eight subjects who received more than one antibiotic agent as empirical therapy were classified as SET on the basis of the isolate being resistant to azithromycin (5 subjects), cefotaxime (2 subjects), or combined ticarcillin-clavulanate potassium (1 subject). Twenty-nine subjects (12.9%) died. A Kaplan-Meier plot of mortality over time for each antibiotic therapy group demonstrated that mortality with the SET group was significantly higher than with the DET group ($p = 0.02$; OR, 3.0 [95% CI, 1.2-7.6]). Even when the DET and MET groups are combined, the mortality was still significantly higher in the SET group ($p = 0.04$; OR, 2.3 [95% CI, 1.0-5.2]). Because only a few subjects received MET and the subjects who received MET were significantly sicker than the other subjects, subsequent analysis is confined to the SET and DET groups.

Because subjects who received SET had a lower predicted mortality than those who received DET, a logistic regression model was used to calculate the OR for death of SET vs. DET adjusted for predicted mortality, which was 6.4 (95% CI, 1.9-21.7). All deaths occurred in patients with a PSI score higher than 90 (PSI classes 4 and 5). In subjects with PSI class 4 or 5 CAP who were given

SET, the predicted mortality-adjusted OR for death was 5.5 (95% CI, 1.7-17.5). Because antibiotic therapy would be expected to have little influence on early deaths, the investigators reanalyzed SET vs. DET groups after excluding all deaths that occurred within 48 hours of presentation (n = 4, 3 in the SET group and 1 in the DET group). Univariate analysis of this subgroup showed a trend to better outcome with DET compared with SET (94% survival vs 85%, respectively; p = 0.06). Multivariate analysis again confirmed that SET was an independent predictor of worse outcome (p = 0.01), with the predicted mortality-adjusted odds ratio for death in subjects given SET being 4.9 (95% CI, 1.6-18.3). Subgroup analysis did not show any significant trends to suggest any advantage or disadvantage of any specific antibiotic agents or combinations of antibiotic agents within the SET or DET groups.

Of the 225 patients with CAP who were identified, 99 were classified as receiving SET, 102 as receiving DET, and 24 as receiving MET. Compared with the other groups, patients who received MET statistically had significantly more severe pneumonia as measured by the PSI score (p = 0.04) and predicted mortality (p = 0.03). Mortality within the SET group was significantly higher than within the DET group (p = 0.02; OR, 3.0 [95% CI, 1.2-7.6]), even when the DET and MET groups (p = 0.04) were combined. In a logistic regression model including antibiotic therapy and clinical risk factors for mortality, SET remained an independent predictor of mortality with a predicted mortality-adjusted odds ratio of death of 6.4 (95% CI, 1.9-21.7). All deaths occurred in patients with a PSI score higher than 90, and the predicted mortality-adjusted odds ratio for death with SET in this subgroup was 5.5 (95% CI, 1.7-17.5).

In comparably matched patients, this group found that SET is associated with a significantly greater risk of death than DET. On the basis of these results, they concluded that monotherapy may be suboptimal for patients with severe bacteremic pneumococcal pneumonia who have PSI scores of greater than 90.[21]

While acknowledging its limitations, the results of this retrospective study strongly suggest that bacteremic patients with pneumococcal CAP who receive at least two effective antibiotic agents within the first 24 hours after presentation to a hospital have a significantly lower mortality than patients who receive only one effective antibiotic agent. In fact, among high-risk patients (PSI classes 4 or

5), receiving only one effective antibiotic agent increases mortality by more than five-fold as compared with patients receiving two effective antibiotic agents.

Although these findings need to be confirmed by a prospective study, the authors suggest that current approaches to the empiric therapy of severe CAP may need to be reevaluated.[21] Accordingly, the ASCAP 2003 Consensus Panel evaluated this study and found its results and conclusions—as well as its clinical implications—to be sufficiently compelling to recommend combination therapy with ceftriaxone plus a macrolide as the initial approach-of-choice in managing moderately-to-severely ill patients suspected of having bacteremia associated with pneumococcal pneumonia.

Further confirmation of the potential improvement in clinical outcomes associated with two-drug therapy, consisting of ceftriaxone plus a macrolide, as compared to monotherapy with an advanced-generation fluoroquinolone, has been reported in abstract form (Abstract L-981) and presented at the Interscience Conference on Antimicrobial Agents and Chemotherapy (San Diego, Sept. 27-30, 2002).[148] Specifically, this retrospective study was designed to compare length of stay (LOS) data for CAP patients treated with single-agent levofloxacin vs. those treated with ceftriaxone/azithromycin.

In a retrospective chart review conducted at two community teaching hospitals, inpatient data from 434 CAP patients were reviewed for LOS, clinical outcomes, and need for additional antibiotic therapy. Patients treated with levofloxacin were carefully matched to patients receiving ceftriaxone/ azithromycin or other single-agent antibiotic therapy according to Fine risk classification. Risk class was designated according to the total number of points assigned for each patient. LOS data were gathered on all patients. Patients were considered treatment failures if signs and symptoms of CAP were still present 48-72 hours after treatment or if additional antibiotics were necessary for CAP treatment during the hospital stay.

The primary comparison was LOS between the levofloxacin and ceftriaxone/azithromycin groups using a two-way ANOVA. All ANOVA F-tests were based on a distribution-normalizing and variance-stabilizing log transformation of days in the hospital. A total of 434 eligible patient charts were identified and reviewed at the two hospital sites. Among these, 225 patients were treated with levofloxacin, 164 patients received ceftriaxone/azithromycin, and 45 patients were treated with other single agent antibiotic therapy (e.g., ceftriaxone, cefotetan, clindamycin, vancomycin). Certain dissimilarities were observed between the treatment groups. A higher percentage of patients in the ceftriaxone/azithromycin group (15.2%) were in the highest risk class (Fine class 5) compared with the levofloxacin group (8.8%). In addition, mean baseline Fine risk scores were 91.0 in the levofloxacin group and 98.0 in the ceftriaxone/azithromycin group, also indicating a higher risk status in the latter group ($p < 0.001$).

The mean LOS was significantly longer among patients treated with levofloxacin compared with patients treated with ceftriaxone/azithromycin, regardless of Fine risk class ($p < 0.001$). Mean LOS in the levofloxacin group was 6.8 days, compared with 4.4 days in the ceftriaxone/azithromycin group. Mean length of stay among patients treated with other single agent antibiotics was 7.2 days. There was no significant treatment x risk interaction effect ($p = 0.459$). LOS data were further analyzed after removing data from any patient who required more than 13 hospital days (outliers). There were 19 outlier patients in the levofloxacin group and none in the ceftriaxone/azithromycin group. This analysis continued to demonstrate a statistical advantage in favor of ceftriaxone/azithromycin relative to levofloxacin ($p < 0.001$). An overall effect of Fine risk class on hospital days also was apparent in this analysis ($p < 0.001$).

Overall, results of the study reveal that at baseline, mean Fine scores were lower (indicating lower severity) in the levofloxacin group (91) compared with the ceftriaxone/azithromycin group (98) ($p < 0.001$). Despite this, mean LOS was longer in the levofloxacin group (6.8 days) than in the ceftriaxone/azithromycin group (4.4 days) ($p < 0.001$). Nineteen patients in the levofloxacin group had a LOS of greater than 13 days; a separate analysis excluding these patients produced similar results. Risk class alone also had a significant effect on LOS ($p < 0.001$). In the levofloxacin group, 36% of patients required additional antibiotics, compared with 8% of ceftriaxone/azithromycin patients. The investigators concluded that despite lower Fine risk scores, levofloxacin was associated with longer hospital stays and more supplemental antibiotic usage compared with ceftriaxone/azithromycin; these both are factors that have the potential for translating into significant cost savings for hospital-based management of CAP.

Despite important limitations of this study (small sample size, retrospective analysis, limited number of sites, and presentation of data in abstract form only), the conclusions are consistent with the study by Waterer et al. This study demonstrated improved outcomes with combination cephalosporin/macrolide therapy, and suggests the need for additional prospective randomized trials to provide confirmation of current trends favoring two-drug therapy for high-risk patients with CAP.[148]

Although all current national guidelines for CAP management, including the IDSA, ATS, ASCAP, and CDC-DRSPWG consensus recommendations, stress the importance of combining cephalosporins such as ceftriaxone with a macrolide, studies demonstrating the favorable effect on mortality rates associated with combined therapy have been published only recently. Further support for a ceftriaxone/azithromycin combination has been strengthened by a recent investigation in which a group retrospectively analyzed all cases of bacteremic *S. pneumoniae* pneumonia in patients 18 and older hospitalized from 1995 to 2000.[149] Standard initial therapeutic regimen in this index institution was cefuroxime ± macrolide from 1995 to 1997, and ceftriaxone + azithromycin from 1998 to 2000.

In total, 95 patients (49 men, 46 women) were included in this study, with a mean age of 63 (range: 20-98). At admission, 30.5% of patients had a leucocyte count greater than 20,000, 11.5% a systolic BP lower than 90 mmHg, 44.2% a respiratory rate greater than 30/min, and 33.6% nausea-vomiting necessitating some form of therapy or that prevented the patient from eating. Interestingly, 16.8% had no fever at admission, and 72.5% became afebrile within 48 hours. Antibiotic resistance was not associated with increased mortality. In total, 15 (15.7%) patients died, four within the first 72 hours. During the 1995-1997 period, only 15% of the patients initially received a macrolide. The mortality rate for the period 1995-1997 (cefuroxime ± macrolide) was 20% and from 1998-2000 (ceftriaxone + azithromycin), it fell to 11%. During this period, PSI scores for evaluated patients were comparable (113-114) and reflected a similar percentage of patients in Fine risk classes 4-5.

The ceftriaxone-azithromycin combination significantly reduced the mortality rate compared to monotherapy (cefuroxime) for the group of patients with CAP that had the highest mortality rate.[149]

EXTENDED SPECTRUM FLUOROQUINOLONES: INTENSIFICATION OF COVERAGE AND PATIENT SELECTION

The extended spectrum quinolones, moxifloxacin, levofloxacin, and gatifloxacin, are indicated for treatment of CAP. Each of these agents is available as an oral and intravenous preparation. Quinolones have been associated with cartilage damage in animal studies; therefore, they are not recommended for use in children, adolescents, and pregnant and nursing women. Upon review of multiple studies, resistance data, and pharmacodynamic data, the ASCAP Consensus Panel has concluded that all advanced generation fluoroquinolones are not "created equally," and that prudent, resistance-sensitive choices require differentiation among the available agents.[150-163]

Moxifloxacin. Among the new fluoroquinolones, moxifloxacin has the lowest MICs against *S. pneumoniae* and more specific gram-positive coverage; therefore, it is recommended by the ASCAP Consensus Panel as the IV or oral fluoroquinolone of choice—when a fluoroquinolone is indicated—for managing patients infected with *S. pneumoniae* and other organisms known to cause CAP. It recently received approval and is indicated for treatment of drug-resistant *S. pneumoniae* (DRSP). Moxifloxacin reaches higher lung fluid concentrations compared to levofloxacin; this is important because quinolones demonstrate concentration-dependent killing.[192,193] Moxifloxacin also is generally well tolerated. In clinical trials, the most common adverse events were nausea (8%), diarrhea (6%), dizziness (3%), headache (2%), abdominal pain (2%), and vomiting (2%). The agent is contraindicated in persons with a history of hypersensitivity to moxifloxacin or any quinolone antibiotic. The safety and effectiveness of moxifloxacin in pediatric patients, pregnant women, and lactating women have not been established.

Although reports of clinical problems are very rare, moxifloxacin has been shown to prolong the QT interval of the electrocardiogram in some patients. The drug should be avoided in patients with known prolongation of the QT interval, patients with uncorrected hypokalemia, and patients receiving Class lA (e.g., quinidine, procainamide) or Class lll (e.g., amiodarone, sotalol) antiarrhythmic agents due to the lack of clinical experience with the drug in these patient populations. Pharmacokinetic studies between moxifloxacin and other drugs that prolong the QT interval such as cisapride, erythromycin, antipsychotics, and tricyclic antidepressants have not been performed. An additive effect of moxifloxacin and these drugs cannot be excluded; therefore, moxifloxacin should be used with caution when given concurrently with these drugs.

The effect of moxifloxacin on patients with congenital prolongation of the QT interval has not been studied; however, it is expected that these individuals may be more susceptible to drug-induced QT prolongation. Because of limited clinical experience, moxifloxacin should be used with caution in patients with ongoing proarrhythmic conditions, such as clinically significant bradycardia or acute myocardial ischemia. As with all quinolones, moxifloxacin should be used with caution in patients with known or suspected CNS disorders or in the presence of other risk factors that may predispose to seizures or lower the seizure threshold.

Gatifloxacin. Gatifloxacin, a broad-spectrum 8-methoxy fluoroquinolone antibiotic, has been approved for the safe and effective treatment of approved indications, including community-acquired respiratory tract infections, such as bacterial exacerbation of chronic bronchitis (ABE/COPD); acute sinusitis; and CAP caused by indicated, susceptible strains of gram-positive and gram-negative bacteria. The recommended dose for gatifloxacin is 400 mg once daily for all individuals with normal renal function. Dosage adjustment is required in patients with impaired renal function (creatinine clearance, < 40 mL/min).

Gatifloxacin is primarily excreted through the kidneys, and less than 1% is metabolized by the liver. In clinical trials, gatifloxacin has been found to be a well-tolerated treatment in 15 international clinical trials at 500 study sites. Gatifloxacin may have the potential to prolong the QTc interval of the electrocardiogram in some patients, and due to limited clinical experience, gatifloxacin should be avoided in patients with known prolongation of the QTc interval, in patients with uncorrected hypokalemia, and in patients receiving Class IA (e.g., quinidine, procainamide) or Class III (e.g., amiodarone, sotalol) antiarrhythmic agents. Gatifloxacin should be used with caution when given together with drugs that may prolong the QTc interval (e.g., cisapride, erythromycin, antipsychotics, tricyclic antidepressants), and in patients with ongoing proarrhythmic conditions (e.g., clinically significant bradycardia or acute myocardial ischemia).

Gatifloxacin should be used with caution in patients with known or suspected CNS disorders or patients who have a predisposition to seizures. The most common side effects associated with gatifloxacin in clinical trials were gastrointestinal. Adverse reactions considered to be drug related and occurring in greater than 3% of patients were: nausea (8%), vaginitis (6%), diarrhea (4%), headache (3%), and dizziness (3%).

Oral doses of gatifloxacin should be administered at least four hours before the administration of ferrous sulfate; dietary supplements containing zinc, magnesium, or iron (such as multivitamins); aluminum/magnesium-containing antacids; or Videx (didanosine, or ddI). Concomitant administration of gatifloxacin and probenecid significantly increases systemic exposure to gatifloxacin. Concomitant administration of gatifloxacin and digoxin did not produce significant alteration of the pharmacokinetics of gatifloxacin; however, patients taking digoxin should be monitored for signs and/or symptoms of digoxin toxicity.

Levofloxacin. Levofloxacin, the S-enantiomer of ofloxacin, is a fluoroquinolone antibiotic that, when compared with older quinolones, also has improved activity against gram-positive organisms, including *S. pneumoniae*. This has important drug selection implications for the management of patients with CAP and exacerbations of COPD. The active stereoisomer of ofloxacin, levofloxacin is available in a parenteral preparation or as a once daily oral preparation that is given for 7-14 days. Levofloxacin is well-tolerated, with the most common side effects including nausea, diarrhea, headache, and constipation. Food does not affect the absorption of the drug, but it should be taken at least two hours before or two hours after antacids containing magnesium or aluminum, as well as sucralfate, metal cations such as iron, and multivitamin preparations with zinc. Dosage adjustment for levofloxacin is recommended in patients with impaired renal function (clearance < 50 mL/min).

Although no significant effect of levofloxacin on plasma concentration of theophylline was detected in 14 health volunteers studied, because other quinolones have produced increases in patients taking concomitant theophylline, theophylline levels should be closely monitored in patients on levofloxacin and dosage adjustments made as necessary. Monitoring patients on warfarin also is recommended in patients on quinolones.

When given orally, levofloxacin is dosed once daily, is well absorbed orally, and penetrates well into lung tissue.[164] It is active against a wide range of respiratory pathogens, including atypical pathogens and many species of *S. pneumoniae* resistant to penicillin.[165,166] In general, levofloxacin has greater activity against gram-positive organisms than ofloxacin and is slightly less active than ciprofloxacin against gram-negative organisms.[167,168]

Levofloxacin is available in both oral and parenteral forms, and the oral and IV routes are interchangeable (i.e., same dose). Levofloxacin is generally well tolerated (incidence of adverse reactions, < 7%). Levofloxacin is supplied in a parenteral form for IV use and in 250 mg and 500 mg tablets. The recommended dose is 500 mg IV or orally qd for 7-14 days for lower respiratory tract infections.

Levofloxacin is indicated for the treatment of adults (> 18 years) with mild, moderate, and severe pulmonary infections, including acute bacterial exacerbations of chronic bronchitis and CAP.[169] It is active against many gram-positive organisms that may infect the lower respiratory tract, including *S. pneumoniae* and *S. aureus*, and it also covers atypical pathogens, including *C. pneumoniae, L. pneumophila*, and *M. pneumoniae*. In addition, it is active against gram-negative organisms, including *E. coli, H. influenzae, H. parainfluenzae, K. pneumoniae*, and *M. catarrhalis*. Although it is active against *Pseudomonas aeruginosa* in vitro and carries an indication for treatment of complicated UTI caused by *Pseudomonas aeruginosa*, levofloxacin does not have an official indication for CAP caused by this gram-negative organism.

Several studies and surveillance data suggest that some newly available, expanded spectrum fluoroquinolones, including levofloxacin (which is approved for DRSP), are efficacious for the treatment of *S. pneumoniae*, including penicillin-resistant strains.[3,17,170] In one study, microbiologic eradication from sputum was reported among all 300 patients with pneumococcal pneumonia treated with oral levofloxacin.[17] In a study of in vitro susceptibility of *S. pneumoniae* clinical isolates to levofloxacin, none of the 180 isolates (including 60 isolates with intermediate susceptibility to penicillin and 60 penicillin-resistant isolates) was resistant to this agent.[170] In addition, a surveillance study of antimicrobial resistance in respiratory tract pathogens found levofloxacin was active against 97% of 9190 pneumococcal isolates and found no cross-resistance with penicillin, amoxicillin-clavulanate, ceftriaxone, cefuroxime, or clarithromycin.

Fluoroquinolones: Resistance Concerns and Over-Extended Spectrum

of Coverage. Despite high level activity against pneumococcal isolates and a formal indication for levofloxacin use in suspected DRSP lower respiratory tract infection, the CDC-DRSPWG recent guidelines do not advocate the use of expanded spectrum fluoroquinolones (among them, levofloxacin) for first-line, empiric treatment of pneumonia.

This is because of the following: 1) their broad, perhaps, over-extended spectrum of coverage that includes a wide range of gram-negative organisms; 2) concern that resistance among pneumococci will emerge if there is widespread use of this class of antibiotics; 3) their activity against pneumococci with high penicillin resistance (MIC = 4 mcg/mL) makes it important that they be reserved for selected patients with CAP; 4) use of fluoroquinolones has been shown to result in increased resistance to *S. pneumoniae* in vitro; and 5) population-based surveillance in the United States has shown a statistically significant increase in ofloxacin resistance among pneumococcal isolates between Jan. 1, 1995, and Dec. 31, 1997 (unpublished data, Active Bacterial Core Surveillance, CDC).[3]

The CDC-DRSPWG concerns about inducing fluoroquinolone resistance not only to *S. pneumoniae*, but also to other pathogenic organisms has support in the medical literature.[171-173] Individual fluoroquinolone use in U.S. hospitals, as measured by inpatient dispensing, is changing over time. Selective pressure exerted by fluoroquinolone use may be causally related to the prevalence of ciprofloxacin resistant *P. aeruginosa*. In fact, databases support growing concern about emerging fluoroquinolone resistance. In this regard, recent NNIS surveillance data indicates that resistance for *P. aeruginosa* to fluoroquinolones is increasing, possibly as a result of increasing use of this drug class.[171-173] To shed light in this possible association, the SCOPE-MMIT network of 35 hospitals tracked inpatient fluoroquinolones dispensing since 1999, and obtained hospital antibiograms to assess for associations between use and resistance rates.

MediMedia Information Technology (MMIT, North Wales, PA) collected data of inpatient-dispensed drugs from each participating hospital information system. Grams of individual fluoroquinolones are converted each quarter to defined daily dose/1000 patient days (DDD/1000PD). Antibiograms (1999) testing susceptibility of *P. aeruginosa* to ciprofloxacin were available from 22 hospitals. The relationship between total fluoroquinolone use and percentage resistance for *P. aeruginosa* to ciprofloxacin was assessed by linear regression. Results indicated that total fluoroquinolone use between 1999 and 2001 remained at ~ 140DDD/1000PD, although mean levofloxacin use increased significantly and ciprofloxacin use declined slightly. There was a significant positive relationship between total fluoroquinolone use and resistance to *P. aeruginosa* ($r = 0.54$, $p = 0.01$).

Investigators concluded that mean total fluoroquinolone dispensing in the 35 hospitals studied was stable, although there were significant differences in use between individual fluoroquinolones. There was a positive relationship between total fluoroquinolone use and resistance to ciprofloxacin for *P. aeruginosa*, but it was not yet possible to determine if the relationship was causal or which fluoroquinolones are most likely responsible. The SCOPE-MMIT network will continue to evaluate the quantitative relationships between antibiotic use and resistance as antibiotic use changes over time, and as resistance rates respond to these changes in selective pressure.[171-173]

Fluoroquinolones and Development of Gram-Negative Resistance.[174] Recent studies also have identified independent risk factors for the development of fluoroquinolone resistance in *E. coli* and *K. pneumoniae* isolates derived from nosocomial infections. Among the risk factors identified were recent fluoroquinolone use, residence in a long-term care facility (LTCF), older age, and recent aminoglycoside use.

This study was a retrospective, blinded, case control study entering patients with *E. coli* and *K. pneumoniae* isolates resistant to fluoroquinolones (using levofloxacin as the index) by NCCLS definitions that were determined to be the cause of nosocomial clinical infection as defined by CDC guidelines. An equal number of controls were randomly selected from the pool of *E. coli* and *K. pneumoniae* isolates that were susceptible to fluoroquinolones. In total, 178 potential cases were identified, of which 42 were ineligible because the isolates represented colonization and/or community-acquired infection. Multivariable analysis was used to determine the association between potential risk factors and fluoroquinolone resistance. Data were collected from Jan. 1, 1998, to June 30, 1999.

Results of the study demonstrated that on multivariable analysis, the following were independent risk factors for fluoroquinolone-resistant infection with these adjusted risk ratios (RRs): Fluoroquinolone use (5.25); LTCF (3.65); prior aminoglycoside use (8.86); and age (1.03). In addition, fluoroquinolone-resistant isolates were more likely to be resistant to other classes of antibiotics than fluoroquinolone-susceptible isolates. Overall, 25% of fluoroquinolone-resistant isolates (cases) had the ESBL phenotype, compared to 4.3% of fluoroquinolone-susceptible isolates (controls). Cases had greater prior antibiotic exposure measured as both number of days of antibiotic therapy and number of antibiotics received. In a subanalysis, 35 of 41 patients (85.4%) who had received a fluoroquinolone in the 30 days prior to infection had a fluoroquinolone-resistant infection.

The results of this study, while interesting, do not shed much light on the best strategies to control fluoroquinolone resistance in nosocomial infections with *E. coli* and *K. pneumoniae*. Risk factors such as prior fluoroquinolone use and older age might lead to the conclusion that a policy of fluoroquinolone restriction is necessary. On the other hand, residence in a LTCF and prior aminoglycoside use suggest horizontal spread that would be better addressed through improved infection control. Prior aminoglycoside use, as well as use of certain other antibiotics, may alter membrane permeability to fluoroquinolones, thereby causing low level resistance and setting the stage for higher level resistance upon exposure to a fluoroquinolone.

Fluoroquinolones and MRSA. Methicillin-resistant *Staphylococcus aureus* (MRSA) is a substantial problem in antibiotic therapy, and its origin is now recognized to be both from the hospital and the community.[2] There are a variety of well-known risk factors for the development of MRSA in the hospital, including extensive prior broad-spectrum antibiotic use, admission to an ICU, prolonged hospitalization, presence of an indwelling catheter, severe comorbid diseases, surgery, and exposure to MRSA-colonized patients. However, a substantial amount of new data has arisen indicating that fluoroquinolones are a risk factor for the increase in MRSA. Given the widespread use of oral fluoroquinolones in the community over the last several years, and the increase in community-acquired MRSA, it is prudent to consider the possibility that fluoroquinolone overuse may be associated with increasing emergence of MRSA.[175]

To address this question, one study evaluated prior antibiotic exposure and the development of nosocomial MRSA bacteremia in patients admitted to a 750-

bed tertiary care hospital.[173] All patients with nosocomial bacteremias from Jan. 1, 1996, to June 30, 1999, were evaluated. For each patient, investigators documented all antibiotics administered prior to the development of the bacteremia. They performed a case-controlled evaluation comparing fluoroquinolone-exposed patients to non-fluoroquinolone-exposed patients in relation to the development of MRSA bacteremia. A chi-squared analysis was conducted and relative risk (RR) calculated.

A total of 514 nosocomial bacteremias occurred over the study period, with 78 (15%) MRSA. The percentage of MRSA bacteremias/nosocomial bacteremias increased from 10% in 1996 to 22% in 1999 ($p < 0.05$). MRSA as a percent of all *S. aureus* clinical isolates increased from 29% to 40%. Prior fluoroquinolone exposure and MRSA bacteremia rose significantly from 25% of cases in 1986 to 65% of cases in 1999 (40% fluoroquinolone alone and 25% fluoroquinolone and other antibiotics) ($p < 0.05$). Cephalosporin exposure and the development of MRSA bacteremia dropped significantly from 50% of cases in 1996 to 0% of cases in 1999 ($p < 0.01$). Overall, 52% of fluoroquinolone-exposed patients developed MRSA bacteremia vs. 8% methicillin-sensitive *S. aureus* (MSSA) bacteremia ($p < 0.05$). In 1996 the RR of fluoroquinolone exposure and the development of MRSA bacteremia was 2.27 (ns), whereas during 1997-1999 the RR of fluoroquinolone exposure was significant, ranging from 3.25 to 4.68 ($p < 0.05$). Fluoroquinolone usage increased hospital-wide over the study period.[173]

The study group noted a significant increase in nosocomial MRSA bacteremias in fluoroquinolone-exposed patients and a significant decrease in patients with cephalosporin exposure over the study period. Fluoroquinolone-exposed patients had 3-4 times greater risk of developing nosocomial MRSA bacteremia than non-fluoroquinolone-exposed patients. Because increasing fluoroquinolone usage may have contributed to the increased selection and development of MRSA bacteremias, the study group implemented policies to limit fluoroquinolone utilization to attempt to control the selection and development of nosocomial MRSA bacteremias in the future.[173]

Selective Fluoroquinolone Use. Based on observational, surveillance, and other published data and emerging trends, from a practical, drug selection perspective, the CDC-DRSPWG has recommended that fluoroquinolones be reserved for selected patients with CAP; these experts have identified specific patient subgroups that are eligible for initial treatment with extended-spectrum fluoroquinolones. For hospitalized patients, these include adults and elderly patients for whom one of the first-line regimens (cephalosporin plus a macrolide) has failed, those who are allergic to the first-line agents, or those who have a documented infection with highly drug-resistant pneumococci (i.e., penicillin MIC = 4 mcg/mL).[109]

Whereas, until recently, fluoroquinolone resistance to *S. pneumoniae* was not considered an urgent clinical issue, the *Morbidity and Mortality Weekly Report* recently covered the appearance of, and increasing levels of, fluoroquinolone resistance to what was once a susceptible organism. Ofloxacin-resistance of 3.1% in 1995 had increased to 4.5% in 1997 (p = 0.02), whereas levofloxacin-resistance of 0.2% in 1998 was reported to be 0.3% in 1999 (p value not significant).[176]

In support of the CDC-DRSPWGs position on restricting fluoroquinolone use, the editors of *Morbidity and Mortality Weekly Report* also cited that while prescriptions in the United States for all antibiotics decreased between 1993 and 1998, the prescriptions for fluoroquinolones increased from 3.1 to 4.6 prescriptions per 100 persons per year, respectively, thus greatly increasing the exposure to these broad spectrum agents.[176]

For this reason, the *Morbidity and Mortality Weekly Report* concluded that, "appropriate use of antibiotics is crucial for slowing the emergence of fluoroquinolone resistance." It is for these reasons, plus concerns for increased gram-negative resistance to fluoroquinolones, that specific recommendations were issued from the CDC-DRSPWG. This recommendation, in essence, reserved fluoroquinolone use for patients who were allergic to first-line therapy, who had failed first-line therapy, or who had proven high level (MIC ≥ 4 mcg/mL) penicillin resistance. This report also does not recommend fluoroquinolone monotherapy for critically ill persons with pneumococcal pneumonia, because its efficacy in such patients has not been established.[176]

ADVANCED GENERATION FLUOROQUINOLONES—MUTANT PROTECTION CONCENTRATIONS, MICs, AND IMPLICATIONS FOR INITIAL DRUG SELECTION

The fluoroquinolone class of antimicrobial agents is being used empirically as initial agents for treatment of outpatient and inpatient management of CAP. Their use is increasing as resistance has developed to the more traditional antimicrobial agents, including macrolides, against which 21-23% of all *S. pneumoniae* isolates now show intermediate or complete resistance. Guidelines now recommend fluoroquinolones as first-line empiric therapy for urinary tract infections in regions were trimethoprim/sulfamethoxazole resistance is greater than 10-20%.[177] And fluoroquinolones are recommended as empiric agents in patients with CAP.[178,179] Though increased use of these agents would be expected to lead to increased resistance, a targeted approach to fluoroquinolone prescribing, emphasizing their appropriate and infection-specific use, may reduce development of antimicrobial resistance and maintain class efficacy.

In this regard, evidence is mounting that suggests a link between inappropriate fluoroquinolone use, development of antimicrobial resistance against the entire fluoroquinolone class, and clinical failure. To maintain the activity of the fluoroquinolone class, clinicians need to implement an evidence-based approach to antimicrobial selection, particularly a strategy in which the most pharmacodynamically potent fluoroquinolone is matched, on an empiric basis when required, to anticipated bacterial pathogens.

The three major factors associated with increasing resistance to fluoroquinolones include the following: 1) underdosing, i.e., use of a marginally potent agent whose MIC is barely reached in serum or infected tissues; 2) overuse of agents known to encourage resistant mutants; and 3) the inability to readily detect and respond to changes in antimicrobial susceptibilities.[150] Traditional reporting of susceptibility data may be misleading and may not readily identify initial changes in resistance patterns or differences between agents of the same class.

The ASCAP 2003 Clinical Consensus Panel has evaluated fluoroquinolones indicated for CAP and recommends that to preserve fluoroquinolone activity, these agents must be continually assessed and used appropriately. They should be tested by hospital laboratories to ensure activity against expected pathogens and local resistance trends must be monitored closely. The individual attributes of a given drug should be matched with the likely pathogen at specific sites of infection. Identifying a single fluoroquinolone that is suitable for all infections is unreasonable, and excessive use of any single fluoroquinolone for all indications will lead to resistance that will adversely affect the entire class. Given the defined strategy of selecting an agent with the best pharmacokinetic and pharmacodynamic profile against the known or suspected pathogen, an appropriate therapeutic choice for most serious infections, such as nosocomial pneumonia in which *P. aeruginosa* is a known or suspected pathogen, would currently include ciprofloxacin in combination with an antipseudomonal beta-lactam or an aminoglycoside.

This recommendation is based on the lower MIC_{90} and mutant prevention concentrations for this fluoroquinolone against *P. aeruginosa* and higher C_{max}/MIC and AUC/MIC ratios compared to other members of the class, including levofloxacin. For CAP infections in which *S. pneumoniae* is anticipated to be the most likely pathogen, moxifloxacin, which currently has the best antipneumococcal pharmacodynamic activity and the lowest mutant prevention concentrations against this organism, would represent the preferred fluoroquinolone. By contrast, levofloxacin's MIC_{90} against *S. pneumoniae* is significantly higher than those of moxifloxacin and gatifloxacin. The AUC/MICs and $C_{max}/MICs$ also are lower for levofloxacin against *S. pneumoniae*, and serum concentrations of a standard dose of levofloxacin for CAP do not reach the mutant prevention concentrations for *S. pneumoniae*.[91]

For these reasons, the ASCAP Consensus Panel has concluded that levofloxacin may not be the best choice for infections caused by *S. pneumoniae*, and has designated it as an alternative agent for this indication. Instead, the panel recommends moxifloxacin as the initial fluoroquinolone of choice when a respiratory fluoroquinolone is deemed appropriate for CAP. Furthermore, recent reports of levofloxacin failures in cases of CAP caused by *S. pneumoniae* are a continuing cause of concern, and other resistance data demonstrating precipitous increases in levofloxacin resistance among *S. pneumoniae* species support the panel's recommendations to avoid levofloxacin as the initial agent selected for empiric management of CAP.

EMPIRIC ANTIBIOTIC COVERAGE FOR CAP: MATCHING DRUGS WITH PATIENT PROFILES

A variety of antibiotics are available for outpatient management of pneumonia. Although the selection process can be daunting, as mentioned, a sensible approach to antibiotic selection for patients with pneumonia is provided by treatment categories for pneumonia generated by the Medical Section of the American Lung Association and published under the auspices of the ATS.[18] This classification scheme helps make clinical assessments useful for guiding therapy, but it also is predictive of ultimate prognosis and mortality outcome.

The most common pathogens responsible for causing CAP, again, include the typical bacteria: *S. pneumoniae, H. influenzae,* and *M. catarrhalis,* as well as the atypical pathogens: *Mycoplasma, Legionella,* and *C. pneumoniae.*[180] *H. influenzae* and *M. catarrhalis* are both found more commonly in patients with COPD. Clinically and radiologically, it is difficult to differentiate between the typical and atypical pathogens; therefore, coverage against all these organisms may be necessary. In patients producing sputum containing polymorphonuclear leukocytes, the sputum gram stain may contain a predominant organism to aid in the choice of empiric therapy. For most patients, though, therapy must be entirely empiric and based on the expected pathogens.[19,181]

Therefore, for the vast majority of otherwise healthy patients who have CAP, but who do not have comorbid conditions and who are deemed well enough to be managed as outpatients, therapy directed toward *S. pneumoniae, H. influenzae, M. pneumoniae, C. pneumoniae, L. pneumophila,* and *M. catarrhalis* is appropriate. From an intensity and spectrum of coverage perspective, coverage of both the aforementioned bacterial and atypical species has become mandatory.

In these cases, one of the newer macrolides should be considered one of the initial agents of choice. The other monotherapeutic agents available consist of the extended spectrum quinolones, which provide similar coverage and carry an indication for initial therapy in this patient subgroup.

For the older patient with CAP who is considered stable enough to be managed as an outpatient, but in whom the bacterial pathogen list also may include gram-negative aerobic organisms, the combined use of a second- or third-generation cephalosporin or amoxicillin-clavulanate plus a macrolide has been recommended. Another option may consist of an advanced generation quinolone.

Use of the older quinolones is not recommended for empiric treatment of community-acquired respiratory infections, primarily because of their variable activity against *S. pneumoniae* and atypical organisms. Although the older quinolones (i.e., ciprofloxacin) generally should not be used for the empiric treatment of CAP, they may provide an important option for treatment of bronchiectasis, particularly when gram-negative organisms such as *Pseudomonas* are cultured from respiratory secretions.[182] In these cases, ciprofloxacin should be used in combination with another anti-pseudomonal agent when indicated.

The most important issue for the emergency physician or pulmonary intensivist is to ensure that the appropriate intensity and spectrum of coverage are provided, according to patient and community/epidemiological risk factors. In many cases, especially when infection with gram-negative organisms is suspected or there is structural lung disease, this will require shifting to and intensifying therapy with an extended spectrum quinolone. However, in most cases of non-ICU patients admitted to the hospital, IV ceftriaxone plus azithromycin IV is recommended, depending on institutional protocols.

Finally, there is an increasing problem in the United States concerning the emergence of *S. pneumoniae* among hospitalized pneumonia patients that is relatively resistant to penicillin and, less commonly, to extended-spectrum cephalosporins. These isolates also may be resistant to sulfonamides and tetracyclines.[18,183,184] Except for vancomycin, the most favorable in vitro response rates to *S. pneumoniae* are seen with extended spectrum quinolones. See Table 2 for a summary of current recommendations for initial management of outpatient and in-hospital management of patients with CAP.

Antimicrobial Therapy and Medical Outcomes. A recent study has helped assess the relationship between initial antimicrobial therapy and medical outcomes for elderly patients hospitalized with pneumonia.[116] In this retrospective analysis, hospital records for 12,945 Medicare inpatients (age 65) with pneumonia were reviewed. Associations were identified between the choice of the initial antimicrobial regimen and three-day mortality, adjusting for baseline differences in patient profiles, illness severity, and process of care. Comparisons were made between the antimicrobial regimens and a reference group consisting of patients treated with a non-pseudomonal third-generation cephalosporin alone.

Of the 12,945 patients, 9751 (75.3%) were community-dwelling and 3194 (24.7%) were admitted from a long-term care facility. Study patients had a mean age of 79.4 years ± 8.1 years, 84.4% were white, and 50.7% were female. As would be expected, the majority (58.1%) of patients had at least one comorbid illness, and 68.3% were in the two highest severity risk classes (IV and V) at initial examination. The most frequently coded bacteriologic pathogens were *S. pneumoniae* (6.6%) and *H. influenzae* (4.1%); 10.1% of patients were coded as having aspiration pneumonia, and in 60.5% the etiologic agent for the pneumonia was unknown.

The three most commonly used initial, empiric antimicrobial regimen in the elderly patient with pneumonia consisted of the following: 1) a non-pseudomonal third generation cephalosporin only (ceftriaxone, cefotaxime, ceftizoxime) in 26.5%; 2) a second generation cephalosporin only (cefuroxime) in 12.3%; and 3) a non-pseudomonal third generation cephalosporin (as above) plus a macrolide in 8.8%. The 30-day mortality was 15.3% (95% CI, 14.6-15.9%) in the entire study population, ranging from 11.2% (95% CI, 10.6-11.9%) in community-dwelling elderly patients to 27.5% (95% CI, 26-29.1%) among patients admitted from a long-term care facility.[116]

As might be predicted, this study of elderly patients with hospitalization for pneumonia demonstrated significant differences in patient survival depending upon the choice of the initial antibiotic regimen. In particular, this national study demonstrated that, compared to a reference group receiving a non-pseudomonal third-generation cephalosporin alone, initial therapy with a non-pseudomonal plus a macrolide, a second generation cephalosporin plus a macrolide, or a fluoroquinolone alone was associated with 26%, 29%, and 36% lower 30-day mortality, respectively. Despite that these regimens are compatible with those recommended by the IDSA and CDC, only 15% of patients received one of the three aforementioned regimens associated with reduced mortality rates.

For reasons that are not entirely clear, patients treated with a beta-lactam/beta-lactamase inhibitor plus a macrolide or an aminoglycoside plus another agent had mortality rates that were 77% and 21% higher than the reference group, respectively.

Role of Specific Pathogens in CAP. Prospective studies evaluating the causes of CAP in elderly adults have failed to identify the cause of 40-60% of cases of CAP, and two or more etiologies have been identified in 2-5% of cases. The most common etiologic agent identified in virtually all studies of CAP in the elderly is *S. pneumoniae*, and this agent accounts for approximately two-thirds of all cases of bacteremic pneumonia.

Other pathogens implicated less frequently include *H. influenzae* (most isolates of which are other than type B), *M. pneumoniae, C. pneumoniae, S. aureus, S. pyogenes, Neisseria meningitidis, M. catarrhalis, K. pneumoniae,* and other gram-negative rods, *Legionella* species, influenza virus (depending on the time of year), respiratory syncytial virus, adenovirus, parainfluenza virus, and other microbes. The frequency of other etiologies (e.g., *Chlamydia psittaci* [psittacosis], *Coxiella burnetii* [Q fever], *Francisella tularensis* [tularemia], and endemic fungi [histoplasmosis, blastomycosis, and coccidioidomycosis]), is dependent on specific epidemiological factors.

The selection of antibiotics, in the absence of an etiologic diagnosis (gram stains and culture results are not diagnostic), is based on multiple variables, including severity of the illness, patient age, antimicrobial intolerance or side effects, clinical features, comorbidities, concomitant medications, exposures, and the epidemiological setting.

OTHER CONSENSUS GUIDELINES FOR ANTIBIOTIC THERAPY

Consensus Report Guidelines: Infectious Disease Society of America. The IDSA, through its Practice Guidelines Committee, provides assistance to clinicians in the diagnosis and treatment of CAP. The targeted providers are internists and family practitioners, and the targeted patient groups are immunocompetent adult patients. Criteria are specified for determining whether the inpatient or outpatient setting is appropriate for treatment. Differences from other guidelines written on this topic include use of laboratory criteria for diagnosis and approach to antimicrobial therapy. Panel members and consultants were experts in adult infectious diseases.

The guidelines are evidence-based where possible. A standard ranking system is used for the strength of recommendations and the quality of the evidence cited in the literature reviewed. The document has been subjected to external review by peer reviewers as well as by the Practice Guidelines Committee, and was approved by the IDSA Council in September 2000. *(See Table 3.)*

Centers for Disease Control Drug-Resistant *Streptococcus pneumoniae* Therapeutic Working Group (CDC-DRSPWG) Guidelines. One of the important issues in selecting antibiotic therapy for the elderly patient is the emerging problem of DRSP. To address this problem and provide practitioners with specific guidelines for initial antimicrobial selection in these patients, the CDC-DRSPWG convened and published its recommendations in May 2000.[3] Some of the important clinical issues they addressed included the following: 1) what empirical antibiotic combinations (or monotherapeutic options) constituted reasonable initial therapy in outpatients, in hospitalized (non-ICU) patients, and in hospitalized intubated or ICU patients; 2) what clinical criteria, patient risk factors, or regional, epidemiological features constituted sufficient trigger points to include agents with improved activity against DRSP as initial agents of choice; and 3) what antibiotic selection strategies were most appropriate for limiting the emergence of fluoroquinolone-resistant strains.

Their conclusions with respect to antibiotic recommendations overlap significantly with the IDSA recommendations and the existing ATS guidelines. The specific differences contained in the CDC-DRSPWG primarily involve the sequence in which antibiotics should be chosen to limit the emergence of fluoroquinolone-resistant strains, a preference for using combination drug therapy, cautionary notes about using fluoroquinolones as monotherapy in critically ill patients, reserving use of fluoroquinolones for specific patient populations, and detailed guidance regarding the comparative advantages among agents in each class. *(See Table 4.)*

Oral macrolide (azithromycin, clarithromycin, or erythromycin) or beta-lactam monotherapy is recommended by the CDC working group as initial therapy in patients with pneumonia who are considered to be amenable to outpatient management. For inpatients not in an ICU (i.e., medical ward disposition), this group recommends for initial therapy the combination of a parenteral beta-lactam (ceftriaxone or cefotaxime) plus a macrolide (azithromycin, erythromycin, etc.).[3] One of the most important, consistent changes among recent recommendations for initial, empiric management of patients with CAP is mandatory inclusion of a macrolide (which covers atypical pathogens and may result in improved mortality if the patient has pneumococcal bacteremia) when a cephalosporin (which has poor activity against atypical pathogens) is selected as part of the initial combination regimen.[21]

For critically ill patients, first-line therapy should include an intravenous beta-lactam, such as ceftriaxone, and an intravenous macrolide, such as azithromycin. The option of using a combination of a parenteral beta-lactam (ceftriaxone, etc.) plus a fluoroquinolone with improved activity against DRSP also is presented. Once again, however, this committee issues clarifying, and sometimes cautionary, statements about the role of fluoroquinolone monotherapy in the critically ill patient, stating that caution should be exercised because the efficacy of the new fluoroquinolones as monotherapy for critically ill patients has not been determined.[3]

Clearly, fluoroquinolones are an important part of the antimicrobial arsenal in the elderly, and the CDC-DRSPWG has issued specific guidelines governing their use in the setting of outpatient and inpatient CAP. It recommends fluoroquinolones be reserved for selected patients with CAP, among them: 1) adults, including elderly patients, for whom one of the first-line regimens (cephalosporin plus a macrolide) has failed; 2) those who are allergic to the first-line agents; or 3) those patients who have a documented infection with highly drug resistant pneumococci (i.e., penicillin MIC > 4 mcg/mL).

Inappropriate Fluoroquinolone Use in Emergency Departments. Increasing resistance to fluoroquinolone antibiotics has been associated with increasing use of these agents. In one recent study, a group from the University of Pennsylvania Hospital System found that in more than 80% of patients who received a fluoroquinolone in two academic EDs, the indication for use was not appropriate when judged by established institutional guidelines.[194]

In this retrospective investigation, 100 consecutive ED patients who received a fluoroquinolone and were subsequently discharged were studied. Appropriateness of the indication for use was judged according to existing institutional guidelines. A case-control study was conducted to identify the prevalence of, and risk factors for, inappropriate fluoroquinolone use.

Among the 100 total patients, 81 received a fluoroquinolone for an inappropriate indication. Of these cases, 43 (53%) were judged inappropriate because another agent was considered first line, 27 (33%) because there was no evidence of infection based on the documented evaluation, and 11 (14%) because of inability to assess the need for antimicrobial therapy. Although the prevalence of inappropriate use was similar across various clinical scenarios, there was a borderline significant association between the hospital in which the ED was located and inappropriate fluoroquinolone use. Of the 19 patients who received a fluoroquinolone for an appropriate indication, only one received both correct dose and duration of therapy.

The investigators concluded that inappropriate fluoroquinolone use in EDs is extremely common and that efforts to limit the emergence of fluoroquinolone resistance must address the high level of inappropriate fluoroquinolone use in EDs. Future studies should evaluate the effect of interventions designed to reduce inappropriate fluoroquinolone use in this setting.[194]

PREVENTION OF DEEP VENOUS THROMBOSIS (DVT)

Background. Although antibiotic therapy, oxygenation, and maintenance of hemodynamic status are the primary triad of emergency interventions in patients with pneumonia, there has been an increasing recognition of the risk for DVT and PE in patients with infections such as pneumonia, especially when accompanied by CHF and/or respiratory failure. Emergency physicians, as well as attending physicians admitting such patients to the hospital, should be aware that the risk of DVT is significant enough to require prophylaxis in patients with CAP who have restricted mobility, most of whom may have such risk factors as obesity, previous history of DVT, cancer, varicose veins, hormone therapy, chronic heart failure (NYHA [New York Heart Association] Class III-IV), or chronic respiratory failure.[185]

From a practical perspective, this subset of patients should be strongly considered for prophylaxis to reduce the risk of DVT. Based on recent studies, the presence of pneumonia in a patient age 75 or older is, in itself, a criterion for prophylaxis against DVT; when these factors are accompanied by CHF (Class III-IV) or respiratory failure, prophylaxis should be considered mandatory if there are no significant contraindications.[185] It should be added that The American College of Chest Physicians (ACCP) guidelines[186] and International Consensus Statement[187] also cite risk factors for DVT and emphasize their importance when assessing prophylaxis requirements for medical patients.

Evidence for Prophylaxis. The data to support a prophylactic approach to

DVT for serious infections are growing. The studies with bid subcutaneous unfractionated heparin (UFH) are inconclusive, although this agent is used for medical prophylaxis. Despite the recognition of risk factors and the availability of effective means for prophylaxis, DVT and PE remain common causes of morbidity and mortality. It is estimated that approximately 600,000 patients per year are hospitalized for DVT in North America.[188] In the United States, symptomatic PE occurs in more than 600,000 patients and causes or contributes to death in up to 150,000 patients annually.[189]

With respect to the risk of DVT in patients with infection, one study group randomized infectious disease patients ages older than 55 years to UFH 5000 IU bid or placebo for three weeks. Autopsy was available in 60% of patients who died. Deaths from PE were significantly delayed in the UFH group, but the six-week mortality rate was similar in both groups. Non-fatal DVT was reduced by UFH. The findings of previous trials of prophylaxis in medical patients have been controversial, as the patient populations and methods used to detect thromboembolism and the dose regimens vary, undermining the value of the findings. Comparative studies with clearly defined populations and reliable end points were, therefore, required to determine appropriate patient subgroups for antithrombotic therapy.[190]

The MEDENOX Trial. In response to the need for evidence to clarify the role of prophylaxis in specific non-surgical patient subgroups, the MEDENOX (prophylaxis in MEDical patients with ENOXaparin) trial was conducted using the low molecular weight heparin (LMWH) enoxaparin in a clearly identified risk group.[185] In contrast to previous investigations, the MEDENOX trial included a clearly defined patient population; the study was designed to answer questions about the need for prophylaxis in this group of medical patients and to determine the optimal dose of LMWH.[185]

Patients in the MEDENOX trial were randomized to receive enoxaparin, 20 or 40 mg subcutaneously, or placebo once daily, beginning within 24 hours of randomization. They were treated for 10 days (4 days in hospital and followed up in person or by telephone contact on day 90 [range, day 83-110]). During follow-up, patients were instructed to report any symptoms or signs of DVT or any other clinical events. The primary and secondary efficacy end points for MEDENOX were chosen to allow an objective assessment of the risk of DVT in the study population and the extent of any benefit of prophylaxis. The primary end point was any venous thromboembolic event between day 1 and day 14. All patients underwent systematic bilateral venography at day 10 or earlier if clinical signs of DVT were observed. Venous ultrasonography was performed if venography was not possible. Suspected PE was confirmed by high probability lung scan, pulmonary angiography, helical computerized tomography, or at autopsy.[185] The primary safety end points were hemorrhagic events, death, thrombocytopenia, or other adverse event or laboratory abnormalities.[185]

A total of 1102 patients were included in the MEDENOX trial, in 60 centers and nine countries. The study excluded patients who were intubated or in septic shock. Overall, the mean age was 73.4, the gender distribution was 50:50 male/female, and the mean body mass index was 25.0. The mean patient ages, gender distribution, and body mass index were similar in all three treatment groups; there were slightly more males than females in the placebo and enoxaparin 20 mg groups, and more females than males in the enoxaparin 40 mg group, but this difference was not significant. The reasons for hospitalization of randomized patients varied.

The majority of patients were hospitalized for acute cardiac failure, respiratory failure, or infection, with pneumonia being the most common infection in those older than age 70. For the study population as a whole, the most prevalent risk factor in addition to the underlying illness was advanced age (50.4%). By day 14, the incidence of DVT was 14.9% in the placebo group and 5.5% in the enoxaparin 40 mg group, representing a significant 63% relative risk reduction (97% CI: 37-78%; $p = 0.0002$) in DVT.

The primary conclusions of the MEDENOX trial can be applied directly to clinical practice. First, acutely ill medical patients with cardiopulmonary or infectious disease are at significant risk of DVT. Second, enoxaparin, given once daily at a dose of 40 mg for 6-14 days reduces the risk of DVT by 63%; and third, the reduction in thromboembolic risk is achieved without increasing the frequency of hemorrhage, thrombocytopenia, or any other adverse event compared with placebo. This study strongly suggests that patients admitted to the hospital with pneumonia should, if there are no contraindications to the use of anticoagulants, be considered candidates for prophylaxis with enoxaparin, 40 mg SC qd, upon admission to the hospital to prevent DVT. The ASCAP 2003 Panel supports this recommendation.

REFERENCES

1. Battleman DS, Callahan M, Thaler HT. Rapid antibiotic delivery and appropriate antibiotic selection reduce length of hospital stay of patients with community-acquired pneumonia: Link between quality of care and resource management. *Arch Int Med* 2002;162:682-688.

2. Sue DY. Community-acquired pneumonia in adults. *West J Med* 1994;161:383-389.

3. Heffelfinger JD, Dowell SF, et al. A report from the Drug-resistant Streptococcus pneumoniae Therapeutic Working Group. Management of community-acquired pneumonia in the era of pneumococcal resistance. *Arch Int Med* 2000;160:1399.

4. Bartlett JG, Mundy M. Community-acquired pneumonia. *N Engl J Med* 1995;333:1618-1624.

5. Fine MD, Smith MA, et al. Prognosis and outcomes of patients with community

Authors: **Year 2003 Antibiotic Selection for Community-Acquired Pneumonia (ASCAP): Gideon Bosker, MD, FACEP,** Panel Moderator and Chairman, Section of Emergency Medicine, Yale University School of Medicine and Oregon Health Sciences University, Editor-in-Chief, *Emergency Medicine Reports.* **Year 2003 ASCAP Panel: Ronald J. DeBellis, PharmD, FCCP,** Associate Professor of Clinical Pharmacy Practice, Massachusetts College of Pharmacy and Health Sciences, Adjunct Assistant Professor of Medicine, University of Massachusetts School of Medicine; **Charles Emerman, MD, FACEP,** Chairman, Department of Emergency Medicine, Cleveland Clinic Hospitals and Metro Health Center, Cleveland, Ohio; **John Gums, PharmD,** Professor of Medicine and Pharmacy, University of Florida, Gainesville, Florida; **Dave Howes, MD, FACEP**, Program Director and Chairman, Residency Program, Department of Emergency Medicine, University of Chicago Hospitals and Clinics, Associate Professor, Pritzker School of Medicine; **Kurt Kleinschmidt, MD, FACEP,** Associate Professor, Department of Emergency Medicine, University of Texas Southwestern Medical School, Parkland Memorial Medical Center, Dallas, Texas; **David Lang, DO, FACEP,** Operational Medical Director, Department of Emergency Medicine, Mt. Sinai Medical Center, Miami, Florida; **Sandra Schneider, MD, FACEP,** Professor and Chairman, Department of Emergency Medicine, University of Rochester/Strong Memorial Hospital, Rochester, New York; **Gregory A. Volturo, MD, FACEP,** Vice Chairman and Associate Professor, Department of Emergency Medicine, University of Massachusetts Medical School, Worcester, Massachusetts.

acquired pneumonia. A meta-analysis. *JAMA* 1996;275:134-141.

6. American Thoracic Society: Guidelines for the Initial Management of Adults with Community-Acquired Pneumonia: Diagnosis, assessment of severity, and initial antimicrobial therapy. *Am Rev Respir Dis* 1993;148:1418-1426.

7. Marrie TJ, Lau CY, Wheeler SL, et al. A controlled trial of a critical pathway for treatment of community-acquired pneumonia. *JAMA* 2000;283:749-755.

8. Marrie TJ. Community-acquired pneumonia: Epidemiology, etiology, treatment. *Infect Dis Clinic North Am* 1998;12:723-740.

9. Bates JH, Campbell AL, et al. Microbial etiology of acute pneumonia in hospitalized patients. *Chest* 1992;101:1005-1012.

10. Fang GD, Fine M, Orloff, et al. New and emerging etiologies for community-acquired pneumonia with implications for therapy-prospective multicenter study of 359 cases. *Medicine* 1990;69: 307-316.

11. Antibiotic Update 1998: Outcome-effective treatment for bacterial infections managed in the primary care and emergency department setting. *Emerg Med Rep* 1997;18:1-24.

12. Fang GD, Fine M, Orloff J, et al. New and emerging etiologies for community-acquired pneumonia with implications for therapy. *Medicine* 1990;69:307-316.

13. Plouffe J, Schwartz DB, Kolokathis A, et al. Clinical efficacy of intravenous followed by oral azithromycin monotherapy in hospitalized patients with community-acquired pneumonia. *Antimicrob Agents Chemother* 2000;44:1796-1802.

14. Vergis EN, Indorf A, et al. Azithromycin vs cefuroxime plus erythromycin for empirical treatment of community-acquired pneumonia in hospitalized patients. A prospective, randomized, multicenter trial. *Arch Int Med* 2000;160:1294-1300.

15. The choice of antibacterial drugs. *Med Lett Drugs Ther* 1996;38: 25-34.

16. Clarithromycin and azithromycin. *Med Lett Drugs Ther* 1992;34: 45-47.

17. File TM, Dunbar L, et al. A multicenter, randomized study comparing the efficacy and safety of intravenous and/or oral levofloxacin versus ceftriaxone and/or cefuroxime in treatment of adults with community-acquired pneumonia. *Antimicrob Agents Chemother* 1997;41:1965-1972.

18. American Thoracic Society, Medical Section of the American Lung Association. *Am Rev Respir Dis* 1993;148:1418-1426.

19. American Thoracic Society. Guidelines for the initial management of adults with community-acquired pneumonia: Diagnosis, assessment of severity, and initial antimicrobial therapy. *Am Rev Respir Dis* 1993;148:1418-1426.

20. Centers for Disease Control and Prevention Web site. http://www.cdc.gov/ncidod/dbmd/diseaseinfo/drugresisstreppneum_t.htm

21. Waterer GW, Somes GW, Wunderink RG. Monotherapy may be suboptimal for severe bacteremic pneumococcal pneumonia. *Arch Intern Med* 2001;161:1837-1842.

22. Niederman MS, McCombs JS, Unger AN, et al. The cost of treating community-acquired pneumonia. *Clin Therapeut* 1998;20:820-837.

23. Medicare and Medicaid statistical supplement, 1995. *Health Care Financ Rev*

1995:16.

24. Fine MJ, Smith MA, Carson CA, et al. Prognosis and outcomes of patients with community-acquired pneumonia. *JAMA* 1995;274: 134-141.

25. Confalonieri M, Potena A, Carbone G, et al. Acute respiratory failure in patients with severe community-acquired pneumonia. A prospective randomized evaluation of non-invasive ventilation. *Am J Respir Crit Care Med* 1999;160:1585-1591.

26. Hoe LK, Keang LT. Hospitalized low-risk community-acquired pneumonia: Outcome and potential for cost-savings. *Respirology* 1999;4:307-309.

27. Dean NC, Suchyta MR, Bateman KA. Implementation of admission decision support for community-acquired pneumonia. A pilot study. *Chest* 2000;117:1368-1377.

28. Davis DA, Thomason MA, Oxman AD, et al. Evidence for the effectiveness of CME. A review of 50 randomized controlled trials. *JAMA* 1992;268:111-1117.

29. Lomas J, Anderson GM, Domnick-Pierre KD, et al. Do practice guidelines guide practice? The effect of a consensus statement on the practice of physicians. *N Engl J Med* 1989;321:1306-1311.

30. Gleicher N. Cesarean section rates in the United States: The short-term failure of the national consensus development conference in 1980. *JAMA* 1984;252:3273-3276.

31. Greco PJ, Eisenberg JM. Changing physician's practices. *N Engl J Med* 1993;329:1271-1273.

32. Mittman BS, Tonesk X, Jacobson PD. Implementing clinical practice guidelines. *Qual Rev Bull* 1992;18:413-422.

33. Tunis SR, Hayward RSA, Wilson MC, et al. Internists' attitudes about clinical practice guidelines. *Ann Intern Med* 1994;120:956-963.

34. Flanders WD, Tucker G, Krishnadasan A, et al. Validation of the pneumonia severity index: Importance of study-specific recalibration. *J Gen Intern Med* 1999;14:333-340.

35. Fine MJ, Auble TE, Yealy DM, et al. A prediction rule to identify low-risk patients with community-acquired pneumonia. *N Engl J Med* 1997;336:243-250.

36. Auble TE, Yealy DM, Fine MJ. Assessing prognosis and selecting an initial site of care for adults with community-acquired pneumonia. *Infect Dis Clin North Am* 1998;2:741-759.

37. Dean NC. Use of prognostic scoring and outcome assessment tools in the admission decision for community-acquired pneumonia. *Clin Chest Med* 1999;20:521-529.

38. Farr BM, Sloman AJ, Fisch MJ. Predicting death in patients hospitalized for community-acquired pneumonia. *Ann Intern Med* 1991;115:428-436.

39. Conte HA, Chen YT, Mehal W, et al. A prognostic rule for elderly patients admitted with community-acquired pneumonia. *Am J Med* 1999;106:20-28.

40. Ewig S, Kleinfeld T, Bauer T, et al. Comparative validation of prognostic rules for community-acquired pneumonia in an elderly population. *Eur Respir J* 1999;14:370-375.

41. Mylotte JM, Naughton B, Saludades C, et al. Validation and application of the pneumonia prognosis index to nursing home residents with pneumonia. *JAGS* 1998;46:1538-1544.

42.   Atlas SJ, Benzer TI, Borowsky LH, et al. Safely increasing the proportion of patients with community-acquired pneumonia treated as outpatients. An interventional trial. *Arch Intern Med* 1998; 158:1350-1356.

43.   Ewig S, Ruiz M, Mensa J, et al. Severe community-acquired pneumonia. Assessment of severity criteria. *Am J Respir Crit Care Med* 1998;158:1102-1108.

44.   Marston BJ, Plouffe JF, et al. Incidence of community-acquired pneumonia requiring hospitalization. Results of a population-based active surveillance study in Ohio. The Community-Based Pneumonia Incidence Study Group. *Arch Int Med* 1997;157:1709-1718.

45.   Marsten. *JAMA* 1997;2780-2080.

46.   Kahn KL, Rogers WH, et al. Measuring quality of care with explicit process criteria before and after implementation of the DRG-based prospective payment system. *JAMA* 1990;264:1969-1973.

47.   McGarvery RN, Harper JJ. Pneumonia mortality reduction and quality improvement in a community hospital. *Qual Rev Bull* 1993;19:124-130.

48.   Meehan TP, Fine MJ, et al. Quality of care, process, and outcomes in elderly patients with pneumonia. *JAMA* 1997;278:2080-2084.

49.   Barker K, Flynn E, et al. Medication Errors observed in 36 health care facilities. *Arch Int Med* 2002:162:1897.

50.   Shah, MN, Meltzer DM. Medication errors in emergency department patients admitted with pneumonia, Abstract 127, American College of Emergency Physicians. ACEP Scientific Assembly, September 2002.

51.   Brentsson E, Lagergard T. Etiology of community-acquired pneumonia in outpatients. *Eur J Clin Microbiol* 1986;5:446-447.

52.   Whitney CG, Barrett N, et al. Increasing prevalence of drug-resistant Streptococcus pneumoniae (DRSP): Implications for therapy for pneumonia. In: Programs and Abstracts of the 36th Annual Meeting of the Infectious Disease Society of America, Nov. 12-15, 1998. IDSA, Abstract 51.

53.   Ball AP. Overview of clinical experience with ciprofloxacin. *Eur J Clin Microbiol* 1986;5:214-219.

54.   Fass RJ. Efficacy and safety of oral ciprofloxacin in the treatment of serious respiratory infections. *Am J Med* 1986;82:202-207.

55.   Davies BI, Maesen FP, Baur C. Ciprofloxacin in the treatment of acute exacerbations of chronic bronchitis. *Eur J Clin Microbiol* 1986;5:226-231.

56.   Hoogkamp-Korstanje JA, Klein SJ. Ciprofloxacin in acute exacerbations of chronic bronchitis. *J Antimicrob Chemother* 1986;18: 407-413.

57.   Maesen FP, Davies BI, Geraedts WH, et al. The use of quinolones in respiratory tract infections. *Drugs* 1987;34(Suppl 1):74-79.

58.   Thys JP. Quinolones in the treatment of bronchopulmonary infections. *Rev Infect Dis* 1988;10(Suppl 1):S212-S217.

59.   Cooper B, Lawlor M. Pneumococcal bacteremia during ciprofloxacin therapy for pneumococcal pneumonia [see comments]. *Am J Med* 1989;87:475.

60.   Gordon JJ, Kauffman CA. Superinfection with Streptococcus pneumoniae during therapy with ciprofloxacin. *Am J Med* 1990; 89:383-384.

61.   Lee BL, Kimbrough RC, Jones SR, et al. Infectious complications with respiratory pathogens despite ciprofloxacin therapy. *N Engl J Med* 1991;325:520-521.

62.   Perez-Trallero E, Garcia-Arenzana JM, Jimenez JA, et al. Therapeutic failure and selection of resistance to quinolones in a case of pneumococcal pneumonia treated with ciprofloxacin. *Eur J Clin Microbiol Infect Dis* 1990;9:905-906.

63.   Ambrose PG, Grasela DM, Grasela TH, et al. Pharmacodynamics of fluoroquinolones against Streptococcus pneumoniae in patients with community-acquired respiratory tract infections. *Antimicrob Agents Chemother* 2001;45:2793-2797.

64.   Craig WA. Pharmacokinetic/pharmacodynamic parameters: Rationale for antibacterial dosing of mice and men. *Clin Inf Dis* 1998; 26:1-12.

65.   MacGowan AC, Bowker RK. The use of in vitro pharmacodynamic models of infection to optimize fluoroquinolone dosing regimens. *J Antimicrob Chemother* 2000;46:163-170.

66.   Wright DH, Brown GH, Peterson ML, et al. Application of fluoroquinolone pharmacodynamics. *J Antimicrob Chemother* 2000;46: 669-683.

67.   Madaras-Kelly KJ, Demasters TA. In vitro characterization of fluoroquinolone concentration/MIC antimicrobial activity and resistance while simulating clinical pharmacokinetics of levofloxacin, ofloxacin, or ciprofloxacin against Streptococcus pneumoniae. *Diagn Microbiol Infect Dis* 2000;37:253-260.

68.   Thorburn CE, Edwards DI. The effect of pharmacokinetics on the bactericidal activity of ciprofloxacin and sparfloxacin against Streptococcus pneumoniae and the emergence of resistance. *J Antimicrob Chemother* 2001;48:15-22.

69.   Gonzalez MA, Uribe F, Moisen SD, et al. Multiple-dose pharmacokinetics and safety of ciprofloxacin in normal volunteers. *Antimicrob Agents Chemother* 1984;26:741-744.

70.   Mazzulli TA, Simor E, Jaeger R, et al. Comparative in vitro activities of several new fluoroquinolones and beta-lactam antimicrobial agents against community isolates of Streptococcus pneumoniae. *Antimicrob Agents Chemother* 1990;34:467-469.

71.   Anzueto A, Niederman MS, Tillotson GS. Etiology, susceptibility, and treatment of acute bacterial exacerbations of complicated chronic bronchitis in the primary care setting: Ciprofloxacin 750 mg b.i.d. versus clarithromycin 500 mg b.i.d. Bronchitis Study Group. *Clin Ther* 1998;20:885-900.

72.   Chodosh S, Schreurs A, Siami G, et al and the Bronchitis Study Group. Efficacy of oral ciprofloxacin vs. clarithromycin for treatment of acute bacterial exacerbations of chronic bronchitis. *Clin Infect Dis* 1998;27:730-738.

73.   Chen D, McGeer A, de Azavedo JC, et al and The Canadian Bacterial Surveillance Network. Decreased susceptibility of Streptococcus pneumoniae to fluoroquinolones

in Canada. *N Engl J Med* 1999;341:233-239.

74. Linares J, De La Campa AG, Pallares R. Fluoroquinolone resistance in Streptococcus pneumoniae [letter]. *N Engl J Med* 1999; 341:1546-1547.

75. Ho PL, Que TL, Tsang DN, et al. Emergence of fluoroquinolone resistance among multiply resistant strains of Streptococcus pneumoniae in Hong Kong. *Antimicrob Agents Chemother* 1999;43: 1310-1313.

76. Ho PL, Yung RW, Tsang DN, et al. Increasing resistance of Streptococcus pneumoniae to fluoroquinolones: Results of a Hong Kong multicentre study in 2000. *J Antimicrob Chemother* 2001; 48:659-665.

77. Goldsmith CE, Moore JE, Murphy PG, et al. Increased incidence of ciprofloxacin resistance in penicillin-resistant pneumococci in Northern Ireland [letter; comment]. *J Antimicrob Chemother* 1998; 41:420-421.

78. Centers for Disease Control. Resistance of Streptococcus pneumoniae to fluoro-quinolones-United States, 1995-1999. *Morbid Mortal Weekly Rep MMWR* 2001;50:800-804.

79. Doern GV, Heilmann KP, Huynh HK, et al. Antimicrobial resistance among clinical isolates of Streptococcus pneumoniae in the United States during 1999-2000, including a comparison of resistance rates since 1994-1995. *Antimicrob Agents Chemother* 2001; 45:1721-1729.

80. Sahm DF, Karlowsky JA, Kelly LJ, et al. Need for annual surveillance of antimicrobial resistance in Streptococcus pneumoniae in the United States: 2-year longitudinal analysis. *Antimicrob Agents Chemother* 2001;45:1037-1042.

81. Sahm DF, Peterson DE, Critchley IA, et al. Analysis of ciprofloxacin activity against Streptococcus pneumoniae after 10 years of use in the United States. *Antimicrob Agents Chemother* 2000;44:2521-2524.

82. Thornsberry C, et al. Longitudinal analysis of resistance among Streptococcus pneumoniae (SP) isolated from 100 geographically distributed institutions in the United States during the 1997-1998 and 1998-1999 respiratory seasons. Abstract of the 39th Interscience Conference on Antimicrobial Agents and Chemotherapy, San Francisco, Sept. 26-29, 1999.

83. Fish DN, Piscitelli SC, Danziger LH. Development of resistance during antimicrobial therapy:A review of antibiotic classes and patient characteristics in 173 studies. *Pharmacotherapy* 1995;15:279-291.

84. Ferraro MJ, Brown S, Harding I. Massachusetts General Hospital, Boston, MA, 2 CMI, Wilsonville, OR, 3 Micron Research, Ely, United Kingdom. Abstract 650 Prevalence of Fluoroquinolone Resistance amongst Streptococcus Pneumoniae Isolated in the United States during the Winter of 2000-01. 42nd ICAAC Abstracts, American Society for Microbiology, Sept. 27-30, 2002, San Diego, CA.

85. Tang P, Green K, et al. Emerging resistance in Respiratory Tract Isolates of Streptococcus peumoniae (SP) in Canada. Abstract L-92. 42nd ICAAC Abstracts, American

Society for Microbiology, Sept. 27-30, 2002, San Diego, CA.

86. Deeks SL, Palacio R, Ruvinsky P, et al. Risk factors and course of illness among children with invasive penicillin-resistant Streptococcus pneumoniae. The Streptococcus pneumoniae Working Group. *Pediatrics* 1999;103:409-413.

87. Straus WL, Qazi SA, Kundi Z, et al. Antimicrobial resistance and clinical effectiveness of co-trimoxazole versus amoxicillin for pneumonia among children in Pakistan. Randomised controlled trial. Pakistan Co-trimoxazole Study Group. *Lancet* 1998;352:270-274.

88. Davidson RJ, Cavalcanti R, Brunton JL, et al Resistance to levofloxacin and failure of treatment of pneumococcal pneumonia. *N Engl J Med* 2002;346:747-750.

89. Weiss K, Restieri C, Laverdiere M, et al. A nosocomial outbreak of fluoroquinolone-resistant Streptococcus pneumoniae. *Clin Inf Dis* 2001;33:517-522.

90. Ho PL, Tse W, Tsang KW, et al. Risk factors for acquisition of levofloxacin-resistant Streptococcus pneumoniae: A case-control study. *Clin Infect Dis* 2001;32:701-707.

91. Scheld WM. Maintaining fluoroquinolone class efficacy: Review of influencing factors. *Emerg Infect Dis* 2003;9:1-5.

92. Iannini PB, Tillotson GS. Impact of quinolone substitution on Pseudomonas aeruginosa resistance, antimicrobial usage and hospital costs: presented at the Antimicrobial Chemotherapy and Clinical Practice meeting, Genova, Italy, Oct. 21-24, 2001. *Pharmacotherapy* 2001;21(Suppl):371. Abstract 111.

93. Fridkin SK, Steward CD, Edwards JR, et al. Surveillance of antimicrobial use and antimicrobial resistance in United States hospitals: project ICARE phase 2. *Clin Infect Dis* 1999;29:245-52.

94. Hill HA, Haber MJ, McGowan JE, et al. A link between quinolone use and resistance in P. aeruginosa?: preliminary data from Project ICARE. Infectious Diseases Society of America 39th Annual Meeting, San Francisco, CA, Oct. 25-28, 2001. Alexandria (VA): Infectious Diseases Society of America; 2001. Abstract 495.

95. Wortmann GW, Bennett SP. Fatal meningitis due to levofloxacin-resistant Streptococcus pneumoniae. *Clin Infect Dis* 1999;29: 1599-1600.

96. Fishman NO, Suh B, Weigel LM, et al. Three levofloxacin treatment failures of pneumococcal respiratory tract infections. 39th Interscience Conference on Antimicrobial Agents and Chemotherapy, San Francisco, CA, Sept. 26-29, 1999. Washington: American Society for Microbiology; 1999. Abstract 825.

97. Kuehnert MJ, Nolte FS, Perlino CA. Fluoroquinolone resistance in Streptococcus pneumoniae. *Ann Intern Med* 1999;131:312-3.

98. Urban C, Rahman N, Zhao X, et al. Fluoroquinolone-resistant Streptococcus pneumoniae associated with levofloxacin therapy. *J Infect Dis* 2001;184:794-8.

99. Empey PE, Jennings HR, Thornton AC, et al. Levofloxacin failure in a patient with pneumococcal pneumonia. *Ann Pharmacother* 2001;35:687-90.

100. Piper J, Couch K, Tuttle D, et al. Epidemiology and clinical outcomes of patients with

levofloxacin resistant pneumococcus. 41st Interscience Conference on Antimicrobial Agents and Chemotherapy, Chicago, IL, Dec. 16-19, 2001. Washington: American Society for Microbiology; 2001. Abstract L-902.

101. Kays MB, Smith DW, Wack MF, et al. Levofloxacin treatment fail-ure in a patient with fluoroquinolone-resistant Streptococcus pneumoniae pneumonia. *Pharmacotherapy* 2002;22:395-9.

102. Ross JJ, Worthington MG, Gorbach SL. Resistance to levofloxacin and failure of treatment of pneumoccal pneumoia. *N Engl J Med* 2002;347:65-67.

103. Davies BI, Maesen FPV. Clinical effectiveness of levofloxacin in patients with acute purulent exacerbations of chronic bronchitis: the relationship with in-vitro activity. *J Antimicrob Chemother* 1999;43(Suppl C):83-90.

104. Sullivan JG, McElroy AD, Honsinger RW, et al. Treating community-acquired pneumonia with once daily gatifloxacin vs once-daily levofloxacin. *J Respir Dis* 1999;20(Suppl):S49-59.

105. Weiss K, Restieri C, Gauthier R, et al. A nosocomial outbreak of fluoroquinolone-resistant Streptococcus pneumoniae. *Clin Infect Dis* 2001;33:517-522.

106. Ho PL, Tse WS, Tsang KWT, et al. Risk factors for acquisition of levofloxacin-resistant Streptococcus pneumoniae: a case-control study. *Clin Infect Dis* 2001;32:701-7.

107. Pallares R, Capdevila O, LiÒares J, et al. Hospital Bellvitge, University of Barcelona, Spain; Clinical Relevance of Current NCCLS Ceftriaxone/Cefotaxime Resistance Breakpoints in non-Meningeal Pneumococcal Infections. Abstract Poster, 2001.

108. Kaplan SL, Mason EO, Barson WJ, et al. Outcome of invasive infections outside the central nervous system caused by Streptococcus pneumoniae isolates nonsusceptible to ceftriaxone in children treated with beta-lactam antibiotics. *Pediatr Infect Dis J* 2001;20:392-396.

109. Cleeland R, Squires E. Antimicrobial activity of ceftriaxone: A review. *Am J Med* 1984;77:3.

110. ASCAP Panel (Antibiotic Selection for Community-Acquired Pneumonia). Jackson, Wyoming, Dec. 6, 2000. A Panel of emergency physicians, internal medicine specialists, and pharmacists assessing treatment guidelines for community-acquired pneumonia.

111. Mandell LA. Antibiotics for pneumonia therapy. *Med Clin N Am* 1994;78:997-1014.

113. Mandell L. Community-acquired pneumonia: Etiology, epidemiology and treatment. *Chest* 1995;108(supp):35S-42S.

112. Edelstein P. Legionnaires' disease. *Clin Infect Dis* 1993;16:741.

114. Garrison D, DeHaan R, Lawson J. Comparison of in vitro antibacterial activities of 7-chloro-7-deoxylincomycin, lincomycin, and erythromycin. *Antimicrob Agents Chemother* 1968;1967:397.

115. Dean NC, Silver MP, Bateman KA, et al. Decreased mortality after implementation of a treatment guideline for community-acquired pneumonia. *Am J Med* 2001;110:451-457.

116. Gleason PP, Meehan TP, Fine JM, et al. Associations between initial antimicrobial

therapy and medical outcomes for hospitalized elderly patients with pneumonia. *Arch Intern Med* 1999;159:2562-2572.

117. Nathwani D, Rubinstein E, Barlow G, et al. Do guidelines for community-acquired pneumonia improve the cost-effectiveness of hospital care? *CID* 2001;32:728 (1 March, 2000).

118. People G, Kapoor WN, Stone RA, et al. Medical outcomes and antimicrobial cost with the use of the American Thoracic Society guidelines for outpatients with community-acquired pneumonia. *JAMA* 1997;278:32-9.

119. Dowell SF. The best treatment for pneumonia: New clues, but no definitive answers. *Arch Intern Med* 1999;159:2511-2512.

120. Canadian Coordinating Office for Health Technology Assessment. Clinical and economic considerations in the use of fluoroquinolones: technology overview. Pharmaceuticals. Ottawa: Canadian Coordinating Office for Health Technology Assessment (CCOHTA), 1997;10:1-13.

121. Al-Eidan FA, McElnay JC, Scott MG, et al. Use of a treatment protocol in the management of community-acquired lower respiratory infection. *J Antimicrob Chemother* 2000;45:387-397.

122. McGarvey RN, Harper IJ. Pneumonia mortality reduction and quality improvement in a community hospital. *QRB Qual Rev Bull* 1993;19:124-130.

123. Dresser LD, Niederman MS, Paladino JA. Cost-effectiveness of gatifloxacin vs ceftriaxone with a macrolide for the treatment of community-acquired pneumonia. *Chest* 2001;119:1439-1448.

124. Kaplan SL, Mason EO Jr, Barson WJ, et al. Outcome of invasive infections outside the central nervous system caused by Streptococcus pneumoniae isolates nonsusceptible to ceftriaxone in children treated with beta-lactam antibiotics. *Pediatr Infect Dis J* 2001;20:392-396.

125. Gums JG. Abstract/poster presentation; American College of Chest Physicians (ACCP), 2001. Antimicrobial susceptibility trends from 1990-2000:Preliminary results of the antimicrobial resistance management (ARM) program. *Pharmacotherapy* 2001;21:1300-1301.

126. Fraschini F, Scaglione F. Study on the relationship between pharmacokinetics and antibacterial activity: Comparison between ceftriaxone and cefotaxime within the respiratory tract. *Chemotherapy* 1989;45:77-82.

127. Browne FA, Clark C, Bozdogan B, et al. Single and multi-step resistance selection study in Streptococcus pneumoniae comparing ceftriaxone with levofloxacin, gatifloxacin and moxifloxacin. *Int J Antimicrob Agents* 2002;20:93-99.

128. Bartlett BG, Dowell SF, Mandell LA, et al. Practice guidelines for the management of community-acquired pneumonia in adults. *Clin Infect Dis* 2000;31:347-82.

129. Appelbaum PC. Antimicrobial resistance in Streptococcus pneu-moniae: A review. *Clin Infect Dis* 1992;15:77_/834.

130. Doern GV, Heilmann KP, Huynh HK, et al. Antimicrobial resistance among clinical isolates of Streptococcus pneumoniae in the United States during 1999-2000, including a comparison of resistance rates since 1994-1995. *Antimicrob Agents Chemother* 2001;45:1721-1729.

131. Jones RN, Pfaller MA. Macrolide and fluoroquinolone (levo-floxacin) resistance among Streptococcus pneumoniae strains: Significant trends from the SENTRY antimicrobial surveillance program (North America, 1997-1999). *J Clin Microbiol* 2001;38:4298-4299.

132. Chen DK, McGeer A, de Azavedo JC, Low DE. Decreased susceptibility of Streptococcus pneumoniae to fluoroquinolone in Canada. Canadian bacterial surveillance network. *N Engl J Med* 1999;22:233-239.

133. Lin ares J, Campa AG, Pallares R. Fluoroquinolone resistance in Streptococcus pneumoniae. *N Engl J Med* 1999;20:1546-1548.

134. Ho P-L, Que Yung RWH, Tsang DNC, et al. Increasing resistance of Streptococcus pneumoniae to fluoroquinolones: results of a Hong Kong multicentre study in 2000. *J Antimicrob Chemother* 2001;48:659-65.

135. Nagai K, Davies TA, Dewasse BE, et al. In vitro development of resistance to ceftriaxone, cefprozil and azithromycin in Streptococcus pneumoniae. *J Antimicrob Chemother* 2000;46:909-915.

136. Enoxacin—A new fluoroquinolone. *Med Lett Drugs Ther* 1992; 34:103-105.

137. Cooper B, Lawer M. Pneumococcal bacteremia during ciprofloxacin therapy for pneumococcal pneumonia. *Am J Med* 1989;87:475.

138. Flynn CM, et al. In vitro efficacy of levofloxacin alone or in combination tested against multi-resistant Pseudomonas aeruginosa strains. *J Chemother* 1996;8:411-415.

139. Dholakia N, et al. Susceptibilities of bacterial isolates from patients with cancer to levofloxacin and other quinolones. *Antimicrob Agents Chemother* 1994;38:848-852.

140. Habib MP, et al. Intersci Conf Antimicrob Agents Chemother 1996;36. Abstract L002. 36th Interscience Conference on Antimicrobial Agents and Chemotherapy. New Orleans, LA. Sept. 15-18, 1996.

141. File TM, et al. Abstr Intersci Conf Antimicrob Agents Chemother 1996;36. Abstract L001 (LM1). 36th Interscience Conference on Antimicrobial Agents and Chemotherapy. New Orleans, LA. Sept. 15-18, 1996.

142. Pfizer, Inc. Azithromycin package insert.

143. Pfizer product monograph. Azithromycin for IV injection.

144. Data on file, Pfizer, Inc. New York, NY.

145. Martinez JA, Horcajada JP, Almela M, et al. Abstract: L-988. Effect of Initial Treatment with a Beta-Lactam plus a Macrolide Compared with a Beta-Lactam Alone on Bacteremic Pneumococcal Pneumonia (BPP) Mortality. Citation: 42nd ICAAC Abstracts, American Society for Microbiology, Sept. 27-30, 2002, San Diego, CA, page 359.

146. de Klerk GJ, van Steijn JH, Lobatto S, et al. A randomised, multicentre study of ceftriaxone versus standard therapy in the treatment of lower respiratory tract infections. *In J Antimicrob Agents* 1999;12:121-127.

147. Mayfield DC, et al. TSN Database, USA, 1996-2000, on file at Roche Laboratories In Vitro Evaluation of Ceftriaxone activity against recent gram negative clinical isolates: results from the TSN Database.

148. Gupta AK, Rai S, Farag B, et al. Comparative analysis of levofloxacin (LV) vs ceftriaxone (CX)/azithromycin (AZ) in the treatment of community-acquired pneumonia (CAP). Length of Stay (LOS)

149. Weiss K, Cortes L, Beaupre A, et al. Clinical Characteristics, Initial Presentation and Impact of Treatment on Mortality in Bacteremic Streptococcus pneumoniae Pneumonia (BSSP). Abstract: L-987.Citation: 42nd ICAAC Abstracts, American Society for Microbiology, Sept. 27-30, 2002, San Diego, CA, page 359.

150. Thomson KS. Minimizing quinolone resistance: are the new agents more or less likely to cause resistance? *J Antimicrob Chemother* 2000;45:719-723.

151. Peterson LR. Quinolone molecular structure-activity relationships: what have we learned about improving antibacterial activity. *Clin Infect Dis* 2001;33(Suppl 3):S180-186.

152. Pestova E, Beyer R, Cianciotto NP, et al. Contribution of topoisomerase IV and DNA gyrase mutations in Streptococcus pneumoniae for resistance to novel fluoroquinolones. *Antimicrob Agents Chemother* 1999;43:2000-2004.

153. Lu T, Zhao X, Drlica K. Gatifloxacin activity against quinolone-resistant gyrase: allele-specific enhancement of bacteriostatic and bactericidal activities by the C-8 methoxy group. *Antimicrob Agents Chemother* 1999;43:2969-2974.

154. Pestova E, Millichap JJ, Noskin GA, et al. Intracellular targets of moxifloxacin: a comparison with other fluoroquinolones. *J Antimicrob Chemother* 2000,45:583-590.

155. M'Zali FH, Hawkey PM, Thomson CJ. The comparative in vitro activity of ciprofloxacin and levofloxacin against clinical strains of Pseudomonas aeruginosa *Clin Microbiol Infect* 2000;6(Suppl 1):91. Abstract WeP122.

156. Dalhoff A, Schubert S, Ullman U. Dissociated resistance among fluoroquinolones. *J Antimicrob Chemother* 2001;47(Suppl 1):33. abstract P67.

157. Nightingale CH. Moxifloxacin, a new antibiotic designed to treat community-acquired respiratory tract infections: a review of microbiologic and pharmacokinetic-dynamic characteristics. *Pharmacotherapy* 2000;20:245-246.

158. Ciprofloxacin (Cipro) package insert. West Haven (CT): Bayer Corporation; 2001.

159. Levofloxacin (Levaquin) package insert. Rarotam (NJ): Ortho-McNeil Pharmaceuticals; 2001.

160. Moxifloxacin (Avelox) package insert. West Haven (CT): Bayer Corporation; 2001.

161. Gatifloxacin (Tequin) package insert. Princeton (NJ): Bristol-Myers-Squibb Pharmaceuticals, Princeton; 2001.

62. Zhao X, Drlica K. Restricting the selection of antibiotic-resistant mutants: a general strategy derived from fluoroquinolone studies. *Clin Infect Dis* 2001;33(Suppl 3):S147-56.

63. Blondeau JM, Zhao X, Hansen G, et al. Mutant prevention concentrations of fluoroquinolones for clinical isolates of Streptococcus pneumoniae. *Antimicrob Agents Chemother* 2001;45:433-438.

64. Levaquin Product Information. Ortho-McNeil Pharmaceuticals. January 1997.

65. Vincent J, et al. Pharmacokinetics and safety of trovafloxacin in healthy male volunteers following administration of single intravenous doses of the prodrug, alatrofloxacin. *J Antimicrob Chemother* 1997;39(supp B):75-80.

66. Spangler SK, et al. Activity of CP 99,219 compared with those of ciprofloxacin, grepafloxacin, metronidazole, cefoxitin, piperacillin, and piperacillin-tazobactam against 489 anaerobes. *Antimicrob Agents Chemother* 1994;38:2471-2476.

67. Child J, et al. The in-vitro activity of CP 99,219, a new naphthyridone antimicrobial agent: A comparison with fluoroquinolone agents. *J Antimicrob Chemother* 1995;35:869-876.

68. Brighty KE, et al. The chemistry and biological profile of trovafloxacin. *J Antimicrob Chemother* 1997;39(supp B):1-14.

69. Mundy LM, et al. Community-acquired pneumonia: Impact of immune status. *Am J Respir Crit Care Med* 1995;152:1309-1315.

70. Kulgman KP, Capper T, et al. In vitro susceptibility of penicillin-resistant S. pneumoniae to levofloxacin, selection of resistant mutants, and time-kill synergy studies of levofloxacin combined with vancomycin, telcoplanin, fusidic acid, and rifampin. *Antimicrob Agents Chemother* 1996;40:2802-2804.

71. Polk R, Johnson C, Clarke J, et al. Virginia Commonwealth University, Richmond, Va; Trends in Fluoroquinolone (FQ) Prescribing in 35 U.S. Hospitals and Resistance for P. aeruginosa: A SCOPE-MMIT Report. MultiMedia Info. Technologies Abstract.

72. Fridkin S, Steward CD, Edwards JR, et al. Surveillance of antimicrobial use and antimicrobial resistance in United States hospitals: project ICARE phase.

73. Project Intensive Care Antimicrobial Resistance Epidemiology (ICARE) hospitals. *Clin Infect Dis* 1999:29:245-252.

74. Lautenbach E, Fishman O, et. al. Risk factors for fluoroquinolone resistance in nosocomial Escherichia coli and Klebsiella pneumoniae infections. *Arch Intern Med* 2002;162:2469-2477.

75. Graham KK, Hufcut RM, Copeland CM, et al. fluoroquinolone exposure and the development of nosocomial MRSA bacteremia. *Infect Cont Hosp Epidemiol* 2000;21:90.

76. Resistance of Streptococcus pneumoniae to fluoroquinolones-United States, 1995-1999. *MMWR Morbid Mortal Wkly Rep* 2001;50:800-804.

77. Warren JW, Abrutyn E, Hebel JR, et al. Guidelines for antimicrobial treatment of

uncomplicated acute bacterial cystitis and acute pyelonephritis in women. Infectious Diseases Society of America (IDSA). *Clin Infect Dis* 1999;29:745-58.

178. American Thoracic Society. Guidelines for the management of adults with community-acquired pneumonia: diagnosis, assessment of severity, antimicrobial therapy, and prevention. *Am J Respir Crit Care Med* 2001;163:1730-1754.

179. Bartlett JG, Dowell SF, Mandell LA, et al. Practice guidelines for the management of community-acquired pneumonia in adults. Infectious Diseases Society of America. *Clin Infect Dis* 2000;31:347-382.

180. Fine MJ, et al. The hospital discharge decision for patients with community-acquired pneumonia. Results from the Pneumonia Patient Outcomes Research Team cohort study. *Arch Intern Med* 1997;157:47-56.

181. Zimmerman T, Reidel KD, Laufen H, et al. Intravenous toleration of azithromycin in comparison to clarithromycin and erythromycin. In: Abstracts of the 36th Interscience Conference on Antimicrobial Agents and Chemotherapy. Washington, DC: American Society Microbiology; 1996:16 Abstract A82.

182. Thys JP, Jacobs F, Byl B. Role of quinolones in the treatment of bronchopulmonary infections, particularly pneumococcal and community-acquired pneumonia. *Eur J Clin Microbiol Infect Dis* 1991;10:304-315.

183. Piscitelli SC, Danziger LH, Rodwold KA. Clarithromycin and azithromycin: New macrolide antibiotics. *Clin Pharm* 1992;11: 137-152.

184. Ortquist A, et al. Oral empiric treatment of community-acquired pneumonia. *Chest* 1996;110:1499-1506.

185. Samama MM, Cohen AT, Darmon JY, et al. A comparison of enoxaparin with placebo for the prevention of thromboembolism in acutely ill medical patients. Prophylaxis in Medical Patients with Enoxaparin Study Group. *N Engl J Med* 1999;341:793-800.

186. Clagett GP, Andersen FA, Heit JA, et al. Prevention of venous thromboembolism. *Chest* 1998;114(5 suppl):531S-560S.

187. Nicolaides AN, Bergquist D, Hull R, et al. Consensus statement. Prevention of venous thromboembolism. *Int Angiol* 1997:16:3-38.

188. Anderson FA, Wheeler HB, Goldberg RJ, et al. A population-based perspective of the hospital incidence and case-fatality rates of deep vein thrombosis and pulmonary embolism. The Worcester DVT study. *Arch Intern Med* 1991;151:933-938.

189. Sandler DA, Martin JF. Autopsy proven pulmonary embolism in hospital patients: Are we detecting enough deep vein thrombosis? *J Royal Soc Med* 1989;82:203-205.

190. Gardund B for the Heparin Prophylaxis Study Group. Randomized, controlled trial of low-dose heparin for prevention of fatal pulmonary embolism in patients with infectious diseases. *Lancet* 1996;347:1357-1361.

191. Neuhauser MM, Weinstein RA, Rydman R, et al. Antibiotic resistance among gram negative bacilli in US intensive care units: Implications for fluoroquinolone use *JAMA* 2003;289:885-888.

192. Andrews JM, Honeybourne D, Jevons G, et al. Concentrations of levofloxacin (HR 355) in the respiratory tract following a single oral dose in patients undergoing fibre-optic bronchoscopy. *J Antimicrob Chemother* 1997;40:573-577.

193. Soman A, Honeybourne D, Andrews J, et al. Concentrations of moxifloxacin in serum and pulmonary compartments following a single 400 mg oral dose in patients undergoing fibre-optic bronchoscopy. *J Antimicrob Chemother* 1999;44:835-838.

194. Lautenbach E, Larosa LA, Kasbekar N, et al. Fluoroquinolone utilization in the emergency departments of academic medical centers. *Arch Intern Med* 2003;163:601-605.

CME QUESTIONS

1. Causative pathogens in community-acquired pneumonia (CAP) are identified in:
   A. fewer than 10% of patients.
   B. fewer than 20% of patients.
   C. fewer than 30% of patients.
   D. fewer than 40% of patients.
   E. fewer than 50% of patients.

2. The American Thoracic Society guideline includes which of the following findings in its criteria for severe pneumonia?
   A. Respiratory rate > 30
   B. Mechanical ventilation
   C. Bilateral or multilobar infiltrates
   D. Shock
   E. All of above

3. The annual incidence of pneumonia in patients older than age 65 is about:
   A. 1%.
   B. 10%.
   C. 15%.
   D. 20%.
   E. None of the above

4. The symptoms of pneumonia may mimic which of the following disorders?
   A. Pulmonary embolism (PE)
   B. Congestive heart failure (CHF)
   C. Lung cancer
   D. COPD
   E. All of the above

5.   At the very least, empiric coverage for CAP in the elderly must provide activity against which of the following pathogens?
     A.   *S. pneumoniae, H. influenzae*, and *M. catarrhalis*
     B.   *Mycoplasma, Legionella*, and *C. pneumoniae*
     C.   *H. influenzae, M. catarrhalis*, and *Mycoplasma*
     D.   *S. pneumoniae, H. influenzae*, and *M. catarrhalis*, as well as against atypical pathogens *Mycoplasma, Legionella*, and *C. pneumoniae*
     E.   None of the above

6.   Which of the following are recommended by the CDC Therapeutic Working Group for Drug Resistant *S. pneumoniae* as first-line, initial empiric monotherapy in individuals with outpatient CAP?
     A.   TMP-SMX
     B.   Macrolides (azithromycin, erythromycin, or clarithromycin)
     C.   Fluoroquinolones (levofloxacin, grepafloxicin, getafloxacin)
     D.   Cephalosporins (cefaclor)
     E.   None of the above

7.   The CDC recommends that fluoroquinolones be reserved for selected patients with CAP, among them those in which of the following group(s)?
     A.   Adults for whom one of the first-line regimens (cephalosporin plus a macrolide) has failed
     B.   Those who are allergic to the first-line agents
     C.   Those patients who have a documented infection with highly drug-resistant pneumococci (i.e., penicillin MIC > 4 mcg/mL)
     D.   All of the above
     E.   None of the above

8.   Studies suggest azithromycin monotherapy is as effective as a combination regimen (i.e., cefuroxime plus erythromycin) for appropriately selected patients with CAP.
     A.   True
     B.   False

For instructions on how to participate in this CME activity, please see the back of this book (page 717).

Urinary Tract Infection: Risk Stratification, Clinical Evaluation, and Evidence-Based Antibiotic Therapy—Year 2003 Update

Clinical Implications of Emerging Resistance Patterns, Medication Compliance Issues, and Pharmacoeconomic Considerations on Antimicrobial Selection

INTRODUCTION

In the constantly shifting landscape of drug resistance, antibiotic options, and pharmacoeconomic considerations, urinary tract infection (UTI) continues to be one of the most frequently diagnosed conditions in patients presenting to the primary care practitioner, emergency department physician, and family medicine specialist.

It is estimated that practitioners manage seven million new cases of cystitis in the United States each year and that, overall, UTIs account for approximately 1 million hospitalizations annually.[1,2] Moreover, UTIs are the leading cause of gram-negative bacteremia in patients of all ages, and are associated with a high risk of morbidity and mortality, especially in the elderly.[3] The total annual cost of treatment is in the billions of dollars.[4]

Among common infections managed in the outpatient setting, few conditions have treatment guidelines, antibiotic selection strategies, or diagnostic

Authors: **Romolo Gaspari, MD, FACEP,** Research Director, Assistant Professor, Department of Emergency Medicine, University of Massachusetts School of Medicine, Worcester, Massachusetts; and **Gideon Bosker, MD, FACEP,** Assistant Clinical Professor, Yale University School of Medicine, New Haven, CT.

protocols that have changed or evolved as rapidly as those used for UTI. Despite a general consensus that empiric treatment of UTI in adult women requires, at the very least, mandatory coverage of *Escherichia coli* and other gram-negative organisms, antibiotic selection strategies—including initial choice of therapy and duration of treatment—vary widely among practitioners and institutions.

There are many reasons for inconsistencies in the current approach to UTI management among hospital-based physicians. Unfortunately, deciphering the strengths and weaknesses of recommendations issued by different authoritative sources can be problematic and confusing, especially since resistance patterns of infecting uropathogens may vary among geographic regions, and because outcome-effectiveness, medication compliance, failure rates, total-resource costs to achieve clinical cure, the risk of recurrent infection, and evolving bacterial resistance issues are not always entered into the drug selection equation.

Because no single set of guidelines is applicable to every patient or hospital practice environment, management guidelines for UTI must be "customized" for the local practice setting and, as always, clinical judgment must prevail. This means taking into account local antibiotic resistance patterns, epidemiological and infection incidence data, and patient demographic features.

Important, new therapeutic options that have been introduced into the antimicrobial armamentarium for uncomplicated UTI offer clinicians compliance-enhancing strategies that can improve clinical outcomes. In this regard, recent introduction of extended release ciprofloxacin (Cipro XR®) has made it possible to enhance medication compliance through once-daily administration of what has been considered to be the "gold standard" antibiotic (ciprofloxacin) for uncomplicated UTI, while at the same time making available a preparation that achieves an AUC that is equivalent to conventional BID ciprofloxacin and achieving a C_{max} that is 40% higher than the conventional BID formulation.

From a practical clinical perspective, because of its potentially compliance-enhancing properties (once-daily dosing and a well-tolerated side effect profile), extended release delivery system, and clinically effective urine concentrations, the extended release formulation represents a risk-management upgrade from BID ciprofloxacin; therefore, it should replace the older formulation as the clinical standard for treatment of uncomplicated UTI when indicated. A well-designed clinical trial comparing the new and conventional formulations supports this shift to the once-daily, extended release formulation and is described in this review.

Even when these factors are considered, a number of important questions about drug selection issues for UTI still remain: 1) What is the appropriate initial, empiric choice for uncomplicated UTI? Once-daily (QD) extended release ciprofloxacin (Cipro XR®) or trimethoprim-sulfamethoxazole (TMP-SMX)? 2) What are the specific "intensification and treatment trigger" criteria that support amplifying initial spectrum of coverage from TMP-SMX to a fluoroquinolone such as extended release ciprofloxacin? 3) How should evolving resistance of *E. coli* to TMP-SMX affect initial antimicrobial therapy? 4) What is the optimal duration of therapy for uncomplicated and complicated UTIs? 5) Which antibiotic currently provides "correct spectrum" coverage, safety, and reliability for outpatient treatment of uncomplicated UTI?

Although optimizing cure rates with so-called convenient, dose- and duration-friendly branded agents that provide appropriate and predictable coverage with a low risk of antimicrobial resistance may be perceived as costly on a drug-acquisition basis, it is important to stress the following point: Antimicrobial agents with more predictable coverage against pathogens implicated in UTI can help avoid the unnecessary costs of treatment failures, disease progression, patient re-evaluations, return visits, patient dissatisfaction, and the pharmacological reservicing costs associated with initiating a second course of antibiotics.[5]

In this sense, antibiotics that lower barriers to clinical cure and provide a predictable spectrum of coverage can be seen as "productivity tools" that improve efficiency of clinical care and potentially reduce the overall costs associated with inpatient and acute outpatient management of UTI.

In light of the important advances, changes, and refinements that have occurred in the area of UTI treatment over the past year, this comprehensive, state-of-the-art review presents a revised and updated set of guidelines outlining UTI epidemiology and management in outpatient and hospital-based settings. Special emphasis has been given to both epidemiological data demonstrating the importance of "correct spectrum" coverage with specific fluoroquinolones, such as ciprofloxacin, and the selection of initial antibiotics for patients deemed suitable for discharge.

In addition, detailed evidence-based analysis comparing ciprofloxacin to TMP-SMX is presented to guide antibiotic selection in patients with uncomplicated UTI and pyelonephritis.[5] Cautionary notes about the overuse of extended-spectrum fluoroquinolones are outlined, and evidence-based studies confirming ciprofloxacin's workhorse role in hospital-based treatment of UTI is discussed. Drawing upon consensus panels, expert opinion, and clinical trials, this clinical consensus report presents antimicrobial protocols and treatment guidelines linked to, and driven by, risk-stratification criteria, evidence-based trials, and specific clinical profiles of patients presenting to the hospital with symptoms and signs suggestive of UTI.

Changing resistance patterns observed with common urinary pathogens have altered the empirical approach to antibiotic selection for both upper and lower UTIs. Previously, decisions regarding antimicrobial therapy have been made based on patient characteristics and the anticipated spectrum of urinary flora. However, increasing levels of resistance to beta-lactams over the past decade has decreased the utility of this drug class for treatment of UTIs. In addition, emerging resistance among *E. coli* species to TMP-SMX also is affecting initial drug selection choices for UTI, a change characterized by the acceptance of such fluoroquinolones as extended release ciprofloxacin as the initial agent of choice for greater than 90% of uncomplicated UTIs seen in the outpatient setting.

EPIDEMIOLOGY

Acute UTI is one of the most common illnesses encountered in adult women, resulting in as many as 8,000,000 office visits per year[6] and at least 100,000 hospital admissions.[7,8] Although the exact frequency of UTI is not known, based on current evidence accumulated from office and hospital surveys it is estimated that there are approximately 7,000,000 episodes of cystitis[9] and 250,000 episodes of pyelonephritis[10] annually in the United States. One prospective study determined the annual incidence of cystitis to be 0.5-0.7% per person-year.[11]

Although many cases of uncomplicated UTI resolve with only transient, mild symptoms, studies suggest considerable morbidity and mortality are associated with all forms of UTI. Two independent studies[12,13] found that asymptomatic bacteriuria in the elderly was associated with an increased mortality rate; however, this is not a universal finding.[14,15] Certain patient populations, in particular those with diabetes and pregnancy, have been found to have a higher level of morbidity.[16,17] Studies reviewing simple cystitis also have revealed substantial morbidity, with limited activity lasting for more than two days.[18] As many as 60% of elderly patients with pyelonephritis will develop bacteremia, and 20% of these cases will result in septic shock.[19] Life-threatening bacteremia as a complication of UTI also has been documented by a number of other investigators.[20-24]

UTIs in women vastly outnumber those in men.[25] This may be related to such factors as the length of the urethra, distance of the urogenital meatus from the anus, and the antibacterial properties of prostatic fluid.[26] Regardless of the reason, the fact that male UTIs are so uncommon has led many authors to classify them as complicated. This is supported by the high degree of virulence found in male UTI isolates, and the high prevalence of non-*E. coli* UTIs.[27]

MICROBIOLOGY AND EMERGING RESISTANCE PATTERNS

For many years, pathogens associated with uncomplicated UTIs remained constant, with *E. coli* identified as the etiologic agent in about 75-90% of infections.[25] Five to fifteen percent of uncomplicated UTIs are caused by *Staphylococcus saprophyticus,*[28,29] with *Klebsiella, Proteus, Enterococcus,* and *Pseudomonas* species seen in much smaller percentages.[30-32]

The emergence of *E. coli* isolates demonstrating resistance to commonly used antibiotics, especially to TMP-SMX, is changing initial drug selection patterns in patients with both uncomplicated and complicated UTIs. The most

Table 1. Most Common Uropathogens Identified in Adult UTI Patients[§]

1)	*Escherichia coli*
2)	*Staphylococcus saprophyticus*
3)	*Klebsiella pneumoniae*
4)	*Proteus mirabilis*
5)	*Enterococcus* faecalis*
6)	*Pseudomonas aeruginosa*
7)	*Enterobacter cloacae*
8)	*Citrobacter*

§ = Listed in order of decreasing frequency

* = Gram-positive organisms

common uropathogens identified in adult patients with UTI include enteric gram-negative bacteria, with *E. coli* being the most common. *(Please see Table 1.)* The remainder of infections are caused by coagulase-negative *Staphylococcus saprophyticus* (10-20%), while *Proteus mirabilis, Klebsiella,* and *Enterococcus* account for less than 5%.[3,33,34] Other aerobic gram-negative bacteria of the Enterobacteriacea family include *Citrobacter, Enterobacter, Serratia,* and *Salmonella.*[35-37] Non-enteric aerobic gram-negative rods such as *Pseudomonas* and aerobic gram-positive cocci such as *Enterococcus* are less prevalent in immunocompetent hosts. *(Please see Table 1).* Group B strepto-cocci infection is observed in neonates secondary to inoculation from a colo-nized mother during delivery through the vaginal canal.

Anaerobic bacteria are rarely pathogenic despite their prevalence in fecal flora. The *Lactobacillus* species, coagulase-negative staphylococci, and *Corynebacterium* are not considered clinically significant isolates in the urine of healthy children between 2 months and 2 years of age.[1,38] *Corynebacterium, Lactobacillus,* and *Streptococcus* species are identified only rarely; when pres-ent, they nearly always represent contamination of the specimen rather than a true pathogen. In complicated UTI, in addition to *E. coli,* there is a higher prevalence of *Pseudomonas, Enterobacter* species, *Serratia, Acinetobacter,*

Klebsiella, and enterococci.[39] There are anecdotal reports of treatment for *Gardnerella vaginalis,* lactobacilli, *Chlamydia trachomatis,* and *Ureaplasma urealyticum* in pregnant women, but it is unclear whether these organisms represent true pathogens in this population.[40,41] Candidal species are now emerging in greater numbers, especially in catheterized patients and those who received previous treatment for enterococcal UTIs.[39]

The high incidence of UTIs in the general population; the potential for complications, especially in high-risk subgroups; and the associated costs of treatment emphasize the importance of appropriate antibiotic therapy. Microbial resistance to nearly all classes of antimicrobials continues to rise despite increasing awareness and concerns worldwide. European studies have shown *E. coli* resistance rates to multiple antibiotics, specifically TMP-SMX, in as many as one-third of patients.[42,43] Similar trends in the United States have prompted a shift to fluoroquinolones such as ciprofloxacin as preferred initial agents for empiric intravenous and/or oral therapy of UTI in both hospital and emergency department settings.[44]

In a cross-sectional survey of urine cultures obtained in the emergency departments of urban tertiary care centers in the United States, microbial resistance was as high as 48% to ampicillin, 25% to tetracycline, 14-28% to TMP-SMX, and 13% to nitrofurantoin.[45] Similar studies have shown that the resistance to ciprofloxacin among common uropathogens, including *E. coli,* frequently encountered in hospital-managed UTI is as low as 1-2%.[46-50]

These epidemiological data have important treatment implications, since recent studies also are already demonstrating outcome differences in clinical efficacy and patient cure rates between UTI patients managed on TMP-SMX and those managed on ciprofloxacin.[51] As would be expected, maintenance of predictable antimicrobial activity by ciprofloxacin against the anticipated spectrum of uropathogens has solidified the role of this antibiotic in treatment pathways for UTI among all institutional settings.

Surveillance and Sensitivity. Hospitals affiliated with managed care organizations also have been prompted to re-evaluate their initial approach to antibiotic selection for UTI. A cross-sectional survey of 4,000 urine cultures obtained from women ages 18 to 50 in an HMO setting between 1992 and

1996 showed *E. coli* prevalence to be 86%, with the resistance rate to TMP-SMX increasing over this period from 9% to 18%. Recent data suggest that in some regions of the country, especially the West, Southwest, and in most major urban centers, the resistance rate to TMP-SMX has risen to as high as 35%.[5,42,43,52-55] The overall resistance to multiple groups of antimicrobials, including the penicillins, cephalosporins, and sulfa drugs, doubled from 8% to 16%.[56] In pregnant patients, *E. coli* resistance to ampicillin, which at one time was a drug of choice for UTI in this population, is now about 20% to 30%.[41]

Fortunately, one class of antimicrobials to which sensitivity rates have remained consistently high is the fluoroquinolone group, of which ciprofloxacin is the most frequently used in the adult population. A two-tiered study from 1989 to 1991 and 1996 to 1997 at an urban sexually transmitted disease clinic evaluated young, sexually active females diagnosed with a UTI and found *E. coli* resistance rates to ampicillin, cephalosporins, or tetracycline in as many as 25% of patients. There was very little change in the low prevalence of organisms resistant to fluoroquinolones.[57]

Additional studies at student health clinics in California over a five-year period demonstrated significant increases in the resistance of *E. coli* to ampicillin (30-45%), tetracycline (29-40%), and TMP-SMX (15-32%), with resistance to fluoroquinolones in less than 5% of organisms.[34] In a recent analysis of young women with uncomplicated pyelonephritis, *E. coli* was isolated in more than 90% of cultures and was resistant to TMP-SMX in 18%, compared with a 0.4% resistance to ciprofloxacin. A significant variance in resistance patterns existed in different geographic regions, with resistance to TMP-SMX as high as 35% on the West Coast of the United States as opposed to 14% in the Midwest and 7% on the East Coast.[51] One caveat regarding bacterial resistance is that in vitro sensitivity results may not correlate with clinical cure rates and in vivo sensitivity. Eradication of a uropathogen depends on the concentration of antibiotics in the urine as opposed to serum, which may be higher than the levels used in in vitro studies.[39]

Recent studies have noted a subtle shift in etiologic agents associated with UTIs. A survey of all UTI pathogens in 1997 found the top four isolates to be *E. coli* (48.6%), *Enterococcus* spp (13.7%), *Klebsiella* spp (12.0%), and

Table 2. Incidence of Urinary Tract Pathogens

PATHOGEN	UNCOMPLICATED CYSTITIS	COMPLICATED UTIs
Escherichia coli	70-95%	40-55%
Klebsiella spp	2-6%	10-17%
Enterobacter spp	0-2%	5-10%
Proteus mirabilis	2-4%	5-10%
Pseudomonas aeruginosa	0-1%	2-10%
Enterococcus spp	2-5%	1-20%
Staphylococcus saprophyticus	5-20%	-------

Modified from references 25,31,63

Pseudomonas aeruginosa (6.2%).[58] More current data from 1998 support these trends.[59] This shift in pathogens may be related to factors such as bladder catheterization or antibiotic use. Another study reported a similar mix of uropathogens in catheter-associated UTIs.[60] Not surprisingly, bacterial isolates found in complicated UTIs follow a similar pattern.[61,62] *(Please see Table 2.)*

Although there are fewer data on patients with pyelonephritis, recently published surveys indicate a similar mix of pathogens, with about 90% of patients with pyelonephritis manifesting infection with *E. coli*.[64,65] Other isolates included those found in lower UTIs. Urethritis is usually caused by *Chlamydia trachomatis, Neisseria gonorrhoeae,* or herpes simplex virus.

***Escherichia coli (E. coli)* Resistance.** The sensitivity of a urinary tract pathogen to a specific antimicrobial agent is defined by measuring the bacteria's ability to grow in the presence of that antibiotic. In the case of *E. coli,* if the strain under evaluation can grow in media containing 2 mcg/mL or greater (mean inhibitory concentration or MIC) of the antibiotic, the strain is considered resistant to that antibiotic. Potential confusion arises when the reported resistance levels are related to the blood concentration of antibiotic and not the urine concentration. As a rule, antibiotics used for UTIs are concentrated in the urine and have higher urine levels then blood levels. Therefore, isolates that are reported resistant to an antibiotic by laboratory testing actually may be eradicated by the antibiotic in the in vivo environment. This concept is clinically relevant and has been demonstrated in a number of studies.[28,66,67]

Due to the consistent, relatively predictable spectrum of pathogens encountered in UTIs, empiric therapy represents an appropriate strategy for the majority of patients, whether they present in the outpatient, emergency department, or in-hospital setting. Historically, empiric therapy using any one of a wide range of agents has proven clinically successful for UTI. Until recently, high cure rates could be expected because a predictable group of urinary pathogens have manifested a low degree of resistance to most antibiotics selected on an empiric basis. However, a number of recent studies have highlighted evolving changes in antimicrobial resistance patterns to *E. coli.* In particular, clinically and microbiologically significant changes in resistance to TMP-SMX among *E. coli* species, and in a small percentage of cases, to fluoroquinolones have been reported in Europe[68,69] and America.[30-32,59,70]

Resistance and Implications for Antibiotic Therapy— Fluoroquinolones Emerge as Initial Agents of Choice. Evolving changes in drug resistance have dramatically altered the approach to empiric therapy of UTI. Although beta-lactams, sulfa-based antibiotics, and fluoroquinolones each have their place in the treatment of UTI, their roles are changing, with fluoroquinolones emerging as initial agents of choice, even for uncomplicated UTI. Penicillin-based antibiotics were once a mainstay of UTI treatment, but current resistance rates among *E. coli* (approaching 40% in many regions) have limited their effectiveness.[30,71,72] Although *E. coli* resistance to fluoroquinolones in America has not reached the levels encountered with other antibiotics,[25,28,72] the level of resistance in other countries is alarming.[73,74] In the United States, however, increasing *E. coli* resistance to TMP-SMX has been accompanied by a paradigm shift in the initial treatment of choice for UTI (please see below).[31,75-78]

The level of *E. coli* resistance to TMP-SMX has more then doubled over the past 12 years and now exceeds 25% in some areas of the country.[79-81] One group of investigators examined a cross-section of urinary isolates from 1992 to 1996 and found an increase of TMP-SMX resistance from 9% to more then 18%.[72]

Subsequent, larger studies have shown similar results.[79-81] Resistance rates in the United States vary from region to region, and knowledge of local resistance rates are important factors when determining initial antibiotic therapy.[31]

Most experts and national association panels concur that sequential selection strategies for antibiotic therapy in UTI, to a significant degree, should depend on the degree of *E. coli* resistance to TMP-SMX in a particular community. In this regard, the Infectious Disease Society of America (IDSA) recommends that alternative antibiotics (i.e., agents other than TMP-SMX) should be used as first-line therapy in areas of the country where TMP-SMX resistance is greater than 10-20%.[78] More specifically, the clinical outcome and pharmacoeconomic implications of fluoroquinolones vs. TMP-SMX therapy have been linked to a 20% *E. coli* drug resistance cut-off point.

With this antibiotic preference issue in mind, two published studies have examined the effect of *E. coli* resistance rates on patient outcomes[75] and economic parameters.[82] One study concluded that the clinical effectiveness of fluoroquinolones such as ciprofloxacin was superior to TMP-SMX when more than 10% of the *E. coli* isolates were resistant to TMP-SMX.[75] At a 20% resistance rate, nitrofurantoin also was superior to TMP-SMX. Another study, using a cost-analytical model, approached the issue of antimicrobial selection from a different angle. Performing a cost analysis of first-line UTI antibiotic options—examining the desirability of one agent vs. another through the prism of increasing antibiotic resistance rates—these investigators found progressive cost savings to the community when a fluoroquinolone was substituted for TMP-SMX as initial agents of choice in areas characterized by a 20% or greater resistance rate among *E. coli* to TMP-SMX.[82] Although authorities identify different resistance rate breakpoints that would favor a shift to a fluoroquinolone as first-line therapy, there is general agreement that the greater the resistance rate, the greater the clinical and pharmacoeconomic benefits to fluoroquinolone use.

It should be stressed that the fluoroquinolones are not immune to the selective pressures causing antibiotic resistance in UTI isolates. Studies in some foreign countries, where there has been heavy use of this class of antibiotics, have shown increasing rates of resistance. A multi-center study found *E. coli* resistance to ciprofloxacin in 36% and 20% of urinary isolates from Portugal and Spain, respectively.[30] However, most studies of urinary isolates in the United States show only a 1-4% resistance rate to fluoroquinolones.[31,59]

Multi-drug resistant uropathogens are becoming increasingly common across America. One retrospective study found that 37% of UTI isolates from emergency department patients were multi-drug resistant.[32] A larger national study of inpatients as well as outpatients looked at almost 39,000 urinary isolates from patients with UTIs and found the number of multi-drug resistant isolates to be 7.1%. Among the resistant strains, 98% were resistant to ampicillin and 93% were resistant to TMP-SMX. The resistance to ciprofloxacin and nitrofurantoin was 39% and 8%, respectively.[79]

URINARY TRACT INFECTIONS IN WOMEN—PRINCIPLES OF MANAGEMENT

Asymptomatic Bacteriuria. Asymptomatic bacteriuria is a well-documented entity that affects women of all ages. A number of large-scale population studies have shown the prevalence of asymptomatic bacteriuria to be directly related to age, with a 1-2% rate in young women, 6-10% in women older than age 60,[83] and 15-20% in women ages 65 and older.[15,84,85] These rates only represent a "snapshot in time," inasmuch as studies have demonstrated a "turnover" of bacteriuria from positive to negative and back again during sequential six-month urine cultures.[86,87]

As a rule, asymptomatic bacteriuria (ASB) should not treated in most patients, since multiple studies have shown that antibiotic therapy does not make a significant impact on long-term outcomes in an otherwise healthy adult population.[88] A recent prospective study of asymptomatic bacteriuria in sexually active young women found prevalence rates of approximately 5%, with 8% of those women developing symptomatic UTI within one week.[89] Specific groups benefiting from antibiotic treatment include pregnant women, neutropenic patients, patients with abnormal renal function, renal transplant recipients in the early post-transplantation period, and men and women planning to undergo urologic procedures.[3,89]

Infants with ASB represent a low-risk population for the development of UTIs, with a tendency toward spontaneous abacteriuria within a few months, and do not generally require antibiotic treatment.[90] School-age children usually are left untreated; however, patients with underlying voiding disorders should be referred appropriately for further evaluation and treatment.

Pregnant women with ASB should be treated with a three- to seven-day course of antibiotics, followed by a subsequent culture to ensure sterilization of urine. Despite increasing resistance rates to ampicillin, amoxicillin and cephalosporins remain a first-line choice in these patients. Ceftriaxone is the preferred agent in pregnant women. Nitrofurantoin is becoming a first-line drug, because it is efficacious, inexpensive, and well-tolerated. The only contraindication to using this drug is in patients with G6PD deficiency, in whom hemolysis can occur. TMP-SMX remains a first-line agent in areas of low resistance, but should be avoided in the first and third trimesters secondary to possible teratogenic effects and the risk of kernicterus from competitive binding of TMP-SMX to bilirubin binding sites. At this time there is no clear evidence to support a single-dose regimen over a typical three- to seven-day course.[40,91,91] A properly sized, randomly controlled trial is recommended for comparison of these regimens, as a single dose has lower cost, fewer adverse effects, and increased compliance compared with longer treatment regimens.[91]

Initial evidence in the elderly population had suggested an increased risk of morbidity and mortality in patients with ASB. More recent studies have challenged these reports, but have failed to identify a connection between ASB and an increase in long-term sequelae such as hypertension or end-stage renal disease. Up to 40% of the elderly will have ASB at some time. Aggressive screening and treatment have little effect on decreasing symptomatic or clinically significant infection and associated complications.[3] Catheterized patients, including those with neurologic disorders or spinal cord injuries, rarely require aggressive work-up and treatment unless symptoms intervene.[93] Interestingly, a recent study of catheterized patients found that catheter-associated UTIs are rarely symptomatic and infrequently cause bacteremia (< 1%). No significant differences were noted between symptomatic and asymptomatic bacteriuria groups with regard to signs and symptoms commonly associated with infection (fever, dysuria, urgency, or flank pain) or leukocytosis.[94] Investigations have noted that both groups are a major reservoir for antibiotic resistant organisms in the hospital setting.

The long-term consequences of asymptomatic bacteriuria have not been fully elucidated, but this condition may have the potential to cause symptomatic UTIs and/or sepsis in a small minority of patients, although such sequelae have not been uniformly substantiated. In addition, the potential for persistent bacteriuria and recurrent UTI to decrease survival continues to be debated, with some investigators finding an association[12,13] while others have not.[14,15] A recent, well-conducted analysis of patients with asymptomatic bacteriuria failed to show an increase in mortality when comorbid factors were accounted for.[95] In summary, most experts currently do not recommend treatment for asymptomatic bacteriuria, except in the high-risk patient populations identified above.[83,96]

Uncomplicated Lower Urinary Tract Infection. The majority of uncomplicated lower UTIs occur in patients who have no functional or anatomical abnormality of their urinary system. Lower UTIs can be categorized into two distinct categories: cystitis and urethritis. In the emergency department, it may be difficult to distinguish between uncomplicated and complicated cystitis. As a rule, however, the clinician will be able to distinguish between cystitis and urethritis on the basis of history and physical exam. Symptoms of urethritis overlap with cystitis, but urethritis usually has a more gradual onset with milder symptoms and little to no urgency or frequency. Associated vaginal discharge or lesions may make the diagnosis more apparent. It usually is reasonable to assume that a young, non-pregnant female with acute onset of dysuria and frequency has a simple cystitis if she has not had any instrumentation or recent antibiotic therapy.

Certain patient populations are at an increased risk for developing a UTI. One group has determined that recent sexual intercourse, diaphragm use, and a history of previous UTIs are independent risk factors for developing a UTI.[11] Although the study population was limited to college age women, other studies that included older women have demonstrated similar risk factors.[97] However, these risk factors are not universally agreed upon and many patients with a confirmed diagnosis of UTI will cite no risk factors.

Complicated Lower Urinary Tract Infections and High Risk Patients.
Complicated UTIs typically occur in patients who have an underlying urinary
tract abnormality causing obstruction. The abnormality may be a physical
obstruction (i.e., kidney stone or bladder catheter), or it may be a functional
abnormality (i.e., neurogenic bladder or vesicoureteral reflux). Infections in
patients with such disease states as diabetes or renal failure, as well as renal
transplantation, also fall into the category of so-called complicated UTI.
(Please see Table 3.) Complicated UTIs encompass patients with a wide variety of syndromes and risk factors that increase the likelihood of poor outcomes. Moreover, studies aimed toward evaluating etiological agents in complicated infections demonstrate a broad range of microbial pathogens, of
which *E. coli* is the most common.[63]

An associated concept is the high-risk patient with UTI, which would
include individuals who are pregnant, immunosuppressed, or those who have
an indwelling catheter. High-risk patients may or may not have a urogenital
abnormality, but the potential sequelae of UTI in these subgroups may overlap
with those encountered in patients with complicated infections; as a result,
some authors use the terms interchangeably. From a clinical perspective, the
important concept is that both patients who have a complicated UTI and those
deemed at high-risk require more prudent management, which includes a
longer duration of therapy, and closer follow up.

Upper Urinary Tract Infection. Upper UTI generally refers to
pyelonephritis, and its potential complications, including perinephric
abscess. Many studies have confirmed that pyelonephritis occurs through
ascending infection from the bladder.[98,99] It is thought that fecal organisms
inoculate the urethra, spread into the bladder, and subsequently ascend the
ureters to the kidney parenchyma. The incidence of pyelonephritis is much
lower then that of cystitis, although the morbidity and mortality are much
greater.[25] Acute pyelonephritis can progress to chronic pyelonephritis or perinephric abscess depending on host factors such as immune status and
obstruction.[100]

Symptoms of pyelonephritis can vary from dysuria to fulminant urosepsis.
Only 20-30% of patients with isolated dysuria will actually have subclinical

Table 3. Patient Subgroups Associated with Complicated Lower Urinary Tract Infection

STRUCTURAL ABNORMALITIES (SURGICAL, CONGENITAL, OR ACQUIRED)

Renal tumors

Urethral or ureteral strictures

Renal cysts

Congenital abnormalities of the urogenital system

Urogenital surgery

FUNCTIONAL ABNORMALITIES

Neurogenic bladder

Vesicoureteral reflux

MECHANICAL OBSTRUCTION TO URINE FLOW

In-dwelling bladder catheterization*

Nephrolithiasis*

Ureteral stents and nephrostomy tubes*

Urogenital instrumentation

HIGH RISK*

Diabetes mellitus*

Pregnancy*

Immunosuppressed*

Sickle cell anemia and trait*

Renal failure*

Modified from references 7, 63

pyelonephritis.[101-103] Patients with subclinical pyelonephritis present with symptoms characteristic of cystitis, but infection is located in the kidney. Subclinical pyelonephritis is impossible to differentiate from cystitis without complicated localization techniques that mostly are used in research studies. Most patients with symptomatic pyelonephritis will present with flank pain, nausea, vomiting, fever, and costovertebral angle tenderness.[104]

DIAGNOSTIC STRATEGIES IN URINARY TRACT INFECTION: URINALYSIS, CULTURE, AND IMAGING STUDIES

The majority of patients with UTI present with unambiguous symptoms and signs suggestive of this disease process, and therefore, present few diagnostic challenges for the astute clinician. However, a minority of infections, especially those encountered in the elderly or immunocompromised individual, may be more clinically challenging. For example, most clinicians would have little difficulty making the diagnosis of UTI in a young woman presenting with one day of dysuria and frequency, whereas diagnostic challenges are likely to surface when UTI causes obtundation in an elderly male. Because a number of modalities are available for diagnostic evaluation, the practitioner must determine which laboratory tests and/or imaging modalities are appropriate and cost-effective in individuals presenting with symptoms suggestive of UTI.

Diagnostic Approach. Clinical experience suggests that most uncomplicated lower UTIs encountered in the outpatient setting can be diagnosed (and cured) without the use of urine cultures.[75] Accordingly, patients who present with symptoms consistent with cystitis or urethritis should undergo a history, physical exam, and urinalysis. The use of dipstick urinalysis and/or microscopic urinalysis provides a diagnostic yield that is sufficiently specific and sensitive to establish the diagnosis of uncomplicated UTI.[105] Due to the increased morbidity and mortality associated with pyelonephritis and UTI in high-risk patients, a urine culture is still recommended for the work-up in this patient subgroup.

Urinalysis. A urinalysis continues to be the "workhorse" laboratory evaluation for establishing the diagnosis of UTI in a broad range of patients; therefore, it is the principal modality employed for the work-up of UTI. The primary utility of a urinalysis is to examine for and document the presence of pyuria, hematuria, nitrates, leukocyte esterase, and bacteria. Although semi-quantitative dipstick and microscopic urinalysis are widely used and have been extensively reviewed in the literature, studies are conflicting as to their accuracy.[105-110]

The presence of red or white cells in the urine can help differentiate the location of the infection. Pyuria is present in almost all patients with urethritis, cystitis, and pyelonephritis. The laboratory/clinical definition of pyuria (number of white cells per high-powered field [hpf]) will affect its sensitivity and specificity for establishing the diagnosis of UTI. One group found that the presence of greater than 5 WBCs per hpf was 85% sensitive for UTI, whereas other authors[111] have reported that greater than 10 WBCs/hpf was a more reliable breakpoint for making the diagnosis.[107] The presence or absence of pyuria should be interpreted within the context of other findings in the urinalysis. Hematuria can be present with cystitis and pyelonephritis but is rarely seen in urethritis.[25] It can be diagnosed semi-quantitatively with a urine dipstick or quantitatively on a microscopic urinalysis. Studies looking at dipstick hematuria have found a sensitivity and specificity of 44% and 88%, respectively.[112] Microscopic analysis of the urine also may demonstrate red cell casts that are indicative of upper tract disease.

Several unique esterases produced by neutrophils in the urine form the basis of one of the screening tests for UTI. The leukocyte esterase can be rapidly detected using a urine dipstick which appears to provide a reliable method for detecting pyuria. Studies have shown that the leukocyte esterase has a sensitivity in the range of 74-96% and a specificity of about 94-98%,[108,113,114] although this may not distinguish the presence of pyuria with this degree of accuracy in clinical practice.[112,115]

The nitrite test on a dipstick urinalysis is a rapid screening test for bacteriuria. It has been found to be 39% sensitive and 93% specific for bacteria in the urine in both prospective and retrospective studies.[105,107,112] One investigation combined nitrate results with the presence of microscopic bacteriuria and/or pyuria (> 10 WBCs per hpf) and found a sensitivity and specificity of in the range of 71-95% and 54-86%, respectively.[107] Other studies have found that the accuracy of this test can be effected by a low level of infection[20] or the type of infecting microorganism.[116]

Urine Culture. Bacteriuria is considered by most clinicians to be the definitive marker of UTI. Studies conducted in the 1950s found that 10^5 colony forming units (cfu) per milliliter was indicative of a UTI.[117,118] However, more recent studies suggest that this level of bacteriuria may miss a large group of UTIs, and support the concept that lower levels (10^2-10^4 cfu) should be considered positive.[7,119] In one provocative study, patients provided urine samples when a diagnosis of UTI was suspected, but they were not treated for two days after onset of symptoms. A repeat urine culture was obtained two days later at which time empiric treatment was started. Interestingly, urine cultures cleared spontaneously in only 5% of the patients who had a low colony-count initially, while 48% now had a colony count of 10^5 or more.[120]

It should be emphasized that lower levels of bacteriuria have been shown to predict UTIs in a variety of settings. Levels greater than 10^2 have shown a sensitivity of 95% and a specificity of 85% for the diagnosis of cystitis in women.[121] Male patients with urine samples growing greater than 10^3 cfu/mL are considered positive for UTI.[26] All patients with pyelonephritis have been found to have a higher level of bacteriuria, with cultures almost uniformly growing at levels greater than 10^4 cfu/mL.[117,122] In summary, studies suggest that antibiotic therapy should be considered for any patient with symptoms of a UTI and a culture positive for 10^3 cfu/mL or greater of a urinary tract pathogen.

Urine Collection. The method by which urine is collected has received little attention in the scientific literature. The most commonly recommended collection technique for women is either a mid-stream clean-catch urine sample, or an in-and-out catheterized specimen. Despite the effort that goes into instruction for a mid-stream clean-catch urine sample, contamination is a frequent problem.[123] There is little rigorous scientific research that supports a mid-stream clean-catch urine sample as the standard for urine collection. In one study, urine samples were randomly collected by one of two techniques. One group received instructions on cleaning and technique for obtaining a mid-stream clean-catch urine specimen. The other group did not clean and no other instructions were given. There was no difference in contamination between the groups. Studies in men revealed similar results.[124,125]

In-and-out sterile catheterization is the most reliable method to obtain a urine sample from women. This procedure has the lowest chance of contamination from vaginal or perineal flora and has a low risk of complications. There is a risk of inducing infection in 1-3% of patients.[126] Catheterizing a male to get a urine sample is not recommended, as any urine sample is usually clean. If the situation demands obtaining a urine sample from a male who cannot cooperate, a catheterized specimen is recommended but a clean "condom" catheter may as useful as bladder catheterization.[127]

Imaging Techniques. Radiographic imaging has no role in the initial work up of most UTIs. Some specific imaging modalities may have utility in identifying upper UTIs or their complications. Ultrasound is relatively poor at identifying infectious conditions of the kidney other than perinephric abscess, infected hydronephrosis, or emphysematous pyelonephritis; fortunately, the conditions are rare.[128] CAT scan has been found to be better for visualizing all infectious conditions of the kidney and has the advantage of identifying alternative, non-infectious conditions.[129,130] The few categories of patients with UTI who should be considered for imaging are patients with recurrent illness or patients who are not improving despite therapy.

ANTIBIOTIC SELECTION FOR UTI: GENERAL PRINCIPLES AND OVERVIEW OF THERAPEUTIC OPTIONS

Because of the relative predictability of uropathogens, and the time delay associated with urine culture results, antibiotic treatment for UTIs relies heavily on empiric therapy. Recent changes in antibiotic resistance trends, however, have forced a reassessment of empiric choices for managing UTI. As is the case for nearly all infections, the ideal antibiotic for UTI is one that provides predictable coverage against all pathogens likely to cause the disease, offers significant penetration of the urinary system and adequate urine concentrations, has few side effects, and shows low resistance rates in the local community to the expected uropathogens. A wide range of treatment options have been extensively studied and reported in the medical literature; however, interpretation of older studies, in particular, must be considered in light of current resistance patterns.

Fluoroquinolones: Current Agents of Choice. With rapidly changing resistance patterns among the common uropathogens, standard first-line treatment (i.e., TMP-SMX) is being replaced in many instances by the fluoroquinolone class. Derivatives of nalidixic acid, fluoroquinolones were discovered accidentally in the early 1960s during the synthesis of the anti-malarial agent, chloroquine.[44] To date, more than 10,000 analogues of nalidixic acid have undergone initial screening, and the first fluoroquinolone antibiotic was approved for clinical use in the late 1980s.[44] These highly effective antimicrobials act on bacterial topoisomerases, a class of enzymes that is essential for maintaining the physicochemical stability and biological activity of bacterial DNA.[44] In general, the newer quinolones have longer serum half-lives, with proven post-antibiotic effects from one to six hours; this allows patient-friendly single- or twice-daily dosing and higher peak levels for maximum bactericidal activity. Recent approval of extended release ciprofloxacin (Cipro XR®)[131] has made available an effective, well-tolerated, and safe once-daily preparation of what most clinicians concur has become the "gold standard" of therapy for UTI (please see below).[44]

In addition, fluoroquinolones are well-absorbed from the gastrointestinal tract, and in the case of ciprofloxacin, equivalent clinical outcomes in selected patient populations with moderate to severe UTI have been established between patient groups who received this drug intravenously and those who received oral therapy.[46,48,132] The fluoroquinolones have excellent penetration into various tissues; they are well-distributed intracellularly, and have the added benefit of eliminating perineal, vaginal, and perirectal reservoirs of uropathogens without altering normal bowel or vaginal flora.[44,133]

As mentioned, the high oral bioavailability of fluoroquinolones allows switching from intravenous to oral therapy without dosage adjustments.[134] Excretion is primarily renal, although some of the compounds have exclusive hepatic metabolism or a combination of the two.[44] They have an extended spectrum of bactericidal activity against gram-negative rods, including *Pseudomonas*, gram-positive cocci, and intracellular pathogens.[133,134] Fluoroquinolones remain classified as category C drugs, requiring practitioners to rule out pregnancy before prescribing them to potentially pregnant patients.[44]

The armamentarium of commonly used fluoroquinolones is expanding at a rapid rate. Ciprofloxacin (Cipro®), which has been a clinically proven gold standard for oral and intravenous-based therapy of UTI has been joined by other agents, many of which also are indicated for community-acquired pneumonia (CAP). The new extended release formulation of ciprofloxacin (Cipro XR®) likely will become the new standard of care for uncomplicated UTI. Other members of this class include gatifloxacin (Tequin®), levofloxacin (Levaquin®), and ofloxacin (Floxin®). Low levels of resistance to fluoroquinolones are beginning to appear through two mechanisms: chromosomal mutations or alterations affecting the ability of fluoroquinolones to permeate the bacterial cell wall.[44] Fortunately, separate isomerases are required to produce this form of resistance; therefore, the emergence of a predictably resistant organism would require a rare double mutation.[44]

An extensive body of clinical research confirms that fluoroquinolones are extremely effective for the treatment of UTIs ranging in severity from uncomplicated cystitis to urosepsis.[135] As would be expected, many studies evaluating newly introduced quinolones compare clinical trial outcomes to the established track record of ciprofloxacin, which has become a standard choice for initial, empiric therapy for most UTIs. In a clinically controlled trial comparing three days of oral ciprofloxacin with seven days of TMP-SMX or nitrofurantoin, bacteriologic cure rates for uncomplicated UTI after 4-6 weeks were 91%, 79%, and 82%, respectively.[136] Clinical cure rates after 4-10 days were similar among the three groups, as was the overall incidence of adverse events. The superior efficacy of ciprofloxacin as compared to TMP-SMX also has been confirmed in patients with acute pyelonephritis.[51]

In certain studies of acute uncomplicated cystitis, levofloxacin has preliminarily been shown to have equal efficacy in single doses as in the standard longer dosing regimens.[137,138] Ciprofloxacin and norfloxacin are effective in either single daily or double dosing regimens in uncomplicated UTI.[139,140] For complicated UTIs, including pyelonephritis, levofloxacin and lomefloxacin have equivalent bacteriologic and clinical cure rates to ciprofloxacin. Of the newer fluoroquinolones, only levofloxacin is approved for both upper and lower UTIs.

Despite the effectiveness of newer fluoroquinolones for UTI, overuse of the extended-spectrum fluoroquinolones (levofloxacin and gatifloxacin) for outpatient and hospital-based management of UTI must be considered in light of recommendations made by the Centers for Disease Control and Prevention (CDC), which has documented concerns about emerging resistance to common pathogens implicated in community-acquired pneumonia (CAP). The fluoroquinolone ciprofloxacin is a preferred oral agent for the treatment of *Pseudomonas aeruginosa* urinary infections.[51] It should be emphasized that although other quinolones may demonstrate activity against, and may be indicated for treatment of gram-negative organisms implicated in UTI, some of these antibiotics, especially those extended-spectrum fluoroquinolones that also are used for initial, empiric treatment of CAP, are active against *Streptococcus pneumoniae.*

Given the recently reported increase in resistance among *S. pneumoniae* species to levofloxacin, attempts should be made to limit selective pressures caused by the overuse of these agents. Consequently, the use of so-called advanced generation fluoroquinolones (AFQs) as initial, first-line agents for UTI should be discouraged because of concerns about emerging resistance among *S. pneumoniae* species implicated in CAP. This cautionary approach is supported by a recent guidelines document issued by the CDCs Drug-Resistant Streptococcus Pneumoniae Therapeutic Working Group.

In this regard, because of significant concerns about, as well as documentation of, emerging resistance to *S. pneumoniae,* the CDC panel has recommended that extended-spectrum fluoroquinolones (i.e., levofloxacin, gatifloxacin, etc.) be "reserved" for selected patients with CAP. In light of this position, which is intended to prevent excessive use of advanced fluoroquinolones and reduce selective pressures against pulmonary pathogens causing CAP, it appears prudent to limit their potential for inducing resistance in the community and reserve such antibiotics as alternative agents in patients with UTI. This approach appears to be justified, especially because an effective and safe fluoroquinolone (i.e., ciprofloxacin extended release) is available for uncomplicated UTI, and does not have significant activity against gram-positive organisms causing CAP. Accordingly, ciprofloxacin is recommended as the initial fluoroquinolone of choice for managing patients with UTI.

OUTCOME-OPTIMIZING AND COMPLIANCE-ENHANCING ANTIMICROBIALS FOR UNCOMPLICATED UTI: GUIDING THE GOLD STANDARD

Optimizing Clinical Outcomes in Uncomplicated UTI. Recent introduction of extended release ciprofloxacin (Cipro XR®) has made it possible to potentially enhance medication compliance through once-daily administration of this "gold standard" antimicrobial for uncomplicated UTI with a preparation that achieves an AUC that is equivalent to conventional BID ciprofloxacin, and a C_{max} that is 40% higher.[131]

The new, extended release formulation features a number of attributes, including absorption that is limited to the upper gastrointestinal tract, and a unique bilayer matrix design that permits about 35% of the dose to be released immediately and the remaining 65% to be released over an extended period. Good urine concentrations are maintained throughout the dosing interval.

Because of its potentially compliance-enhancing properties (once-daily dosing and a well tolerated side effect profile), extended release delivery system, and clinically effective urine concentrations, the extended release formulation represents a risk-management upgrade as compared to BID ciprofloxacin; therefore, it should replace the older formulation as the clinical standard for treatment of uncomplicated UTI when indicated. A well-designed clinical trial (please see below) supports this shift to the once-daily, extended release formulation.

Clinical Studies. To evaluate the clinical usefulness and possible advantages of extended release ciprofloxacin, a study was designed to compare the efficacy and safety of extended release ciprofloxacin 500 mg QD to conventional immediate-release ciprofloxacin 250 mg BID for women with uncomplicated UTI. This study design, which represented the U.S. pivotal trial, was a double-blind, randomized phase III study enlisting adult, non-elderly, non-pregnant outpatient women with acute uncomplicated UTI.[131]

With 422 total evaluable patients, the two treat arms compared a three (3)-day course of extended release (Cipro XR®) 500 mg once-daily vs. conventional 250 mg twice-daily administration. Efficacy of these regimens, which included assessment of bacteriological eradication and clinical cure, was measured at 4-11 Days (test-of-cure visit) and at 25-50 days (late follow-up visit) following completion of therapy. In addition, adverse event monitoring, which included documentation of possible drug-related adverse events as well as laboratory parameter evaluation, was included in the study design.

To ensure the study population reflected "real world" patients with uncomplicated UTI, inclusion criteria required that at least two of the following signs and symptoms of uncomplicated UTI be present: dysuria, frequency, urgency, or suprapubic pain. An infectious etiology for this symptom complex was confirmed on the basis of a positive mid-stream clean-catch urine culture, demonstrating a uropathogen 10^5 cfu/mL or greater, and pyuria (≥ 10 leukocytes/mm^3). The study excluded individuals with asymptomatic bacteriuria, evidence of complicated UTI, three or more UTIs in the previous year, or anatomic/medical factors predisposing to UTIs.

Baseline Characteristics. The extended release ciprofloxacin (500 mg QD x 3 days) and conventional ciprofloxacin (250 mg BID x 3 days) treatment groups were well-matched with respect baseline characteristics. The mean age of patients in the ciprofloxacin extended release (CipXR) group was 34.3 years, and 35.1 years in the ciprofloxacin conventional group (CipBID). Eighty-nine percent of the CipXR patients had a duration of infection lasting for two or more days, and 82% of those in the CipBID group had a duration of two or more days prior to treatment.

Clinical Cure and Bacteriologic Eradication Rates. The causative organism at time of enrollment was *E. coli* in about 80% of patients in both treatment groups, with *E. faecalis, K. pneumoniae, P. mirabilis,* and *S. saprophyticus* each being encountered in less than 10% of cases. Overall, 99% of the pre-therapy isolates were susceptible to ciprofloxacin. Clinical cure rates were 95% for CipXR vs. 93% for CipBID for efficacy-valid comparisons. Intent-to-treat results were similar, with a 90% cure rate for QD CipXR vs. 93% for CipBID. Clinical response at late follow-up visits also were reported in this study, and revealed that continued clinical cure rates were 89% for CipXR vs. 87% for CipBID. Failures were seen in only 9% of QD CipXR and in 16% of patients in the CipBID treatment arms.[131]

With respect to bacteriologic eradication by organism, CipXR and CipBID

Table 4. Ciprofloxacin Extended Release (Cipro XR®) vs. Ciprofloxacin BID in Patients with Uncomplicated UTI

SIDE EFFECT, SAFETY, AND TOLERABILITY PROFILES		
	CIP EXT-REL (N = 444)	**CIP BID** (N = 447)
Drug-related Adverse Events (AEs)	46 (10%)	41 (9%)
Headache	7 (2%)	3 (< 1%)
Nausea	12 (3%)	4 (< 1%)
Vaginal moniliasis	4 (< 1%)	10 (2%)
Vaginitis	4 (< 1%)	7 (2%)
Serious drug-related AEs	0 (0%)	0 (0%)
Drug-related AEs leading to premature discontinuation	1 (< 1%)	0 (0%)

Modified from reference 131

demonstrated comparable results at the test-of-cure visit. Overall, 97% of *E. coli* were eradicated in both groups, with comparable rates of bacteriologic eradication, ranging from 79% to 98%, observed for both formulations among such uropathogens as *E. faecalis, P. mirabilis, S. saprophyticus,* and *K. pneumoniae.* Continued eradication was reported for 86% of QD CipXR and 81% of CipBID patients. Recurrence was reported at a similar rate in both treatment groups (8% each).

Drug-Related Adverse Events. The extended release formulation, CipXR, demonstrated a side effect, safety, and tolerability profile that was comparable to CipBID, with an overall drug-related adverse event rate of 10% (46/444 patients) for the extended release formulation and 9% (41/447) for the conventional formulation. *(Please see Table 4.)* No serious drug-related adverse events were seen in either treatment arm.

Conclusions. This study demonstrated that once-daily extended release ciprofloxacin achieved bacteriologic eradication and clinical cure in greater than 94% of patients had a comparable safety profile to ciprofloxacin BID, and was as effective as ciprofloxacin BID in treating women with uncomplicated UTI.

DISEASE-SPECIFIC URINARY TRACT INFECTION SYNDROMES: ANTIMICROBIAL MANAGEMENT

Asymptomatic Bacteriuria. Treatment recommendations for asymptomatic bacteriuria are consistent for most patient populations. There is little evidence that attempting to eradicate bacteria from the urine of most patients who are asymptomatic has any clinical benefit. The largest potential risk when repeatedly treating asymptomatic bacteriuria is in the selection of more virulent or resistant pathogens. The one patient subgroup for which treatment is uniformly recommended is in pregnancy. Pregnant women with asymptomatic bacteriuria should be treated with three days of a beta-lactam, nitrofurantoin, or in unusual cases, TMP-SMX.[141] However, TMP-SMX should not be used during the first trimester or near term. Treatment is not recommended for asymptomatic bacteriuria in non-pregnant patients.

Acute Bacterial Cystitis. Available therapies for uncomplicated acute bacterial cystitis include a wide range of antibiotic options and treatment durations. Fortunately, guidelines issued by the Infectious Disease Society of America in 1999 provide a practical, evidence-based guide for the practitioner.[78] Additional research and focus on resistance issues have helped refine the clinical approach to management of UTI.

The appropriate length of treatment for uncomplicated UTI has received a considerable amount on attention, with recommended treatment regimens ranging from 1-14 days of duration. A review of the literature suggests that three days of therapy with appropriate antibiotics is more effective then one day, but equally effective as longer courses.[78] It should be noted that, despite its widespread use, the commonly employed three-day treatment course with TMP-SMX does not currently carry a formal FDA indication for the treatment of cystitis. Some antibiotics, such as the beta-lactams and nitrofurantoin, may be less effective when given for three days as compared to longer periods of time.[142,143] However, three days of therapy with approved fluoroquinolones is sufficient for the treatment of acute uncomplicated cystitis.

A variety of antimicrobial agents can be used in the treatment of uncomplicated lower UTIs. Among the most commonly used are beta-lactams, fluoroquinolones, TMP-SMX, nitrofurantoin, and fosfomycin. Beta-lactams were used extensively in the 1970s but increasing resistance has led to the dependence on other antibiotics. Recent studies, however, demonstrate that 40% of the most common uropathogens are resistant to beta-lactams.[30,72] Nevertheless, beta-lactams are still the drug of choice in some patient populations, including in pregnant women and individuals with UTIs caused by enterococcus. Recommended therapy for cystitis during pregnancy is a three-day course with either amoxicillin 500 mg PO TID; cephalexin 250 mg PO QID; or a 10-day treatment course with nitrofurantoin 100 mg PO QHS.[141] Sulfonamides may interfere with bilirubin binding and cause hyperbilirubinemia in newborns; therefore, they are not recommended near term.

Trimethoprim-sulfamethoxazole (TMP-SMX) has been used extensively over the last decade for the treatment of lower UTIs, and was considered the antibiotic of choice until recently.[25] A meta-analysis encompassing several studies evaluating the efficacy of TMP-SMX indicates a cure rate of 93% using a three-day course.[78] The slightly increased relapse rate of the three-day vs. the seven-day treatment course was counterbalanced by the decrease in side effects. The three-day regimen for TMP-SMX is 160/800 mg orally every 12 hours.

As stressed earlier, the use of TMP-SMX for first-line therapy in cystitis has been affected by recent recognition of increasing resistance rates in most areas of the United States.[29-31] The current recommendations are to use TMP-SMX as the first-line agent for cystitis in areas where TMP-SMX resistance is less then 10-20% as there is evidence that other antibiotics are more effective, from both a clinical and cost perspective when the resistance rates exceed 10-20%.[78] In one important analysis, Le and Miller conducted a cost analysis for uncomplicated UTIs that supported switching from empiric treatment with TMP-SMX to ciprofloxacin when community resistance to TMP-SMX surpassed 20%.[82]

Nitrofurantoin is a well-established urinary tract antibiotic that, to a great degree, has fallen out of favor because of its four times daily dosing schedule. A newer formulation permits twice-daily dosing. Nitrofurantoin is highly concentrated in the urine and achieves minimal tissue levels, making it an ideal antibiotic for UTIs. Unfortunately, the cure rates for this antibiotic can be as low as 80%.[143,144] The newer formulation is given 100 mg BID for 7-10 days. Nitrofurantoin remains a second- or third-line therapy in most patient populations.

Fosfomycin tromethamine is a newer antibiotic that has been approved for single-dose therapy of uncomplicated UTI. Although some trials have found that fosfomycin is as effective as other first-line agents,[145] this is not universally accepted. A study in 1999 evaluating fosfomycin in UTI found a clinical cure rate of 80%.[146] Two other small studies found fosfomycin to be as effective as norfloxacin, but with a higher rate of side effects.[147,148] The clinical data on fosfomycin is still evolving and further information is needed before it can be advocated as a first-line agent.

In most areas of the country, fluoroquinolones have become the first-line agent of choice for uncomplicated lower UTI. Of the fluoroquinolones, ofloxacin, norfloxacin, ciprofloxacin, gatifloxacin, and levofloxacin all are either partially or totally cleared by the kidneys and cover the majority of uropathogens.[149] Some of the newer fluoroquinolones have little or no renal penetration and are not suitable for treating UTIs. As a group, the fluoroquinolones have been found to be highly effective for treatment of UTI. As outlined earlier, the recently introduced extended release formulation of ciprofloxacin should replace the older formulation as the clinical standard for treatment of uncomplicated UTI when indicated. *(Please see Table 5.)*

The suprapubic discomfort or dysuria common to UTI can be treated with oral analgesics (Tylenol, Motrin) or phenazopyridine (Pyridium) with a TID dose of 100-200 mg for no more than 48 hours.[38] Elderly females with lower UTI symptoms and no systemic complications may be treated for three days with similar regimens as prescribed for younger women.[150] In patients suspected of having a complicated UTI, including patients with symptoms lasting longer than one week, diabetic patients, immunocompro-

Table 5. Antibiotic Therapy for Acute Uncomplicated UTI in Adults

CYSTITIS (3-DAY REGIMEN)

AGENT OF CHOICE:

Fluoroquinolone (initial agent of choice)

> Ciprofloxacin extended release (Cipro® XR) 500 mg po QD x 3 days

ALTERNATIVE FIRST-LINE AGENTS:

Fluoroquinolones (alternative)

> Levofloxacin 250 mg po QD x 3 days
>
> Ofloxacin 200 mg po BID x 3 days
>
> Norfloxacin 400 mg po BID x 3 days

> Trimethoprim/sulfamethoxazole* 160/800 mg po bid x 3 days

SECONDARY ALTERNATIVES:

> Amoxicillin 500 mg po TID x 7-10 days (known enterococcus infection only)
>
> Nitrofurantoin 100 mg po BID x 7 days
>
> Amoxicillin-clavulanic acid 250 mg po QID x 7 days
>
> Fosfomycin One 3-g sachet orally

*Only if *E. coli* resistance is < 10-20% in patient population (based on regional resistance surveillance data).

mised individuals, and nontoxic febrile patients without evidence of acute pyelonephritis, the treatment duration should be between five and seven days.[39] Because these patients are less able to tolerate treatment failures and are more susceptible to recurrent infection, ciprofloxacin is recommended as the initial agent of choice. Moreover, in these patients, a urine culture is recommended prior to administration of antibiotics to ensure proper management and identification of the uropathogen in the event of treatment failure or recurrence.[39]

COMPLICATED URINARY TRACT INFECTIONS

Adult patients with pyelonephritis can be managed on an inpatient or outpatient basis, depending upon clinical severity. A retrospective comparison of inpatient and outpatient management of pyelonephritis suggested that general guidelines for admission should include the following: 1) underlying anatomical urinary tract abnormality; 2) an immunocompromised host (diabetes mellitus, cancer, sickle cell disease, transplant patients); 3) urinary tract obstruction; 4) failed outpatient management of pyelonephritis; 5) progression of uncomplicated UTI; 6) persistent vomiting; 7) renal failure; 8) suspected urosepsis; 9) age older than 60; 10) poor social situation; and 11) inadequate access to follow-up.[151] If these criteria are used for making in-hospital dispositions, it is estimated that 70% of all patients who are treated for pyelonephritis can be managed as outpatients.[152]

The general consensus for emergency department management of pyelonephritis is to begin parenteral therapy with a fluoroquinolone (ciprofloxacin) intravenously in patients who meet admission criteria.[153] Nontoxic patients with uncomplicated pyelonephritis suitable for outpatient management may receive oral ciprofloxacin for a total of 7-14 days, depending on clinical judgment and hospital protocols.[153] Other parenteral therapies include a combination of ampicillin or a third-generation cephalosporin plus an aminoglycoside in extended-interval dosing (i.e., every 24-48 hours).[41,154-156] The extended-spectrum cephalosporins, such as ceftriaxone, should be considered for serious urinary infections because of the high urinary concentrations that are achieved.[157]

If gram-positive cocci are the causative organism, ampicillin/ sulbactam with or without an aminoglycoside is recommended.[158] Admitted patients with suspected enterococci may require extended-spectrum penicillins (Timentin® or Zosyn®) or alternative therapies, including nitrofurantoin to treat isolated vancomycin-resistant enterococci (VRE). Because multi-drug resistance is common in VRE isolates, susceptibility testing is recommended for ampicillin, aminoglycosides, chloramphenicol, fluoroquinolones, minocycline (a tetracycline), and rifampin.[157] UTI caused by *Pseudomonas* often will require double antimicrobial coverage.

Acute Pyelonephritis. Patients with pyelonephritis are generally more ill then those with uncomplicated cystitis. As would be expected for a more invasive infection, the recommended treatment duration is significantly longer. Although some studies have shown a shorter duration of therapy may be effective,[65,159,160] most authors recommend a seven- to 14-day treatment course for pyelonephritis.[25,78] Intravenous therapy is commonly administered to patients with more severe illness, with oral therapy reserved for outpatient treatment. However, there are few data demonstrating superiority of intravenous over oral antibiotics. Even for patients who will be managed in the out-of-hospital environment, many physicians will give at least one dose of IV antibiotic, followed by oral therapy for the duration of the treatment course.

To evaluate the efficacy and cost of antibiotics used in pyelonephritis, a randomized, double-blind, multicenter trial analyzed 255 women with acute uncomplicated pyelonephritis. These patients received either ciprofloxacin 500 mg BID for seven days, or TMP-SMX 160/180 mg BID for 14 days.[51] More than 90% of UTI culture isolates from both groups were *E. coli*. Bacteriologic and clinical cure rates were greater at 4-11 days in the ciprofloxacin group (99% and 96%, respectively) than the TMP-SMX group (89% and 83%, respectively). At 22-28 days, bacteriologic and clinical cure rates were 84% vs. 74% and 82% and 74%, respectively. Bacterial and clinical cure rates with TMP-SMX in patients found to be infected with resistant *E. coli* were only 50% and 35%, respectively. Adverse effects were similar among groups, occurring in 24% with ciprofloxacin and in 33% with TMP-SMX. Health care resource use and estimated total treatment costs were calculated, from initial evaluation to "prescription pad" to "cure," including needed hospitalization, lab testing, office visits, and other procedures. Mean total cost per patient was 29% higher for TMP-SMX-treated patients than for ciprofloxacin-treated patients.[51]

Because of additional interventions and antibiotic prescriptions required in the TMP-SMX group to achieve a cure, the mean cost per cure also was 25% higher in the TMP-SMX group than in the ciprofloxacin-treated patients. These studies help confirm that knowledge of local resistance rates is imperative in deciding which antibiotics should be used in the treatment of UTI. They support the use of ciprofloxacin as a first-line agent in the management of uncomplicated pyelonephritis. With the current outcome- and cost-sensitive environment of managed care, clinicians must make informed choices in the management of their patients.[51,158] A related randomized trial found that oral and intravenous ciprofloxacin were equally effective in the empiric treatment of severe pyelonephritis or complicated UTIs, provided that severe sepsis, obstruction, and focal renal suppuration are not present.[161] Since all patients in this study were hospitalized, a direct comparison between inpatient and outpatient treatment with ciprofloxacin is still needed.

In pregnant women, pyelonephritis tends to occur more commonly during the second half of pregnancy.[2] In general, outpatient treatment is not the standard of care for pregnant women. Inpatient treatment with intravenous antibiotics and close monitoring are usually required to maximize outcomes. Treatment options are similar to other adult regimens, including ampicillin with gentamicin, cephalosporins, and extended-spectrum penicillins or aztreonam.[2] Patients may be discharged safely and parenteral therapy stopped after defervescence within 48-72 hours of admission.[162] Persistent fever or symptoms require further evaluation and consultation.

A study of more than 100 women with uncomplicated pyelonephritis at less than 24 weeks' gestation found that almost 10% of those treated initially as outpatients eventually required hospitalization.[163] Two additional studies suggest that, in very carefully selected patients, outpatient treatment may be a safe option.[164,165] However, without concise, evidence-based protocols or guidelines to guide this decision, the acceptable and prudent choice in pregnant women is to admit them for initial parenteral antibiotics and supportive care. In both non-pregnant adults and pregnant patients, failure to respond to appropriate antibiotics requires emergent radiologic studies, including ultrasound and possible CT scan, to evaluate for obstruction, masses, and renal and perirenal abscess. All patients should have follow-up urine cultures 1-2 weeks after completion of therapy to ensure eradication of infection. *(Please see Table 6.)*

UTI MANAGEMENT IN HIGH-RISK POPULATIONS

Catheterized Patients (Indwelling and Intermittent). A significant per-

Table 6. Antibiotic Treatment of Pyelonephritis (10-14 Day Treatment Duration)

FIRST-LINE AGENTS	
Fluoroquinolones	10-14 day course
Ciprofloxacin	(preferred) 500 mg Q 12 hours PO, IV
ALTERNATIVE FIRST-LINE AGENTS	
Levofloxacin	250 mg Q 24 hours PO, IV
Ceftriaxone	1-2 g Q 24 hours IV
Ofloxacin	200-300 mg Q 12 hours PO, IV
Norfloxacin	400 mg Q 12 hours PO
SECOND-LINE AGENTS	
TMP-SMX	160/800 mg Q 12 hours PO, IV
Ampicillin/sulbactam	3 g Q 6 hours IV
Amoxicillin/clavulanate	875/125 mg Q 12 hours PO
Piperacillin/Tazobactam	4.5 g Q 8 hours IV
Gentamicin	3-5 mg/kg/day divided q 6 hours IV

Modified from references 25, 78

centage of complicated UTIs originate in patients with chronic indwelling bladder catheterization. Studies show that following initial indwelling bladder catheterization, 5% of patients per day will develop bacteriuria.[166] Patients with long-term catheterization are invariably bacteriuric.[167,168] Prophylactic antibiotics lower the incidence of bacteriuria,[169,170] at the expense of selecting out more virulent organisms.[171-173] Currently, prophylactic antibiotics in catheterized patients are not recommended.[63]

A small percentage of patients with bacteriuria will progress to symptomatic UTI.[171] However, the vast majority will clear spontaneously.[96] Warren and colleges conducted an autopsy study comparing catheterized and uncatheterized patients.[174] Catheterized patients were seven times more likely to have renal inflammation or pyelonephritis. Although smaller studies have shown an increased mortality associated with nosocomial UTIs,[167,175] definitive investigations in this area have not yet been conducted.

Intermittent bladder catheterization may substitute for chronic indwelling catheters in some patient populations. Injury to the spinal cord (SCI) can cause a "neurogenic bladder," resulting in functional obstruction during urination. These patients have a much higher rate of UTI,[176] and the value of intermittent catheterization has been well established.[177-179] Donovan and colleges followed daily urine culture and analysis for 60 days of intermittent catheterization and found a total of 178 episodes of bacteriuria from 25,780 catheterizations.[180]

The consequences of and approach to asymptomatic bacteriuria in spinal cord injury (SCI) patients is not universally agreed upon as some authors believe that bacteria in the urine serves as a reservoir for more serious infections.[181] Studies reviewing various methods of ridding SCI patients of bacteria in their urine have showed mixed results.[176,182,183] Using antibiotics to prevent UTI does not seem to have any lasting effect and may pre-select out more virulent pathogens. One consensus panel of experts in the field recommends no treatment of asymptomatic bacteriuria in this population.[184]

Urinary Tract Infection in Men. UTIs in young men are uncommon and, consequently, they are classified as complicated by some authors.[25] The significant difference in UTI rates between men and women of the same age are thought to be due to anatomical differences between the sexes. Among other factors, the length of the urethra, a drier environment surrounding the meatus, and antibacterial properties of prostatic fluid contribute to a lower rate of infection in men.[26] Some of the risk factors that have been identified in men are homosexuality,[184] sex with an infected partner,[185] prostatic hypertrophy,[26] and lack of circumcision,[187] but this is not universally agreed upon.[188]

Some of these differences between UTIs in men and women support the classification of male UTIs as complicated. *E. coli* has been found to be the most common infectious agent in male UTIs, with a distribution of pathogens closer to that found in complicated female UTIs.[26,188] Although uropathogens in men show an increased virulence as compared to those seen in women,[27] the symptoms of male cystitis are similar to those seen in women.[188] A urine culture is recommended in the work up of male patients with dysuria, with 103 cfu/mL considered to be positive.

Because of the relatively small number of clinical studies on UTIs in men, treatment recommendations in this population are based on studies in women.[189] As a rule, seven days of antibiotic therapy are recommended for the treatment of a lower UTI, and 14 days for pyelonephritis. Recurrent UTIs require a six-week regimen.[26] Studies in men have shown that asymptomatic bacteriuria in men does not require treatment.[190,191]

Prostatitis always must be considered in the differential diagnosis. The male urethra courses through the center of the prostate on its way to the bladder. This relationship allows for invasion of urinary tract pathogens into the prostate, causing acute bacterial prostatitis. Patients with prostatitis will present with symptoms of a UTI and a large tender prostate.[126] The enlarged prostate also may cause symptoms of bladder obstruction by physically blocking urine flow. The agents that cause prostatitis are the same gram-negative agents that cause UTI. Treatment for acute bacterial prostatitis may include TMP-SMX or a fluoroquinolone and should last four weeks. Ciprofloxacin is recommended for treatment for chronic prostatitis and requires a treatment duration of 6-12 weeks.[192]

Renal Stones and UTIs. Although not common, the coexistence of nephrolithiasis and infection may have serious consequences. Renal stones associated with infection are usually one of two types: struvite or apatite, although any type of renal stone may be associated with infection. Struvite stones usually are found in women with recurrent infections and are associated with urease-producing organisms such as *Proteus mirabilis* and *Providencia stuartii*.[193] Apatite renal stones also are commonly associated with infection and are formed of calcium phosphate. Many of the struvite stones form what are called "staghorn calculi" with large branching stones located within the renal pelvis. Smaller calcium phosphate stones (typical renal stones) also may become associated with infection, but this is even less common.

Patients with infected renal stones do not usually present with signs of renal colic. The growth of these stones is slow and insidious and patients may present with chronic complaints. Such symptoms may include fever, hematuria, vague abdominal pain, recurrent UTIs, or urosepsis.[193] The exception to this is the infection of a "typical" calcium phosphate stone, which may present with renal colic. Complications of infected renal stones include recurrent stones, renal failure, sepsis, and death.

Treatment for most infected stones focuses on removal of the stone, but advanced disease may require nephrectomy.[193] Studies evaluating conservative treatment versus surgical removal found a higher rate of kidney failure and mortality in patients managed conservatively.[194,195] Although antibiotics are recommended in patients with stones, if significant obstruction is present, the antibiotic will not be filtered by that kidney and will be unable to penetrate to the source of infection.[196] For smaller non-obstructing stones, antibiotics and close follow-up for stone passage may be acceptable.

Pregnancy. UTIs in pregnancy are associated with a number of serious side effects generally not encountered in the general population. The most important risk stems from the effect of the infection on the unborn fetus. Multiple studies have shown that untreated UTI increases the rate of prematurity as well as fetal morbidity and mortality. In one study of pregnant women with pyelonephritis, 15% of the newborns were 2500 grams or less.[197] A retrospective study looking at 41,000 matched pregnant women with and without UTIs found an increased rate of fetal death as well as developmental delay later in life.[17]

Although pregnancy does not predispose a patient to acquire bacteriuria, it is associated with an increased incidence of pyelonephritis.[198] The reasons for this are most likely related to the hormonal effects on the ureters and mechanical effects of the uterus.[141] Accordingly, most cases of pyelonephritis occur in the second and third trimesters. A small minority (1-2%) of these patients may present in septic shock.[194] The physical exam and most laboratory findings are similar to non-pregnant patients with pyelonephritis. One important difference, however, is that a urinalysis may be inaccurate in pregnant patients and should not be relied on for diagnosing a UTI.[200]

The treatment of pregnant patients with UTIs differs from non-pregnant patients. Due to the consequences UTI in pregnancy, treatment of asymptomatic bacteriuria is recommended for all patients. A three-day course of a beta-lactam, nitrofurantoin, or a sulfonamide is recommended for both cystitis and asymptomatic bacteriuria.[141] Follow-up is critical for these patients, as one third of them will become reinfected during their pregnancies. Urine cultures also are recommended due to the high levels of beta-lactam resistance (up to 40%) seen in most communities. The length of treatment for both asymptomatic bacteriuria and cystitis is controversial and can range from three to seven days.

The treatment of pyelonephritis is more aggressive in pregnant patients. All pregnant patients with pyelonephritis should be hospitalized for at least 24 hours. Hydration is critical, as many of the patients will be dehydrated from vomiting. Beta-lactams are considered the agent of choice until culture results return. Ceftriaxone is one recommended agent of choice for initial empiric therapy. *(Please see Table 7.)*

Diabetes. Women with diabetes mellitus are more likely to have UTIs than those without this condition.[16] Moreover, diabetic women with asymptomatic bacteriuria also are more likely to progress to pyelonephritis.[202] One study reviewing UTIs in diabetics found that the greatest risk factors for developing complicated UTI were the presence of bacteriuria and recent sexual intercourse. Diabetics also are at increased risks for certain complications. About 75% of patients with perinephric abscess and 85-100% of those with emphysematous pyelonephritis have diabetes as a comorbid condition.[128]

To complicate matters further, diabetes also may be a risk factor for single and multi-drug resistance. One study of multi-drug resistance in the emergency department found that non-catheterized diabetic patients were 2.4 times more likely to have a two-drug resistant urinary pathogen.[32] However, increased uropathogen resistance in diabetic patients has not been found by all investigators.[203] All diabetic patients with a UTI require a culture and close follow-up.

SUMMARY

UTIs encompass a wide range of disorders, from asymptomatic bacteria to fulminant sepsis. Historically, the treatment of UTI has proven successful with

Table 7. Antibiotic Options for UTI During Pregnancy

Ceftriaxone	1-2 g Q24 h IV	Class B
Cephalexin	250 mg BID-QID	Class B
Amoxicillin	500 mg TID	Class B
Nitrofurantoin	100 mg BID	Class B
Amoxicillin-clavulanic acid	250 mg QID	Class B
Fosfomycin	One 3 g sachet	Class B
Or		
Nitrofurantoin	100 mg QHS for 10 d	Class B

Note: TMP-SMX should not be used during 1st trimester or at term.

Modified from references 141, 201

empiric antibiotic therapy. Although the range of pathogens has remained relatively constant over time, the changing spectrum of resistance has altered the treatment landscape dramatically. Antibiotic agents, especially TMP-SMX, which has been a mainstay of therapy cannot be considered the treatment of choice in areas in which *E. coli* resistance to TMP-SMX surpasses 10-20%; resistance rates of this magnitude are now reported in all regions of the United States except New England.

New formulations of antimicrobials that historically have been shown to be effective and safe for management of uncomplicated UTI are now available and represent first-line therapy. In this regard, extended release ciprofloxacin (Cipro XR®) has potentially compliance-enhancing properties (once-daily dosing and a well-tolerated side effect profile), an extended release delivery system, and produces clinically effective urine concentrations in patients with uncomplicated UTI. As such, it represents a risk-management upgrade as compared to BID ciprofloxacin and should replace this older formulation as the clinical standard for treatment of uncomplicated UTI when indicated. A well-designed, real world clinical trial supports the shift to the once-daily, extended release formulation.

REFERENCES

1. Lifshitz E, Kramer L. Outpatient urine culture: Does collection technique matter? *Arch Intern Med* 2000;160:2537-2540.

2. Roberts JA. Management of pyelonephritis and upper urinary tract infections. *Urol Clin North Am* 1999;26:753-763.

3. Orenstein R, Wong ES. Urinary tract infections in adults. *Am Family Phys* 1999;59:1225-1234.

4. Saint S, Scholes D, Fihn SD, et al. The effectiveness of a clinical practice guideline for the management of presumed uncomplicated urinary tract infection in women. *Am J Med* 1999;106:636-641.

5. Talan DA, Stamm WE, Hooton TM, et al. Comparison of ciprofloxacin (7 days) and trimethoprim-sulfamethoxazole (14 days) for acute uncomplicated pyelonephritis in women. *JAMA* 2000;283:12.

6. The National Kidney and Urologic Diseases Advisory Board 1990 long-range plan—window on the 21st century. Bethesda, MD: National Institutes of Health; 1990.

7. Johnson JR, Stamm WE. Urinary tract infections in women: diagnosis and treatment. *Ann Intern Med* 1989;111:906-917.

8. Patton JP, Nash DB, Abrutyn E. Urinary tract infection: Economic considerations. *Med Clin North Am* 1991;75:495-513.

9. Schappert SM. National Ambulatory Medical Care Survey: 1992 summary. *Adv Data* 1994(253):1-20.

10. Stamm WE, et al. Urinary tract infections: From pathogenesis to treatment. *J Infect Dis* 1989;159:400-406.

11. Hooton TM, et al. A prospective study of risk factors for symptomatic urinary tract infection in young women. *N Engl J Med* 1996;335:468-474.

12. Sourander LB, Kasanen A. A 5-year follow-up of bacteriuria in the aged. *Gerontol Clin* (Basel) 1972;14:274-281.

13. Dontas AS, et al. Bacteriuria and survival in old age. *N Engl J Med* 1981;304:939-943.

14. Nicolle LE, et al. The association of bacteriuria with resident characteristics and survival in elderly institutionalized men. *Ann Intern Med* 1987;106:682-686.

15. Nordenstam GR, et al. Bacteriuria and mortality in an elderly population. *N Engl J Med* 1986;314:1152-1156.

16. Geerlings SE, et al. Consequences of asymptomatic bacteriuria in women with diabetes

mellitus. *Arch Intern Med* 2001;161:1421-1427.

17. McDermott S, et al. Perinatal risk for mortality and mental retardation associated with maternal urinary-tract infections. *J Fam Pract* 2001;50:433-437.

18. Foxman B, Frerichs RR. Epidemiology of urinary tract infection: I. Diaphram use and sexual intercourse. *Am J Public Health* 1985;75:1308-1313.

19. Gleckman RA, et al. Bacteremic urosepsis: A phenomenon unique to elderly women. *J Urol* 1985;133:174-175.

20. Freid MA, Vosti KL. The importance of underlying disease in patients with gram-negative bacteremia. *Arch Intern Med* 1968;121:418-423.

21. Roberts FJ. A review of positive blood cultures: Identification and source of microorganisms and patterns of sensitivity to antibiotics. *Rev Infect Dis* 1980;2:329-339.

22. Krieger JN, Kaiser DL, Wenzel RP. Urinary tract etiology of bloodstream infections in hospitalized patients. *J Infect Dis* 1983;148:57-62.

23. Kreger BE, et al. Gram-negative bacteremia. III. Reassessment of etiology, epidemiology and ecology in 612 patients. *Am J Med* 1980;68:332-343.

24. Bryan CS, Reynolds KL. Hospital-acquired bacteremic urinary tract infection: Epidemiology and outcome. *J Urol* 1984;132:494-498.

25. Hooton TM, Stamm WE. Diagnosis and treatment of uncomplicated urinary tract infection. *Infect Dis Clin North Am* 1997;11:551-581.

26. Lipsky BA. Urinary tract infections in men. Epidemiology, pathophysiology, diagnosis, and treatment. *Ann Intern Med* 1989;110:138-150.

27. Ulleryd P, et al. Virulence characteristics of Escherichia coli in relation to host response in men with symptomatic urinary tract infection. *Clin Infect Dis* 1994;18:579-584.

28. McCarty JM, et al. A randomized trial of short-course ciprofloxacin, ofloxacin, or trimethoprim/sulfamethoxazole for the treatment of acute urinary tract infection in women. Ciprofloxacin Urinary Tract Infection Group. *Am J Med* 1999;106:292-299.

29. Gupta K, Scholes D, Stamm WE. Increasing prevalence of antimicrobial resistance among uropathogens causing acute uncomplicated cystitis in women. *JAMA* 1999;281:736-738.

30. Kahlmeter G. The ECO*SENS Project: A prospective, multinational, multicentre epidemiological survey of the prevalence and antimicrobial susceptibility of urinary tract pathogens-interim report. *J Antimicrob Chemother* 2000;46(Suppl A):15-22.

31. Gupta K, et al. Antimicrobial resistance among uropathogens that cause community-

acquired urinary tract infections in women: A nationwide analysis. *Clin Infect Dis* 2001;33:89-94.

32.   Wright SW, et al. Prevalence and risk factors for multidrug resistant uropathogens in ED patients. *Am J Emerg Med* 2000;18:143-146.

33.   Lutters M, Vogt N. Antibiotics duration for treating uncomplicated, symptomatic lower urinary tract infections in elderly women. *Cochrane Database of Systematic Rev* 2000;2.

34.   Anderson R. Management of lower urinary tract infections and cystitis. *Urol Clin North Am* 1999;26:729-735.

35.   Steele RW. The epidemiology and clinical presentation of urinary tract infections in children 2 years of age through adolescence. *Pediatr Ann* 1999;28:653-658.

36.   American Academy of Pediatrics. Practice parameter: The diagnosis, treatment, and evaluation of the initial urinary tract infection in febrile infants and young children. *Pediatrics* 1999;103:843-852.

37.   Jacobson SH, Eklof O, Eriksson CG, et al. Development of hypertension and uremia after pyelonephritis in childhood: 27 year follow up. *BMJ* 1989;299:703-706.

38.   Shaw KN, Gorelick MH. Urinary tract infection in the pediatric patient. *Pediatr Clin North Am* 1999;46:1111-1124.

39.   Wood CA, Abrutyn E. Urinary tract infection in older adults. *Clin Geriatr Med* 1998;14:267-283.

40.   Connoly AM, Thorp JM. Urinary tract infections in pregnancy. *Urol Clin North Am* 1999;26:779-787.

41.   Delzell JE, Lefevre ML. Urinary tract infection in pregnancy. *Am Fam Phys* 2000;61:713-721.

42.   Newell A, Riley P, Rogers M. Resistance patterns of urinary tract infections diagnosed in a genitourinary medicine clinic. *Int J STD AIDS* 2000;11:499-500.

43.   Baerheiy A, Digranes A, Hunskar S. Are resistance patterns published by microbiological laboratories valid for general practice? *APMIS* 1999;107:676-680.

44.   O'Donnell JA, Gelone SP. Antibacterial therapy: Fluoroquinolones. *Infect Dis Clin North Am* 2000;14:489-513,xi.

45.   Marco CA, Parker K. Antimicrobial resistance among organisms causing urinary tract infections [letter]. *Acad Emerg Med* 1997;4:159-160.

46.   Mombelli G, Pezzoli R, Pinoja-Lutz G, et al. Oral vs. intravenous ciprofloxacin in the

initial empirical management of severe pyelonephritis or complicated urinary tract infections. A prospective randomized clinical trial. *Arch Intern Med* 1999;159:53-8.

47. Flanagan PG, Davies EA, Stout RW. A comparison of single-dose vs. conventional-dose antibiotic treatment of bacteriuria in elderly women. *Age Aging* 1991;20:206-211.

48. Wiseman LR, Balfour JA. Ciprofloxacin, a review of its pharmacological profile and therapeutic use in the elderly. *Drugs & Aging* 1994;(4)(2):145-173.

49. Li-McLeod J, Cislo P, Gomolin IH. Cost analysis of ciprofloxacin oral suspension vs. trimethoprim/sulfamethoxazole oral suspension for treatment of acute urinary tract infections in elderly women. Presented at the American Society of Consultant Pharmacists Annual Meeting, Nov. 1-4, 2000; Boston, MA. Abstract #3.

50. Stapleton A, Stamm WE. Prevention of urinary tract infection. *Infect Dis Clin North Am* 1997;11:719-733.

51. Talan DA, Stamm WE, Hooton TM, et al. Comparison of ciprofloxacin (7 days) and trimethoprim-sulfamethoxazole (14 days) for acute uncomplicated pyelonephritis in women. *JAMA* 2000;283:1583-1590.

52. Blaine WB, Yu W, Summe JP. Epidemiology of hospitalization of elderly Medicare patients for urinary tract infections, 1991-1996, Abstract L-87, Presented at the 38th Interscience Conference on Antimicrobial Agents and Chemotherapy; Sept. 15-18, 1996; San Diego, CA.

53. Patton JP, Nash DB, Abrutyn E. Urinary tract infection: Economic considerations. *Med Clin North Am* 1991;75:495-513.

54. Haley RW, Culver DH, White JW. The nationwide nosocomial infection rate: A new need for vital statistics. *Am J Epidemiol* 1985;121:159-167.

55. Boscia JA, Kobasa WD, Knight RA, et al. Epidemiology of bacteriuria in an elderly population. *Am J Med* 1986;80:208-214.

56. Simon D, Trenholme G. Antibiotic selection for patients with septic shock. *Crit Care Clin* 2000;16:215-231.

57. Gupta K, Hooton TM, Wobbe CL, et al. The prevalence of antimicrobial resistance among uropathogens causing acute uncomplicated cystitis in young women. *Int J Antimicrob Agents* 1999;114:305-308.

58. Jones RN, et al. Characteristics of pathogens causing urinary tract infections in hospitals in North America: Results from the SENTRY Antimicrobial Surveillance Program, 1997. *Diagn Microbiol Infect Dis* 1999;35:55-63.

59.   Mathai D, Jones RN, Pfaller MA. Epidemiology and frequency of resistance among pathogens causing urinary tract infections in 1,510 hospitalized patients: A report from the SENTRY Antimicrobial Surveillance Program (North America). *Diagn Microbiol Infect Dis* 2001;40:129-136.

60.   Harding GK, et al. How long should catheter-acquired urinary tract infection in women be treated? A randomized controlled study. *Ann Intern Med* 1991;114:713-719.

61.   Nicolle LE, et al. Treatment of complicated urinary tract infections with lomefloxacin compared with that with trimethoprim-sulfamethoxazole. *Antimicrob Agents Chemother* 1994;38:1368-1373.

62.   Cox CE, Holloway WJ, Geckler RW. A multicenter comparative study of meropenem and imipenem/cilastatin in the treatment of complicated urinary tract infections in hospitalized patients. *Clin Infect Dis* 1995;21:86-92.

63.   Nicolle LE. A practical guide to the management of complicated urinary tract infection. *Drugs* 1997;53:583-592.

64.   Johnson JR, et al. Therapy for women hospitalized with acute pyelonephritis: A randomized trial of ampicillin versus trimethoprim-sulfamethoxazole for 14 days. *J Infect Dis* 1991;163:325-330.

65.   Talan DA, et al. Comparison of ciprofloxacin (7 days) and trimethoprim-sulfamethoxazole (14 days) for acute uncomplicated pyelonephritis pyelonephritis in women: a randomized trial. *JAMA* 2000;283:1583-1590.

66.   Nicolle LE, et al. Comparison of three days' therapy with cefcanel or amoxicillin for the treatment of acute uncomplicated urinary tract infection. *Scand J Infect Dis* 1993;25:631-637.

67.   Masterton RG, Bochsler JA. High-dosage co-amoxiclav in a single dose versus 7 days of co-trimoxazole as treatment of uncomplicated lower urinary tract infection in women. *J Antimicrob Chemother* 1995;35:129-137.

68.   Goettsch W, et al. Increasing resistance to fluoroquinolones in Escherichia coli from urinary tract infections in the netherlands. *J Antimicrob Chemother* 2000;46:223-228.

69.   Sotto A, et al. Risk factors for antibiotic-resistant Escherichia coli isolated from hospitalized patients with urinary tract infections: A prospective study. *J Clin Microbiol* 2001;39:438-444.

70.   Steinke DT, et al. Prior trimethoprim use and trimethoprim-resistant urinary tract infection: A nested case-control study with multivariate analysis for other risk factors. *J*

Antimicrob Chemother 2001;47:781-787.

71. Dyer IE, Sankary TM, Dawson JA. Antibiotic resistance in bacterial urinary tract infections, 1991 to 1997. *West J Med* 1998;169:265-268.

72. Gupta K, Stamm WE. Pathogenesis and management of recurrent urinary tract infections in women. *World J Urol* 1999;17:415-420.

73. Iqbal J, Rahman M, Kabir MS. Increasing ciprofloxacin resistance among prevalent urinary tract bacterial isolates in Bangladesh. *Jpn J Med Sci Biol* 1997;50:241-250.

74. Garcia-Rodriguez JA. Bacteriological comparison of cefixime in patients with non-complicated urinary tract infection in Spain. Preliminary results. *Chemotherapy* 1998;44(Suppl 1):28-30.

75. Gupta K, Hooton TM, Stamm WE. Increasing antimicrobial resistance and the management of uncomplicated community-acquired urinary tract infections. *Ann Intern Med* 2001;135:41-50.

76. Stamm WE. An epidemic of urinary tract infections? *N Engl J Med* 2001;345:1055-1057.

77. Hooton TM, Levy SB. Antimicrobial resistance: A plan of action for community practice. *Am Fam Physician* 2001;63:1087-1098.

78. Warren JW, et al. Guidelines for antimicrobial treatment of uncomplicated acute bacterial cystitis and acute pyelonephritis in women. Infectious Diseases Society of America (IDSA). *Clin Infect Dis* 1999;29:745-758.

79. Sahm DF, et al. Multidrug-resistant urinary tract isolates of Escherichia coli: Prevalence and patient demographics in the United States in 2000. *Antimicrob Agents Chemother* 2001;45:1402-1406.

80. Zhanel GG, et al. Antibiotic resistance in respiratory tract isolates of Haemophilus influenzae and Moraxella catarrhalis collected from across Canada in 1997-1998. *J Antimicrob Chemother* 2000;45:655-662.

81. Newell A, Riley P, Rodgers M. Resistance patterns of urinary tract infections diagnosed in a genitourinary medicine clinic. *Int J STD AIDS* 2000;11:499-500.

82. Le TP, Miller LG. Empirical therapy for uncomplicated urinary tract infections in an era of increasing antimicrobial resistance: A decision and cost analysis. *Clin Infect Dis* 2001;33:615-621.

83. Nicolle LE. Asymptomatic bacteriuria in the elderly. *Infect Dis Clin North Am* 1997;11:647-662.

84. Boscia JA, et al. Epidemiology of bacteriuria in an elderly ambulatory population. *Am J Med* 1986;80:208-214.

85. Kasviki-Charvati P, et al. Turnover of bacteriuria in old age. *Age Ageing* 1982;11:169-174.

86. Abrutyn E, et al. Epidemiology of asymptomatic bacteriuria in elderly women. *J Am Geriatr Soc* 1991;39:388-393.

87. Boscia JA, Abrutyn E, Kaye D. Asymptomatic bacteriuria in elderly persons: treat or do not treat? *Ann Intern Med* 1987;106:764-766.

88. Nicolle LE. Asymptomatic bacteriuria-important or not? *N Engl J Med* 2000;343:1037-1039.

89. Hooton TM, Scholes D, Stapleton AE, et al. A prospective study of asymptomatic bacteriuria in sexually active young women. *N Engl J Med* 2000;343:992-997.

90. Rushton HG. Urinary tract infections in children: Epidemiology, evaluation and management. *Pediatr Urol* 1997;44:1133-1167.

91. Villar J, Lydon-Rochelle MT, Gülmezoglu AM, et al. Duration of treatment for asymptomatic bacteriuria during pregnancy (Cochrane Review). In: The Cochrane Library, Issue 3, 2000. Oxford: Update Software.

92. Vazques JC, Villar J. Treatments for asymptomatic urinary tract infections during pregnancy (Cochrane Review). In: The Cochrane Library, Issue 3, 2000. Oxford: Update Software.

93. Alrajhi AA. Urinary tract infection in spinal cord injury patients. *Saudi Med J* 1999;20:24-28.

94. Tambyah PA, Maki DG. Catheter-associated urinary tract infection is rarely symptomatic: A prospective study of 1497 catheterized patients. *Arch Intern Med* 2000;160:678-682.

95. Abrutyn E, et al. Does asymptomatic bacteriuria predict mortality and does antimicrobial treatment reduce mortality in elderly ambulatory women? *Ann Intern Med* 1994;120:827-833.

96. Warren JW, et al. Fever, bacteremia, and death as complications of bacteriuria in women with long-term urethral catheters. *J Infect Dis* 1987;155:1151-1158.

97. Geerlings SE, et al. Risk factors for symptomatic urinary tract infection in women with diabetes. *Diabetes Care* 2000;23:1737-1741.

98. O'Hanley P, et al. Molecular basis of Escherichia coli colonization of the upper urinary

tract in BALB/c mice. Gal-Gal pili immunization prevents Escherichia coli pyelonephritis in the BALB/c mouse model of human pyelonephritis. *J Clin Invest* 1985;75:347-360.

99. Sobel JD. Pathogenesis of urinary tract infection. Role of host defenses. *Infect Dis Clin North Am* 1997;11:531-549.

100. Svanborg Eden C, et al. Host-parasite interaction in the urinary tract. *J Infect Dis* 1988;157:421-426.

101. Stamm WE, Hooton TM. Management of urinary tract infections in adults. *N Engl J Med* 1993;329:1328-1334.

102. Ronald A, Nicolle LE, Harding G. Single dose treatment failure in women with acute cystitis. *Infection* 1992;20(Suppl 4):S276-S279.

103. Busch R, Huland H. Correlation of symptoms and results of direct bacterial localization in patients with urinary tract infections. *J Urol* 1984;132:282-285.

104. Jones SR, Smith JW, Sanford JP. Localization of urinary-tract infections by detection of antibody-coated bacteria in urine sediment. *N Engl J Med* 1974;290:591-593.

105. Sultana RV, et al. Dipstick urinalysis and the accuracy of the clinical diagnosis of urinary tract infection. *J Emerg Med* 2001;20:13-19.

106. Jenkins RD, Fenn JP, Matsen JM. Review of urine microscopy for bacteriuria. *JAMA* 1986;255:3397-3403.

107. Bailey BL Jr. Urinalysis predictive of urine culture results. *J Fam Pract* 1995;40:45-50.

108. Komaroff AL. Urinalysis and urine culture in women with dysuria. *Ann Intern Med* 1986;104:212-218.

109. Morgan MG, McKenzie H. Controversies in the laboratory diagnosis of community-acquired urinary tract infection. *Eur J Clin Microbiol Infect Dis* 1993;12:491-504.

110. Lammers RL, et al. Comparison of test characteristics of urine dipstick and urinalysis at various test cutoff points. *Ann Emerg Med* 2001;38:505-512.

111. Stamm WE. Measurement of pyuria and its relation to bacteriuria. *Am J Med* 1983;75(1B):53-58.

112. Blum RN, Wright RA. Detection of pyuria and bacteriuria in symptomatic ambulatory women. *J Gen Intern Med* 1992;7:140-144.

113. Kusumi RK, Grover PJ, Kunin CM. Rapid detection of pyuria by leukocyte esterase activity. *JAMA* 1981;245:1653-1655.

114. Gelbart SM, Chen WT, Reid R. Clinical trial of leukocyte test strips in routine use. *Clin*

Chem 1983;29:997-999.

115. Winkens RA, et al. The validity of urine examination for urinary tract infections in daily practice. *Fam Pract* 1995;12:290-293.

116. Holloway J, Joshi N, O'Bryan T. Positive urine nitrite test: An accurate predictor of absence of pure enterococcal bacteriuria. *South Med J* 2000;93:681-682.

117. Kass EH. Asymptomatic infections of the urinary tract. *Trans Assoc Am Physicians* 1956;69:56.

118. Kass EH. Bacteriuria and the diagnosis of infections of the urinary tract. *Arch Intern Med* 1957;100:709-714.

119. Kunin CM, White LV, Hua TH. A reassessment of the importance of "low-count" bacteriuria in young women with acute urinary symptoms. *Ann Intern Med* 1993;119: 454-460.

120. Arav-Boger R, Leibovici L, Danon YL. Urinary tract infections with low and high colony counts in young women. Spontaneous remission and single-dose vs multiple-day treatment. *Arch Intern Med* 1994;154:300-304.

121. Stamm WE, et al. Diagnosis of coliform infection in acutely dysuric women. *N Engl J Med* 1982;307:463-468.

122. Fairley KF, et al. Site of infection in acute urinary-tract infection in general practice. *Lancet* 1971;7725:615-618.

123. Stamm WE, et al. Causes of the acute urethral syndrome in women. *N Engl J Med* 1980;303:409-415.

124. Lipsky BA, et al. Is the clean-catch midstream void procedure necessary for obtaining urine culture specimens from men? *Am J Med* 1984;76:257-262.

125. Lipsky BA, et al. Diagnosis of bacteriuria in men: specimen collection and culture interpretation. *J Infect Dis* 1987;155:847-854.

126. Harwood-nuss A, Etheredge W, McKenna I. Urological Emergencies. In: *Emergency Medicine Concepts and Clinical Practice.* Barkin, Ed. St. Louis: Mosby; 19982227-2261.

127. Nicolle LE, et al. Urine specimen collection with external devices for diagnosis of bacteriuria in elderly incontinent men. *J Clin Microbiol* 1988;26:1115-1119.

128. Kawashima A, Sandler CM, Goldman SM. Imaging in acute renal infection. *BJU Int* 2000;86(Suppl 1):70-79.

129. Hoddick W, et al. CT and sonography of severe renal and perirenal infections. *AJR Am J Roentgenol* 1983;140:517-520.

130. June CH, et al. Ultrasonography and computed tomography in severe urinary tract infection. *Arch Intern Med* 1985;145:841-845.

131. Henry DC, Riffer E, Haverstock DC, et al. Once-daily extended release ciprofloxacin vs. conventional twice-daily ciprofloxacin for the treatment of uncomplicated urinary tract infections. 42nd Interscience Conference on Antimicrobial Agents and Chemotherapy, Sept. 27-30, 2002; San Diego, CA. Abstract L-1800 (oral presentation, E. Riffer, Sept. 30, 2002).

132. Gomolin IH, Siami P, Haverstock D, et al. Efficacy and safety of oral ciprofloxacin suspension vs. TMP/SMX for treatment of community- and nursing home-residing elderly women with acute urinary tract infection. Presented at the 6th International Symposium on New Quinolones; Nov. 15-17, 1998; Denver, Colorado.

133. San Joaquin VH, Stull TL. Antibacterial agents in pediatrics. *Infect Dis Clin North Am* 2000;14:341-355,viii.

134. Langtry HD, Lamb HM. Levofloxacin: Its use in infections of the respiratory tract, skin, soft tissues and urinary tract. *Drugs* 1998;56:487-415.

135. Ronald A. The quinolones and renal infection. *Drugs* 1999;58(suppl 2):96-98.

136. Iravani A, Klimberg I, Briefer C, et al. A trial comparing low-dose, short-course ciprofloxacin and standard 7 day therapy with co-trimoxazole or nitrofurantoin in the treatment of uncomplicated urinary tract infection. *J Antimicrob Chemother* 1999;43 (suppl A):67-75.

137. Koyama Y, Mikami O, Matsuda T, et al. [Efficacy of single-dose therapy with levofloxacin for acute cystitis: Comparison to three day therapy.] [Japanese] *Hinyokika Kiyo* 2000;46(1):49-52.

138. Perry CM, Barman-Balfour JA, Lamb HM. Gatifloxacin. *Drugs* 1999;58:683-696.

139. Krcmery S, Naber KG. Ciprofloxacin once vs. twice daily in the treatment of complicated urinary tract infections. German Ciprofloxacin UTI Study Group. *Int J Antimicrob Agents* 1999;11:133-138.

140. Pimentel FL, Dolgner A, Guimaraes J, et al. Efficacy and safety of norfloxacin 800 mg once-daily vs. norfloxacin 400 mg twice-daily in the treatment of uncomplicated urinary tract infections in women: A double blind, randomized clinical trial. *J Chemother* 1998;10:122-127.

141. Gilstrap LC 3rd, Ramin SM. Urinary tract infections during pregnancy. *Obstet Gynecol Clin North Am* 2001;28:581-591.

142. Pitkajarvi T, et al. Pivmecillinam treatment in acute cystitis. Three versus seven days study. *Arzneimittelforschung* 1990;p40:1156-1158.

143. Spencer RC, Moseley DJ, Greensmith MJ. Nitrofurantoin modified release versus trimethoprim or co-trimoxazole in the treatment of uncomplicated urinary tract infection in general practice. *J Antimicrob Chemother* 1994;33(Suppl A):121-129.

144. Hooton TM, et al. Randomized comparative trial and cost analysis of 3-day antimicrobial regimens for treatment of acute cystitis in women. *JAMA* 1995;273:41-45.

145. Stein GE. Fosfomycin tromethamine: Single-dose treatment of acute cystitis. *Int J Fertil Womens Med* 1999;44:104-109.

146. Stein GE. Comparison of single-dose fosfomycin and a 7-day course of nitrofurantoin in female patients with uncomplicated urinary tract infection. *Clin Ther* 1999;21:1864-1872.

147. Boerema JB, Willems FT. Fosfomycin trometamol in a single dose versus norfloxacin for seven days in the treatment of uncomplicated urinary infections in general practice. *Infection* 1990;18(Suppl 2):S80-S88.

148. de Jong Z, Pontonnier F, Plante P. Single-dose fosfomycin trometamol (Monuril) versus multiple-dose norfloxacin: results of a multicenter study in females with uncomplicated lower urinary tract infections. *Urol Int* 1991;46:344-348.

149. O'Donnell JA, Gelone SP. Fluoroquinolones. *Infect Dis Clin North Am* 2000;14:489-513, xi.

150. Satlan M, Kaye D. Antibacterial therapy: Antibiotic agents in the elderly. *Infect Dis Clin North Am* 2000;14(2):

151. Safrin S, Siegel D, Black D. Pyelonephritis in adult women: Inpatient vs. outpatient therapy. *Am J Med* 1988;85:793-798.

152. Lutters M, Herrmann F, Dayer P, et al. [Antibiotic utilization in a university geriatric hospital and drug formularies]. [French] *Schweiz Med Wochenschr* 1998;128:268-271.

153. Klimberg IW, Cox CE II, Fowler CL, et al. A controlled trial of levofloxacin and lomefloxacin in the treatment of complicated urinary tract infections. *Urology* 1998;51:610-615.

154. Anonymous. A meta-analysis of studies on the safety and efficacy of aminoglycosides given either once daily or as divided doses. In: Database of Abstracts of Reviews of Effectiveness, Volume 1, 2000. NHS Center for Reviews and Dissemination.

155. Anonymous. A meta-analysis of extended-interval dosing vs. multiple daily dosing of

aminoglycosides. In: Database of Abstracts of Reviews of Effectiveness, Volume 1, 2000. NHS Center for Reviews and Dissemination.

156. Anonymous. A meta-analysis of the relative efficacy and toxicity of single daily dosing vs. multiple daily dosing of aminoglycosides. In: Database of Abstracts of Reviews of Effectiveness, Volume 1, 2000. NHS Center for Reviews and Dissemination.

157. Virk A, Steckelberg JM. Clinical aspects of antimicrobial resistance [symposium on antimicrobial agents-part XVII]. *Mayo Clin Proc* 2000;75:200-214.

158. Bosker GB. *Pharmatecture: Minimizing medications to maximize results: A systematic approach to outcome-effective drug selection.* St. Louis, Missouri: Facts and Comparisons; 1999.

159. Bailey RR, Peddie BA. Treatment of acute urinary tract infection in women. *Ann Intern Med* 1987;107:430.

160. Bailey RR. Duration of antimicrobial treatment and the use of drug combinations for the treatment of uncomplicated acute pyelonephritis. *Infection,* 1994;22(Suppl 1):S50-S52.

161. Mombelli G, Pezzoli R, Pinoja-Lutz G, et al. Oral vs intravenous ciprofloxacin in the initial empirical treatment of severe pyelonephritis or complicated urinary tract infections: A prospective randomized clinical trial. *Arch Intern Med* 1999;159:53-58.

162. Engel JD, Schaeffer AJ. Office management of urologic problems: Evaluation of and antimicrobial therapy for recurrent urinary tract infections in women. *Urol Clin North Am* 1998;25:685-701.

163. Millar LK, Wing DA, Paul RH, et al. Outpatient treatment of pyelonephritis in pregnancy: A randomized controlled trial. *Obstet Gynecol* 1995;86:560-564.

164. Wing DA, Hendershott CM, Debuque L, et al. A randomized trial of three antibiotic regimens for the treatment of pyelonephritis in pregnancy. *Obstet Gynecol* 1998;92:249-253.

165. Wing DA, Hendershott CM, Debuque L, et al. Outpatient treatment of acute pyelonephritis in pregnancy after 24 weeks. *Obstet Gynecol* 1999;94:633-638.

166. Garibaldi RA, et al. An evaluation of daily bacteriologic monitoring to identify preventable episodes of catheter-associated urinary tract infection. *Infect Control* 1982;3:466-470.

167. Warren JW. Catheter-associated urinary tract infections. *Infect Dis Clin North Am* 1987;1:823-854.

168. Warren JW, et al. A prospective microbiologic study of bacteriuria in patients with chronic indwelling urethral catheters. *J Infect Dis* 1982;146:719-723.

169. Garibaldi RA, et al. Factors predisposing to bacteriuria during indwelling urethral catheterization. *N Engl J Med* 1974;291:215-219.

170. Hustinx WN, et al. Impact of concurrent antimicrobial therapy on catheter-associated urinary tract infection. *J Hosp Infect* 1991;18:45-56.

171. Stark RP, Maki DG. Bacteriuria in the catheterized patient. What quantitative level of bacteriuria is relevant? *N Engl J Med* 1984;311:560-564.

172. Warren JW, et al. Cephalexin for susceptible bacteriuria in afebrile, long-term catheterized patients. *JAMA* 1982;248:454-458.

173. Alling B, et al. Effect of consecutive antibacterial therapy on bacteriuria in hospitalized geriatric patients. *Scand J Infect Dis* 1975;7:201-207.

174. Warren JW, Muncie HL Jr, Hall-Craggs M. Acute pyelonephritis associated with bacteriuria during long-term catheterization: A prospective clinicopathological study. *J Infect Dis* 1988;158:1341-1346.

175. Platt R, et al. Mortality associated with nosocomial urinary-tract infection. *N Engl J Med* 1982;307:637-642.

176. Reid G, Howard L. Effect on uropathogens of prophylaxis for urinary tract infection in spinal cord injured patients: preliminary study. *Spinal Cord* 1997;35:605-607.

177. Walsh JJ. Further experience with intermittent catheterisation. *Paraplegia* 1968;6:74-78.

178. Stover SL, Miller JM 3rd, Nepomuceno CS. Intermittent catheterization in patients previously on indwelling catheter drainage. *Arch Phys Med Rehabil* 1973;54:25-30.

179. Donovan WH, Kiviat MD, Clowers DE. Intermittent bladder emptying via urethral catheterization or suprapubic cystocath: A comparison study. *Arch Phys Med Rehabil* 1977;58:291-296.

180. Donovan WH, et al. Bacteriuria during intermittent catheterization following spinal cord injury. *Arch Phys Med Rehabil* 1978;59:351-357.

181. Montgomerie JZ, et al. Low mortality among patients with spinal cord injury and bacteremia. *Rev Infect Dis* 1991;13:867-871.

182. Reid G, et al. Cranberry juice consumption may reduce biofilms on uroepithelial cells:P pilot study in spinal cord injured patients. *Spinal Cord* 2001;39:26-30.

183. Sandock DS, Gothe BG, Bodner DR. Trimethoprim-sulfamethoxazole prophylaxis

against urinary tract infection in the chronic spinal cord injury patient. *Paraplegia* 1995;33:156-160.

184. The prevention and management of urinary tract infections among people with spinal cord injuries. National Institute on Disability and Rehabilitation Research Consensus Statement. Jan. 27-29, 1992. *J Am Paraplegia Soc* 1992;15:194-204.

185. Barnes RC, et al. Urinary-tract infection in sexually active homosexual men. *Lancet* 1986;1(8474):171-173.

186. Wong ES, Stamm WE. Sexual acquisition of urinary tract infection in a man. *JAMA* 1983;250:3087-3088.

187. Spach DH, Stapleton AE, Stamm WE. Lack of circumcision increases the risk of urinary tract infection in young men. *JAMA* 1992;267:679-681.

188. Krieger JN, Ross SO, Simonsen JM. Urinary tract infections in healthy university men. *J Urol* 1993;149:1046-1048.

189. Lipsky BA. Managing urinary tract infections in men. *Hosp Pract* (Off Ed). 2000;35:53-59; discussion 59-60; quiz 144.

190. Nicolle LE, et al. Bacteriuria in elderly institutionalized men. *N Engl J Med* 1983;309:1420-1425.

191. Mims AD, et al. Clinically inapparent (asymptomatic) bacteriuria in ambulatory elderly men: Epidemiological, clinical, and microbiological findings. *J Am Geriatr Soc* 1990;38:1209-1214.

192. Lipsky BA. Prostatitis and urinary tract infection in men: What's new; what's true? *Am J Med* 1999;106:327-334.

193. Gleeson MJ, Griffith DP. Struvite calculi. *Br J Urol* 1993;71:503-511.

194. Rous SN, Turner WR. Retrospective study of 95 patients with staghorn calculus disease. *J Urol* 1977;118:902-904.

195. Koga S, et al. Staghorn calculi—long-term results of management. *Br J Urol* 1991;68:122-124.

196. Manthey DE, Teichman J. Nephrolithiasis. *Emerg Med Clin North Am* 2001;19:633-654, viii.

197. Gilstrap LC, et al. Renal infection and pregnancy outcome. *Am J Obstet Gynecol* 1981;141:709-716.

198. Gilstrap LC 3rd, Cunningham FG, Whalley PJ. Acute pyelonephritis in pregnancy: An anterospective study. *Obstet Gynecol* 1981; 57:409-413.

199. Cunningham FG, Morris GB, Mickal A. Acute pyelonephritis of pregnancy: A clinical review. *Obstet Gynecol* 1973;42:112-117.

200. Tincello DG, Richmond DH. Evaluation of reagent strips in detecting asymptomatic bacteriuria in early pregnancy: Prospective case series. *BMJ* 1998;316:435-437.

201. Delzell JE Jr., Lefevre ML. Urinary tract infections during pregnancy. *Am Fam Physician* 2000;61:713-721.

202. Geerlings SE, et al. Asymptomatic bacteriuria may be considered a complication in women with diabetes. Diabetes Mellitus Women Asymptomatic Bacteriuria Utrecht Study Group. *Diabetes Care* 2000;23:744-749.

203. Wright SW, Wrenn KD, Haynes ML. Trimethoprim-sulfamethoxazole resistance among urinary coliform isolates. *J Gen Intern Med* 1999;14:606-609.

CME QUESTIONS

9. The most common uropathogen in adult patients with urinary tract infections (UTIs) is:
A. *Proteus mirabilis*
B. *E. coli*
C. *Klebsiella*
D. enterococci

10. In acute cystitis, which of the following antibiotics is now recommended as a first-line agent in most adult populations with resistance rates to TMP-SMX in excess of 10-20%?
A. TMP-SMX
B. Amoxicillin/clavulanic acid
C. Nitrofurantoin
D. Fluoroquinolone (extended release ciprofloxacin, Cipro XR®)

11. Acute urinary tract infection (UTI) results in as many as 8,000,000 office visits per year and at least 100,000 hospital admissions.
A. True
B. False

12. The majority of uncomplicated lower UTIs occur in patients who have a functional or anatomical abnormality of their urinary system.

A. True

B. False

13. The level of *E. coli* resistance to TMP-SMX has more then doubled over the past 12 years and now exceeds 25% in some areas of the country.

A. True

B. False

14. As a rule, symptomatic bacteriuria (ASB) should be treated in most patients, since multiple studies have shown that antibiotic therapy makes a significant impact on long-term outcomes in an otherwise healthy adult population.

A. True

B. False

15. The advantages of extended release (once-daily) ciprofloxacin over ciprofloxacin BID potentially include which of the following?

A. Extended release ciprofloxacin is potentially compliance-enhancing because of its once-daily dosing and a well-tolerated side effect profile.

B. The extended release delivery system delivers clinically effective urine concentrations.

C. The extended release formulation represents a risk-management upgrade as compared to BID ciprofloxacin, and should replace the older formulation as the clinical standard for treatment of uncomplicated UTI when indicated.

D. A well-designed clinical trial supports this shift to the once-daily, extended release formulation based on features cited above.

E. All of the above

For instructions on how to participate in this CME activity, please see the back of this book (page 717).

Outpatient Management of Bacterial Infections in the Respiratory Tract (OMBIRT): Diagnosis, Evaluation, and Antibiotic Selection in the Primary Care Setting

Assessment and Therapeutic Strategies for Evaluating and Managing Outpatients with Community-Acquired Pneumonia (CAP) and Acute Bacterial Exacerbations of Chronic Obstructive Pulmonary Disease (ABE/COPD)

INTRODUCTION

Antibiotic guidelines for treatment of community-acquired pneumonia (CAP) and acute bacterial exacerbations of chronic obstructive pulmonary disease (ABE/COPD) vary from institution to institution, and depending upon antimicrobial resistance patterns, such protocols also may vary from region to region. The variability among antimicrobial strategies is exemplified by the somewhat different approaches advocated by national associations, infectious disease experts, and published reviews in the medical literature. As a general rule, however, outcome-effective antibiotic selection, which is the subject of this consensus review, means taking into account local antibiotic resistance patterns, epidemiological and infection incidence data, and patient demographic features; then, against the background of clinical judgment, it also means determining the most appropriate agent for an individual patient.

To address these complex issues, the OMBIRT (Outpatient Management of Bacterial Infections in the Respiratory Tract) Consensus Panel and Scientific Roundtable met in August 2001 to review, analyze, and interpret published, evidence-based trials assessing the safety and efficacy of antibiotic therapy for managing ABE/COPD and CAP. In addition, the OMBIRT Panel was charged with developing strategies that would ensure appropriate use of antibiotics in this patient population, and with making recommendations for how patients with respiratory infections should be evaluated in the outpatient setting.

Treatment guidelines generated by the OMBIRT Panel were based on evidence presented from well-designed clinical trials, and focused on out-of-hospital management by the primary care practitioner. An update of the Panel's recommendations has been prompted by recent introduction of drug dosing and duration of therapy regimens that are likely to promote even greater patient compliance and acceptability, in particular, approval of a three-day course of azithromycin (500 mg PO once-daily x 3 days) to treat acute exacerbations of COPD precipitated by *Streptococcus pneumoniae, Haemophilus influenzae,* and *Moraxella catarrhalis.* In addition to new drug formulations, the panel conducted a detailed analysis of national consensus guidelines issued by the American Thoracic Society (ATS), Infectious Disease Society of America (IDSA), CDC Drug-Resistant Streptococococcus pneumonaie Working Group (CDCDRSP-WG), and the Antibiotic Selection in Community-Acquired Pneumonia (ASCAP) Panel to identify advances in the decision-making process for outpatient management of respiratory tract infections.

With these objectives in clear focus, the purpose of this comprehensive review, which includes the OMBIRT Panel guidelines, assessment strategies, and treatment recommendations, is to provide a state-of-the-art clinical resource outlining, in precise and practical detail, clinical protocols for acute management of CAP and ABE/COPD. To achieve this goal, all of the critical aspects entering into the equation for maximizing outcomes while minimizing costs, including systematic patient evaluation, disposition decision trees, and outcome-effective antibiotic therapy, will be discussed in detail. In addition, because appropriate disposition of patients with CAP and ABE/COPD has become essential for cost-effective patient management, this review includes critical pathways and treatment tables that incorporate risk stratification protocols and intensification-of-treatment trigger (IOTT) criteria that can be used to identify those patient subgroups that are suitably managed in the outpatient setting and those more appropriately admitted to the hospital for more intensive care.

OVERVIEW

Evaluating advantages and disadvantages among recommendations and protocols issued by different authoritative sources can be problematic and confusing, to say the least. And although management guidelines for CAP must be "customized" for the local practice environment and for the individual patient, there appears to be a consensus regarding one aspect of CAP management: the outpatient with CAP generally requires treatment with an antibiotic that provides adequate coverage against *S. pneumoniae, H. influenzae, M. catarrhalis, Mycoplasma pneumoniae, Chlamydia pneumoniae,* and *Legionella pneumophila*. In contrast, the uncomplicated outpatient with ABE/COPD typically requires coverage against *S. pneumoniae, H. influenzae*, and *M. catarrhalis*. In both conditions, antibiotics that provide activity against these organisms may be considered "correct spectrum" coverage. Accordingly, those agents—most important among them, advanced generation macrolides and advanced generation fluoroquinolones—that provide this range of coverage within the framework of monotherapy, represent appropriate, initial choices for these conditions.

Unfortunately, no single set of guidelines or critical pathways is applicable to every patient or practice environment; therefore, clinical judgment must take in account other factors that suggest the need for "intensifying" therapy with antibiotics whose spectrum extends beyond the six aforementioned organisms and includes other gram-negative species. In this regard, when patients with CAP present with risk factors or historical features that strongly suggest the likelihood of infection with such gram-negative organisms as *Klebsiella pneumoniae* (chronic alcoholism) or *Escherichia coli* (infection acquired in a nursing home), it is appropriate to use an agent (an advanced generation fluoroquinolone) providing this spectrum of coverage. However, a cautionary note is in order. When, in the setting of CAP, the probability of gram-negative infection with *E. coli, Pseudomonas* species, or other enterobacteria is relatively low, using an extended spectrum quinolone as initial therapy may represent "over-extended" coverage, in the sense that resistance pressure may be exerted against organisms not typically implicated in such infections, among them *E. coli, Pseudomonas,* and other enterobacteria.

Identifying treatment trigger points and historical features that support amplifying spectrum of coverage from a "correct spectrum" macrolide to an "extended spectrum" fluoroquinolone are essential for outcome-effective antibiotic use. As a rule, clinical results in ABE/COPD and CAP can be optimized by using risk-stratification criteria. Such clinical findings as hypotension, tachypnea, impaired oxygen saturation, multi-lobar involvement, elevated blood urea nitrogen, and altered level of consciousness are predictive of more serious disease in CAP, as is acquisition of CAP in a nursing home environment. These patients generally will need to be treated as inpatients.

With these antibiotic selection issues in clear focus, the OMBIRT Panel will review current strategies for evaluating and managing oupatients with bacterial infection of the respiratory tract and present a set of consensus guidelines outlining antibiotic selection for these patients.

ACUTE BACTERIAL EXACERBATIONS OF CHRONIC OBSTRUCTIVE PULMONARY DISEASE (ABE/COPD)— GENERAL PRINCIPLES

Acute bacterial exacerbations of chronic obstructive pulmonary disease (ABE/COPD) are common, costly, and above all, complex to manage. In fact, few conditions produce such a broad range of outcomes, require such customized approaches, or present so many options for treatment.[1,2]

Although there have been important advances in patient assessment techniques and therapeutics, including pulmonary function testing, capnometry, pulse oximetry, disposition support tools, and antimicrobial therapy, ABE/COPD continues to be a leading cause of morbidity and mortality in the United States.[2] From patient disposition to antimicrobial selection, optimizing management of these patients requires the clinician to integrate a number of clinical, laboratory, radiologic, and etiologic factors, and then initiate a course of action that accounts for all the risks, costs, and benefits of an individualized treatment plan.

Despite a number of guidelines and the availability of new, targeted spectrum antibiotics, the management of ABE/COPD in the outpatient setting remains extremely challenging. More than ever, it requires a multifactorial analysis of myriad clinical, historical, and laboratory parameters that predict success or possible failure for each individual case. In this regard, clinical decision-making in ABE/COPD can be problematic for the primary care physician.

Achieving optimal patient outcomes for this common and debilitating condition requires the primary care physician to consider several features of each individual case. (*Please see Table 1.*) Factors that must be considered include the patient's age, response to medical therapy, overall pulmonary function, character and severity of previous exacerbations, bacterial colonization status of the patient, previous requirements for mechanical ventilation, and local antimicrobial resistance patterns. With this in mind, a Severity-of-Exacerbation and Risk Factor (SERF) pathway can be employed to help guide patient disposition, empiric antibiotic selection, and necessity for additional diagnostic investigation. (*Please see Table 2.*)

The antibiotic selection process for ABE/COPD in the office-based setting offers multiple options. Currently, the pathogens most often responsible for causing "uncomplicated and typical" cases of ABE/COPD that can be treated in the outpatient environment include the bacterial organisms, *S. pneumoniae, H. influenzae,* and *M. catarrhalis.* Because it may be difficult, if not impossible, to identify a specific pathogen at the time of initial patient assessment, empiric antimicrobial coverage against all expected pathogens usually is necessary to minimize treatment failures. Patients with advanced disease and multiple risk factors may have exacerbations caused by *Klebsiella* species, *Pseudomonas aeruginosa,* and other gram-negative species. As will be discussed below, these patients may require intensification of therapy with agents that are active against gram-negative organisms.

In this vein, the development of advanced generation macrolides (e.g., azithromycin), as well as extended spectrum quinolones, has made it possible to treat most patients using monotherapy. Finally, because there is a growing

Table 1. Factors Influencing Patient Disposition in ABE/COPD

- Age of patient
- Overall respiratory status
- Respiratory rate
- O_2 saturation
- Degree of hypercarbia
- Patient's status compared to baseline
- Mental status
- Home environment
- Likelihood of acceptable medication compliance
- Nighttime emergency department visit
- Previous pattern of frequent relapse
- Pulmonary function tests
- FEV_1 less than 40% of predicted normal
- Multiple ED courses of aerosolized beta-agonists

incidence of resistance among common bacterial agents that cause CAP (in some areas of the United States, intermediate-to-complete resistance to penicillin among *S. pneumoniae* is reported to be greater than 25%), antibiotic selection must be guided by local and/or regional resistance patterns.

ACUTE BACTERIAL EXACERBATIONS OF COPD— OMBIRT PANEL OVERVIEW AND RECOMMENDATIONS

Although certain recommendations can be made regarding management of patients with ABE/COPD, the OMBIRT Panel noted that the number, quality, and design of studies evaluating and comparing effectiveness of and indications for antibiotic therapy are less than optimal, and in general, inferior to those available for CAP. In addition, upon review of multiple studies comparing advanced generation macrolides (azithromycin or clar-

Table 2. The SERF Risk-Stratification Pathway for Antibiotic Selection in ABE/COPD

SEVERITY OF EXACERBATION AND RISK FACTOR (SERF) SUPPORT TOOL

RATIONALE

The need for intensification and amplification of antimicrobial coverage in patients with acute exacerbations of chronic obstructive pulmonary disease (ABE/COPD) depends on:

- Likelihood of infection with gram-negative enterobacteria
- Colonization status
- Patient's history of exacerbations and antimicrobial treatment response record
- Ability of patient to tolerate a treatment failure given his or her respiratory status
- Other factors requiring sound clinical judgment.

THE SERF PATHWAY

- Based on evidence-based trials and consensus opinion
- Designed as a clinical decision support tool to help guide empiric antibiotic therapy for outpatients with ABE/COPD.

Final decisions regarding drug selection should be made by the clinician on a patient-by-patient basis using on a comprehensive database including history, physical examination, and other diagnostic information.

ithromycin) and advanced generation fluoroquinolones, no significant differences in clinical outcomes could be observed in outpatients managed with these antibiotic regimens.

The tendency to overuse antibiotics in patients with ABE/COPD should be recognized by primary care practitioners, and only patients meeting clinical criteria for antibiotic therapy should receive antibiotics for their exacerbations. The OMBIRT Panel recommendations for outpatient management of ABE/COPD are summarized in this section, and supportive evidence, analysis of clinical trials, and adjunctive approaches to managing ABE/COPD are discussed in subequent sections.

Appropriate Use of Antibiotics. As a rule, the clinical criteria for initiating antibiotic therapy in patients with a documented history of COPD, and who are suspected of having ABE/COPD, include the presence of at least two of the following three symptoms: increasing purulence of sputum, increasing volume of sputum production, and increasing cough and/or dyspnea. In contrast, patients with symptoms of acute tracheobronchitis who have no previous history of COPD initially should not be treated with antibiotics, since antibiotics have not been shown to improve outcomes in this patient population.

However, it was recognized by the panel that in real world practice a significant percentage of patients fall into a clinical gray zone. In particular, those outpatients with persistent (i.e., > 10-14 days) symptoms of acute tracheobronchitis, and who have no previous history of COPD may be considered appropriate candidates for antibiotic therapy, especially if clinical assessment suggests that persistent symptoms may be due to infection with such atypical organisms as *C. pneumoniae* or *M. pneumoniae*.

Appropriate use of antibiotics in ABE/COPD requires clinical confirmation of the diagnosis, which is usually made on the basis of symptom exacerbation and clinical history. As a rule, chest x-ray is not recommended or encouraged for typical cases of ABE/COPD, but should be considered in patients who present with an atypical presentation and in whom CAP is suspected.

Appropriate antibiotic use and selection is designed to accomplish the following: 1) return patient's respiratory status (FEV_1, oxygenation, respiratory rate, symptoms, etc.) back to baseline; 2) reduce the number and frequency of exacerbations; and 3) prevent hospitalization. The principal respiratory tract pathogens that must be covered on an empiric basis in individuals with moderate-to-severe ABE/COPD in the outpatient setting include S. *pneumoniae, H. influenzae, M. catarrhalis, Haemophilus parainfluenzae,* and *Staphylococcus aureus*. Some patients, especially those with severe disease, a recent history of mechanical ventilation and hospitalization, and/or high-dose chronic steroid therapy are more susceptible to infection with *Pseudomonas* species.

Treatment. The majority of double-blinded, prospective clinical trials comparing new generation macrolides (azithromycin and clarithromycin) vs. new generation fluoroquinolones (moxifloxacin, gatifloxacin, and levofloxacin) demonstrate comparable outcomes in terms of clinical cure and bacteriologic eradication rates at days 7, 14, and 28 in outpatients with either moderate or severe ABE/COPD. Emergence of resistance among *S. pneumoniae* to new generation fluoroquinolones has been reported in a number of geographic regions, including the United States, Hong Kong, and Canada. Given the emergence of such strains and the presence of numerous studies demonstrating comparable effectiveness between macrolides and advanced generation fluoroquinolones, the OMBIRT Panel supports cautious, restrictive use of fluoroquinolones for appropriately selected patients with ABE/COPD, and recommends the advanced generation macrolide, azithromyzin, as the initial agent of choice for managing appropriately risk-stratified outpatients with ABE/COPD. (*Please see Table* 3.)

The frequency of drug-resistant *S. pneumoniae* (DRSP) causing ABE/COPD is not known, but is presumed to be less than or equal to the incidence of DRSP causing outpatient CAP. There currently is no evidence to support initial outpatient therapy directed at DRSP for patients with ABE/COPD. As it does in the management of CAP, the panel cautions against overuse of new generation fluoroquinolones as initial agents in outpatients with ABE/COPD, and recommends their use as alternative agents when: 1) first-line therapy with advanced generation macrolides such as azithromycin fails; 2) patients are allergic to first-line agents; or 3) patients have documented or suspected infection with gram-negative organisms.

Given concerns about antibiotic overuse, the potential for emerging resistance among DRSP to fluoroquinolones, the panel concurs with other guideline panels specifying advanced generation macrolides as initial therapy for outpatient ABE/COPD and use of fluoroquinolones as alternative agents in patients who fail therapy or who have risk factors predictive of gram-negative infection. Patients who do not respond to oral therapy with one class of antibiotics (relapse) may be treated with a course of antibiotics with different gaps in coverage. Reinfections should be treated with antibiotics that have been shown to be effective in previous exacerbations.

Table 3. OMBIRT Consensus Panel Antiboitic Treatment*† Recommendations for ABE/COPD

SERF** CATEGORY A

CONDITION • SEVERITY • SUSPECTED PATHOGENS

Acute Bacterial Exacerbation of COPD (ABE/COPD)

Mild severity based on SERF (severity of exacerbation and risk factors) pathway and IOTT (intensity of treatment triggers) criteria

— Suspected pathogens: *Streptococcus pneumoniae, Haemophilus influenzae, Moraxella catarrhalis*

Initial (preferred agent, any class) first-line therapy: Azithromycin 500 mg PO qd x 3 days

Alternative first-line agents (macrolides): Clarithromycin 500 mg PO qd x 7 days

Alternative first-line agents (fluoroquinolones): Moxifloxacin (preferred) 400 mg PO qd x 5 days; Gatifloxacin 400 mg PO qd x 7 days; Levofloxacin 500 mg PO qd x 7 days

Alternative first-line agents (other classes, including generic formulations): Amoxicillin-clavulanate 875 mg PO q 12 hours x 10 days; Doxycycline 100 mg PO bid x 7-14 days; Trimethoprim-sulfamethoxazole 1 DS tablet PO bid x 7-14 days

SERF CATEGORY B

CONDITION • SEVERITY • SUSPECTED PATHOGENS

Moderate-to-severe bacterial exacerbation of COPD (ABE/COPD)

Severity based on SERF pathway and IOTT criteria

— Suspected pathogens: *Streptococcus pneumoniae, Haemophilus influenzae, Moraxella catarrhalis*

Initial (preferred agent, any class) first-line therapy: Azithromycin 500 mg PO qd x 3 days

Alternative first-line agents (macrolides): Clarithromycin 500 mg PO qd x 7 days

Alternative first-line agents (fluoroquinolones): Moxifloxacin (preferred) 400 mg PO qd x 5 days; Gatifloxacin 400 mg PO qd x 7 days; Levofloxacin 500 mg PO qd x 7 days

Alternative first-line agents (other classes): Amoxicillin-clavulanate 875 mg PO q 12 hours x 10 days

† OMBIRT Panel recommendations and preferences are based on a critical analysis and evaluation of published clinical trials, FDA indications, association guidelines, and pharmatectural criteria including cost, spectrum of coverage, compliance parameters (daily dose frequency, duration of therapy, and side effects), pregnancy category, and risk of drug-drug and/or drug-disease interactions.

** SERF - Severity of Exacerbation and Risk Factor clinical assessment strategy.

SERF CATEGORY C

CONDITION • SEVERITY • SUSPECTED PATHOGENS

Severe and/or frequently recurrent (ABE/COPD)

Severity based on SERF pathway and IOTT criteria

— Associated risk factors and historical features: Recent hospitalization for ABE/COPD and documented infection with gram-negative organisms such as: *Klebsiella, Pseudomonas,* and other enterobacteria; patients with structural lung disease (bronchiectasis); or patients who have failed first-line macrolide therapy.

— Suspected pathogens: *Streptococcus pneumoniae, Haemophilus influenzae,* and *Moraxella catarrhalis,* in addition to possible infection with gram-negative organisms known to cause exacerbations in patients who are risk-stratified to a more severe category (see above)

Initial (preferred agent, any class) first-line therapy: Moxifloxacin (preferred) 400 mg PO qd x 5 days; Gatifloxacin 400 mg PO qd x 7 days; Levofloxacin 500 mg PO qd x 7 days

Alternative first-line agents (fluoroquinolones): Ciprofloxacin 500 mg PO bid x 10 days (Although effective in clinical trials and recommended for acute, documented gram-negative exacerbations of COPD, ciprofloxacin is not the agent of choice when ABE/COPD is thought to be secondary to *S. pneumoniae* infection)

Alternative agents (other classes): Amoxicillin-clavulanate 875 mg PO q 12 hours x 10 days

* Approved indications for recommended antimicrobial agents:

Azithromycin: Indicated for acute bacterial exacerbations of COPD caused by susceptible species of *Streptococcus pneumoniae, Moraxella catarrhalis,* and *Haemophilus influenzae.*

Clarithromycin: Indicated for acute bacterial exacerbations of COPD caused by susceptible species of *Streptococcus pneumoniae, Moraxella catarrhalis, Haemophilus influenzae,* and *Haemophilus parainfluenzae.*

Moxifloxacin: Indicated for acute bacterial exacerbations of COPD caused by susceptible species of *Streptococcus pneumoniae, Moraxella catarrhalis, Haemophilus influenzae, Staphylococcus aureus, Klebsiella pneumoniae,* and *Haemophilus parainfluenzae.*

Gatifloxacin: Indicated for acute bacterial exacerbations of COPD caused by susceptible species of *Streptococcus pneumoniae, Moraxella catarrhalis, Haemophilus influenzae, Staphylococcus aureus,* and *Haemophilus parainfluenzae.*

Levofloxacin: Indicated for acute bacterial exacerbations of COPD caused by susceptible species of *Streptococcus pneumoniae, Moraxella catarrhalis, Haemophilus influenzae, Staphylococcus aureus,* and *Haemophilus parainfluenzae.*

Unfortunately, limited data exist to guide physicians in the cost-effective treatment of acute exacerbation of chronic bronchitis (ABE/COPD). One important study, however, attempted to determine the antimicrobial efficacy of various agents and compared total outcome costs for patients with ABE/COPD. For the purpose of this analysis, a retrospective review was performed of 60 outpatient medical records of individuals with a diagnosis of COPD associated with acute episodes seen in the pulmonary clinic of a teaching institution. Empirical antibiotic choices were divided into first-line (amoxicillin, co-trimoxazole, tetracyclines, erythromycin); second-line (cephradine, cefuroxime, cefaclor, cefprozil); and third-line (azithromycin, amoxicillin-clavulanate, ciprofloxacin) agents.

In this study, patients receiving first-line agents (amoxicillin, co-trimoxazole, tetracyclines, erythromycin) failed significantly more frequently (19% vs 7%; $p < 0.05$) than those treated with third-line agents (azithromycin, amoxicillin-clavulanate, ciprofloxacin). Moreover, patients prescribed first-line agents were hospitalized significantly more often for ABE/COPD within two weeks of outpatient treatment as compared with patients prescribed third-line agents (18.0% vs 5.3% for third-line agents; $p < 0.02$). Time between subsequent ABE/COPD episodes requiring treatment was significantly longer for patients receiving third-line agents compared with first-line and second-line agents ($p < 0.005$).

Two advanced generation macrolides—azithromycin and clarithromycin—are available for treating ABE/COPD. Based on outcome-sensitive criteria and pharmatectural considerations such as cost, daily dose frequency, duration of therapy, side effects, and drug interactions, the OMBIRT Panel recommends azithromycin as first-line, preferred initial therapy in moderate-to-severe, non-hospitalized patients, with clarithromycin or doxycycline as an alternative agent; and, as second-line therapy, moxifloxacin, gatifloxacin, or levofloxacin. Amoxillin-clavulanate is another alternative agent. When historical or clinical factors in the SERF (Severity of Exacerbation and Risk Factor) pathway suggest the presence of gram-negative infection, a new generation fluoroquinolone would be considered the agent of choice. Physicians are urged to prescribe antibiotics in ABE/COPD at the time of diagnosis and to encourage patients to fill and begin taking their prescriptions on the day of diagnosis.

Primary care physicians are discouraged from using antibiotics for "chronic prophylaxis" against ABE/COPD, since studies do not support the efficacy of this strategy for preventing acute exacerbations. Patients should be instructed about issues related to the importance of medication compliance, and in the case of short (5-day) courses of therapy, they should be educated that although they are only consuming medications for a five-day period, such antibiotics as azithromycin remain at the tissue site of infection for about nine days and continue to deliver therapeutic effects during that period.

Either verbal or on-site, re-evaluation of patients is recommended within a three-day period following diagnosis and initiation of antibiotic therapy. Follow-up in the office or clinic within three days is recommended in certain risk-stratified patients, especially the elderly, those with co-morbid illness, signifcantly impaired FEV_1, and those in whom medication compliance may be compromised.[3] More urgent follow-up may be required in patients with increasing symptoms, including dyspnea, fever, and other systemic signs or symptoms. Follow-up chest x-rays generally are not recommended in patients with outpatient ABE/COPD, except in certain high-risk groups.

ANTIBIOTIC THERAPY FOR ABE/COPD: THE SERF (SEVERITY OF EXACERBATION AND RISK FACTOR) PATHWAY FOR OUTCOME-EFFECTIVE DRUG SELECTION

Patients in whom exacerbation of COPD is associated with acute respiratory infection are at high risk for relapse unless treated.[3] Patients with acute bronchitis that is unrelated to COPD probably do not benefit from antibiotic therapy. It should be noted, however, that for patients with COPD, antibiotics appear to have a role in the treatment of exacerbations caused by bacterial bronchitis (i.e., ABE/COPD). The outpatient with an increase in sputum quantity and/or a change in character or color, especially if accompanied by increasing cough and dyspnea, should be treated with a course of outpatient antibiotics.

It should be stressed that many patients with COPD have colonization of their tracheal tract with *S. pneumoniae, H. influenzae,* or *M. catarrhalis*.[4] Other organisms, such as *Klebsiella* species, *M. pneumoniae, Pseudomonas, S. aureus, Proteus* species, or *Chlamydia* TWAR also may be seen. Unfortunately, making an etiologic bacteria-specific diagnosis in ABE/COPD usually is not possible. Consequently, most patients will require empiric therapy directed at the most likely etiologic organisms.

Although a number of clinical decision support tools, consensus guidelines, and recommendations have been issued, none has universal support. In large part, this is because the etiologic agents responsible for ABE/COPD, the outcome-effectiveness of various antibiotics, and risk-stratification parameters are not as thoroughly elaborated as they are for CAP. Consequently, several authors have argued that there is an immediate need for guidelines on antibiotic use in COPD. The OMBIRT Panel has reviewed published trials and generated a set of guidelines based on evidence-based trials. Several attempts to formulate such protocols have resulted in broadly similar recommendations. Although the guidelines inevitably have been hampered by the lack of well-designed prospective studies, they have taken a practical approach that seems to be logical and can be used in the primary care setting. It must be emphasized, however, that the concepts on which the guidelines are based have not yet been verified by prospective clinical trials.[5-7]

Antibiotics. A number of relatively inexpensive, well-tolerated antibiotics are available, including amoxicillin, trimethoprim-sulfamethoxazole, doxycycline, and tetracycline. Antimicrobial resistance, particularly involving *H. influenzae, M. catarrhalis,* and *S. pneumoniae,* has become an increasing problem with many of these agents, specifically with older members of each of these drug classes. There is an increase in amoxicillin-resistant, beta-lactamase-producing *H. influenzae.* New agents are providing solutions to these difficulties. The azalide antibiotic azithromycin has the advantage of an appropriate spectrum of coverage, an acceptable safety profile, reasonable cost, and a patient-dosing schedule that improves patient compliance.

The newer fluoroquinolones, moxifloxacin, gatifloxacin, and levofloxacin, are advantageous when gram-negative bacteria predominate;

ciprofloxacin is an excellent choice in this subgroup, especially for those with structural lung disease such as bronchiectasis and documented infection with gram-negative species (e.g., *Pseudomonas* species). Amoxicillin-clavulanate also has in vitro activity against beta-lactamase-producing *H. influenzae* and *M. catarrhalis*, as well as *S. pneumoniae*; moreover, the agent's clinical efficacy in lower respiratory tract infection attributable to enzyme-producing strains has been demonstrated.

Severity of Exacerbation and Risk Factors Pathway. The Severity of Exacerbation and Risk Factors (SERF) pathway for antibiotic selection in outpatients with ABE/COPD is a clinical decision, consensus-driven support tool based on epidemiology, efficacy, and prognostic data generated by many published clinical trials.[5,23] In general, the need for intensification and amplification of antimicrobial coverage in patients with acute exacerbations of chronic obstructive pulmonary disease (ABE/COPD) depends on the likelihood of infection with gram-negative enterobacteria, colonization status, the patient's history of exacerbations and antimicrobial treatment response record, the patient's ability to tolerate a treatment failure given his or her respiratory status, and other factors.

The SERF Pathway (*please see Table 2*), which is based on evidence-based trials and consensus opinion, is designed as a clinical support tool to help guide empiric antibiotic therapy for outpatients with ABE/COPD. Final decisions regarding drug selection should be made by the clinician on a patient-by-patient basis using a comprehensive database including history, physical examination, and other diagnostic information. Specifically, the SERF pathway identifies a number of IOTT criteria that have been generated from consensus reports, reviews, and prospective trials in ABE/COPD. These factors should be considered when selecting an antibiotic for empiric outpatient treatment of ABE/COPD. The OMBIRT Panel notes there is ample support in the medical literature for using clinical parameters identified in the SERF pathway and using IOTT criteria. (*Please see Tables 2 and 4.*)

Approximately one-half of all exacerbations of COPD can be attributed to bacterial infection, and antibiotic therapy has been demonstrated to improve clinical outcomes and accelerate clinical and physiologic recovery. The major pathogen continues to be *H. influenzae,* and resistance to beta-lactam antibiotics such as ampicillin can be expected in 20-40% of isolated strains.[24] Certain high-risk patients, in whom the cost of clinical treatment failure is high, can be identified by simple clinical criteria.

Studies suggest, for example, that patients with significant cardiopulmonary comorbidity, frequent purulent exacerbations of COPD, advanced age, generalized debility, malnutrition, chronic corticosteroid administration, long duration of COPD, and severe underlying lung function may be more likely to fail therapy with older drugs, such as ampicillin, and that early relapse can be expected.[24] Treatment directed toward resistant pathogens using appropriate agents may be expected to lead to improved clinical outcomes and overall lower costs, particularly if hospital admissions and respiratory failure can be prevented. Future studies examining the role of antibiotics should enroll these high-risk patients to determine if new therapies have significant clinical, quality-of-life, and economic advantages over older agents.[24]

Other authors have proposed different classification schemes. There is general agreement that acute exacerbations of chronic bronchitis (AECB) can be defined as the presence of increases in cough/sputum, sputum purulence, and dyspnea. However, recent investigations suggest that the severity of AECB also may be divided into three stages based on the history of the patient: 1) previously healthy individuals; 2) patients with chronic cough and sputum and infrequent exacerbations; and 3) persons with frequent exacerbations or more severe chronic airflow limitation.

Comparative Trials of Antibiotic Efficacy in Acute Bacterial Exacerbations of COPD. The goals of therapy for ABE/COPD are to resolve the infection expeditiously, maintain an infection-free interval for as long as possible, and select an antibiotic with the fewest adverse effects and most favorable compliance profile. Because patients with COPD frequently are on complicated, multi-modal drug therapy (consumption of many medications with a complicated dosing schedule is not uncommon), identifying effective, compliance-enhancing regimens for ABE/COPD is an important clinical objective. (*Please see Table 5.*) Moreover, because the key meta-analysis study supporting the efficacy of antibiotics in ABE/COPD was based on older trials

Table 4. SERF Pathway: Intensification of Treatment Trigger (IOTT) Criteria for Risk-Stratification in ABE/COPD

INTENSIFICATION-OF-TREATMENT TRIGGER (IOTT) CRITERIA SHOULD BE CONSIDERED WHEN SELECTING AN ANTIBIOTIC FOR EMPIRIC OUTPATIENT TREATMENT OF ABE/COPD.

WHEN IOTT CRITERIA ARE PRESENT, CLINICIANS SHOULD CONSIDER NEWER AGENTS WITH EVIDENCE-BASED SUPPORT AS INDICATED AND RECOGNIZE POSSIBLE LIMITATIONS OF OLDER AGENTS SUCH AS SULFONAMIDES, PENICILLINS, AND TETRACYCLINES

IOTT criteria include the following:

- History of multiple bacterial exacerbations of COPD within a short time period (more than 3 exacerbations in < 4 months)

- Multiple antimicrobial treatment exposures

- Documentation of gram-negative (enterobacteria, pseudomonas, Klebsiella, etc.) respiratory tract colonization

- History of requiring mechanical ventilation after treatment failure of ABE/COPD

- History of gram-negative nosocomial lower respiratory tract infection

- Chronic, systemic corticosteroid use

- Multiple emergency department visits with relapse within a 10-day period

- Supplemental home oxygen

- Smoking

- High prevalence (documented) S. pneumoniae resistance to penicillin

- Chronic alcoholism associated with history of gram-negative (Klebsiella) lower respiratory tract infection

- Serious co-morbidity (immunosuppression, HIV, underlying malignancy, etc.)

with "older" agents, it is important that practitioners are aware of more recent studies evaluating effectiveness of newer antibiotics for this condition.

One randomized, multicenter, investigator-blinded, parallel-group study compared a five-day, once-daily course of azithromycin (two 250 mg capsules on day 1, followed by one 250 mg capsule on days 2-5) with a 10-day, three-times-daily course of amoxicillin-clavulanate (one 500 mg tablet tid) in 70 patients with ABE/COPD.[23] At the end of therapy, all 29 (100%) efficacy-assessable patients treated with azithromycin were cured or improved, compared with 25 (93%) of 27 assessable patients given amoxicillin-clavulanate (p = NS). Bacteriologic eradication rates were 86% (25 of 29 isolates) with azithromycin and 87% (20 of 23 isolates) with the comparative agent. Azithromycin was well tolerated; adverse events considered related or possibly related to treatment were reported in 28% of azithromycin recipients, compared with 39% of amoxicillin-clavulanate recipients (p = NS). The authors concluded that the five-day, once-daily regimen of azithromycin is comparable to a standard agent in the treatment of patients with ABE/COPD.[23]

The results of this study indicated that the administration of azithromycin once daily for five days is comparable to amoxicillin-clavulanate in the treatment of patients with ABE/COPD. The dosing schedule of azithromycin described in this trial is among the the shortest and simplest regimens among commonly prescribed oral antibiotics for ABE/COPD.[23] Because reduced frequency of dosing and shorter therapy duration may improve patient compliance, and potentially outcomes, practitioners should be aware of differences among effective agents as they relate to these compliance-sensitive parameters.

The safety and efficacy of macrolides vs. fluoroquinolones have been compared in clinical trials; all of them demonstrated, in a rather consistent manner, comparable clinical outcomes in patients with ABE/COPD.[49,50] In one study, 986 patients were randomized to receive either moxifloxacin 400 mg PO qd for either 5 or 10 days, or clarithromycin 500 mg PO bid for 10 days.[49] The main outcome measures were bacteriologic response rate at the end of therapy (post-therapy, days 0-6) and at follow-up (post-therapy, days 7-17), as well as overall clinical response. Two patient populations were analyzed: efficacy-

Table 5. Multi-Modal Pharmacotherapy for ABE/COPD: Checklist of Agents Requiring Consideration

- Beta-agonists (selective agents preferred)
- Anticholinergic drug
- Home oxygen
- Systemic corticosteroids
- Inhaled corticosteroids
- Antibiotics (advanced generation macrolides and quinolones preferred)
- Theophylline (efficacy is controversial)

valid (i.e., those with a pretherapy pathogen) and intent-to-treat (all subjects who took a drug).

In 420 efficacy valid patients, overall clinical resolution was 89% for five days of moxifloxacin vs. 91% for 10 days of moxifloxacin, vs. 91% for 10 days of clarithromycin. Bacteriologic eradication rates at the end of therapy were 94% and 95% for five-day moxifloxacin and 10-day moxiflloxacin, respectively, and 91% for the clarithromycin group. Overall, moxifloxacin 400 mg once daily was found to be clinically and bacteriologically equivalent to a 10-day course of clarithromycin for treatment of ABE/COPD.[49]

A safety and efficacy study comparing moxifloxacin, an oral advanced generation fluoroquinolone, with azithromycin was conducted between October 1998 and April 1999. In all, 576 patients with ABE/COPD were enrolled in 37 centers across the United States and Canada; 280 (49%) of those enrolled had acute bacterial exacerbations of chronic bronchitis (i.e., pretherapy pathogen). Patients were randomized to receive either moxifloxacin 400 mg administered once daily for five days or azithromycin for five days (500 mg qd x 1, then 250 qd x 4). For the purposes of study blinding, all patients received encapsulated tablets.[25]

The main outcome measure was clinical response at the test-of-cure visit (14-21 days post-therapy). Three patient populations were analyzed for efficacy: clinically-valid, microbiologically-valid (i.e., those with a pretherapy pathogen), and intent-to-treat (i.e., received at least 1 dose of the study drug).

For the efficacy-valid group, clinical response at the test-of-cure was 88% for patients in each treatment group. In 237 microbiologically-valid patients, corresponding clinical resolution rates were 88% for five-day moxifloxacin vs. 86% for five-day azithromycin. Bacteriological eradication rates at the end of therapy were 95% for five-day moxifloxacin and 94% for the azithromycin. Corresponding eradication rates at the test-of-cure visit were 89% and 86%, respectively. Among the 567 intent-to-treat patients (283 moxifloxacin and 284 azithromycin), drug-related events were reported for 22% and 17%, respectively. Diarrhea and nausea were the most common drug-related events reported in each group.

The investigators concluded that a five-day course of azithromycin was clinically and bacteriologically equivalent to moxifloxacin 400 mg once daily for five days for treatment of patients with ABE/COPD of proven bacterial etiology.[25] Similar results and conclusions were reached in a prospective, multicenter, phase IIIb clinical trial evaluating patients with signs and symptoms of ABE/COPD. Patients randomly received either a five-day oral course of azithromycin (500 mg qd x 1, then 250 qd x 4) or moxifloxacin (400 mg once-daily), and rates of clinical success were assessed at follow-up 14-21 days after completion of therapy. Clinical resolution at 14-21 days was 85% for the moxifloxacin- and 81% for the azithromycin-treated patients (95% CI, -6.0% to 14%).[26]

In another prospective, multicenter, double-blind study, the efficacy of ciprofloxacin was compared with that of clarithromycin as therapy for patients with ABE/COPD from whom a pretherapy pathogen was isolated; the efficacy was measured by the infection-free interval. Patients randomly received either ciprofloxacin or clarithromycin (500 mg twice a day for 14 days). Three hundred seventy-six patients with acute exacerbations of chronic bronchitis were enrolled in the study, 234 of whom had an ABE/COPD. Clinical resolution was observed in 90% (89 of 99) of ciprofloxacin recipients and 82% (75 of 91) of clarithromycin recipients for whom efficacy could be evaluated. The median infection-free interval was 142 days for ciprofloxacin recipients and 51 days for clarithromycin recipients ($p = 0.15$). Bacteriologic eradication rates were 91% (86 of 95) for ciprofloxacin recipients and 77% (67 of 87) for clarithromycin recipients (p = 0.01). The investigators concluded that compared with clarithromycin, treatment of ABE/COPD with ciprofloxacin was associated with a trend toward a longer infection-free interval and a statistically significantly higher bacteriologic eradication rate.[32]

Three-Day Therapeutic Regimens—Recently Introduced Regimens for Management of ABE/COPD. In a randomized, double-blind controlled clinical trial of acute exacerbation of chronic bronchitis (AECB), azithromycin (500 mg once daily for 3 days) was compared with clarithromycin (500 mg twice daily for 10 days). The primary end point of this trial was the clinical cure rate at day 21-24. For the 304 patients analyzed in the modified intent to treat analysis at the day 21-24 visit, the clinical cure rate for three days of azithromycin was 85% (125/147), compared to 82% (129/157) for 10 days of clarithromycin.

The following outcomes were the clinical cure rates at the day 21-24 visit for the bacteriologically evaluable patients by pathogen:

Pathogen	Azithromycin (3 Days)	Clarithromycin (10 Days)
S. pneumoniae	29/32 (91%)	21/27 (78%)
H. influenzae	12/14 (86%)	14/16 (88%)
M. catarrhalis	11/12 (92%)	12/15 (80%)

In the safety analysis of this study, the incidence of treatment-related adverse events, primarily gastrointestinal, were comparable between treatment arms (25% with azithromycin and 29% with clarithromycin). The most common side effects were diarrhea, nausea, and abdominal pain, with comparable incidence rates for each symptom of 5-9% between the two treatment arms. In adults given 500 mg/day for three days, the discontinuation rate due to treatment-related side effects was 0.4%. Overall, the most common treatment-related side effects in adult patients receiving multiple-dose regimens of azithromycin were related to the gastrointestinal system, with diarrhea/loose stools (4-5%), nausea (3%), and abdominal pain (2-3%) being the most frequently reported.

No other treatment-related side effects occurred in patients on the multiple-dose regimens of azithromycin with a frequency of greater than 1%.

Infectious Precipitants of ABE/COPD. The role of bacterial and viral-mediated infection as precipitants of acute respiratory decompensation in the setting of COPD has been controversial. Certainly, numerous studies have confirmed the role of viral infection in acute exacerbations of COPD.[33-35] In one study, 32% of patients with an acute exacerbation had evidence of viral infection.[34] In these and other investigations evaluating the role of viral infection, the most common agents identified include influenza virus, parainfluenzae, and respiratory syncytial (RSV) virus.[33-37]

Interestingly, although many treatment guidelines for ABE/COPD do not mandate empirical antimicrobial coverage of atypical organisms (e.g., *M. pneumoniae, C. pneumoniae*, and *Legionella*) for patients with ABE/COPD, studies show that atypical organisms such as *Mycoplasma* or *Chlamydia* occasionally may be associated with decompensation in patients with COPD. In fact, many patients with COPD have serologic evidence of previous *Chlamydia* infection. On the other hand, recent studies suggest that acute *C. pneumoniae* infection occurs in only about 5% of acute exacerbations of COPD.[35,36]

Epidemiology. The precise role of bacterial infection is more difficult to ascertain, and equally problematic to confirm in the individual patient. Nevertheless, it is clear that bacterial precipitants play an important etiologic role in ABE/COPD. In one Canadian study enrolling 1687 patients (80% of which had ABE/COPD), sputum cultures were obtained in 125 patients (7.4%). Normal flora was found in 76 of 125 sputum specimens (61%), and a pathogen was found in 49 (39%). Of all the patients having sputum cultures, *H. influenzae* was the most common pathogen, occurring in 24 cases (19%), followed by *S. pneumoniae* in 15 (12%) and *M. catarrhalis* in 10 (8%).[4] Complicating confirmation of a linkage between acute bacterial infection and clinical deterioration in COPD is the fact that patients with COPD have chronic colonization of the respiratory tree with such organisms as *S. pneumoniae, H. influenzae,* and *H. parainfluenzae.*[37] In addition, *M. catarrhalis* is being recognized with increasing frequency.

Role of Antibiotics. It should be noted that many studies were performed prior to the availability of more potent, compliance-enhancing agents, many of which, such as azithromycin and the new generation fluoroquinolones, are not only active against atypical organisms, but also against beta-lactamase-producing *H. influenzae* and *M. catarrhalis*. Furthermore, the failure rate of older antibiotics may be as high as 25%.[39,40]

One approach to delineating the precise role of bacterial infection in ABE/COPD is to evaluate the efficacy of antibiotics in producing symptomatic and functional improvement in patients during an acute exacerbation of COPD. A number of trials have been performed to assess the relationships between antibiotic treatment and resolution of symptoms, many of them using tetracycline as the therapeutic agent.[33] Some of these studies demonstrated a role for antibiotics during the acute exacerbation, while others did not find a significant advantage.

However, a landmark meta-analysis of nine studies performed between 1957 and 1992 confirms that there is a small, but statistically significant benefit when antibiotics are used for acute exacerbations of COPD.[38] The benefits are relatively greater for those patients with ABE/COPD who require hospitalization.

Clinical studies of acute exacerbations of COPD are difficult to interpret because of the heterogeneous nature of COPD, diffuse symptoms that can vary spontaneously, and difficulties in defining clinical response both in the short and long term. Although the role of bacterial infection—and as a result, empiric use of antibiotics—in COPD is somewhat controversial, the most currently available evidence shows that bacterial infection has a significant role in acute exacerbations, but its role in disease progression is less certain. Moreover, based on the preponderance of published evidence, antibiotic therapy is recommended in all patients with ABE/COPD who present with infectious symptoms (i.e., increased sputum production, change in character of the sputum, increased coughing, and shortness of breath), suggesting that antimicrobial therapy will produce a better outcome.[4,41-44]

Upper respiratory tract commensals, such as nontypable *H. influenzae*, cause most bronchial infections by exploiting deficiencies in the host defenses.[41] Some COPD patients are chronically colonized by bacteria between exacerbations, which represents an equilibrium in which the numbers of bacteria are contained by the host defenses but not eliminated. When an exacerbation occurs, this equilibrium is upset and bacterial numbers increase, which incites an inflammatory response. Neutrophil products can further impair the mucosal defenses, favoring the bacteria, but if the infection is managed, symptoms resolve. However, if the infection persists, chronic inflammation may cause lung damage. About 50% of exacerbations involve bacterial infection, but these patients are not easy to differentiate from those who are uninfected, which means that antibiotics should be given empirically to the majority of patients who present with ABE/COPD. Further research is needed to characterize those patients in whom bacterial infection may play a more important role and in whom more intensive antibiotic coverage is required.

Old vs. New Agents. The antibiotic arsenal available for treatment of acute bacterial exacerbations of COPD includes a wide range of older and newer agents representing several drug classes. Although many of the studies confirming efficacy of antibiotics in ABE/COPD were performed with such older agents as amoxicillin and tetracycline, usage patterns are changing in favor of newer agents such as macrolides and advanced generation fluoroquinolones with a broader spectrum of coverage and compliance-enhancing features.

There is evidence-based justification for this evolution in prescribing practices.[4,41-43] In the past, antibiotics such as amoxicillin, ampicillin, tetracycline, erythromycin, and co-trimoxazole were widely employed. Many of the meta-analysis trials demonstrating the usefulness of antibiotics drew upon studies using these agents. But resistance patterns have changed.[41-46] In particular, during the last 10 years, there has been a steady rise in the frequency of beta-lactamase production by *H. influenzae* and *M. catarrhalis*, and more recently, strains of penicillin-resistant pneumococci have emerged.[41-47]

Fortunately, these older antibiotics have been joined by newer agents with either a wider spectrum of activity in vitro, better pharmacokinetics, lower incidence of side effects, more convenient dosing, and/or a shorter duration of therapy. Among the antibiotics approved for acute bacterial exacerbations of COPD, and which also have evidence-based support for their effectiveness in this condition, the azalide azithromycin; the macrolide clarithromycin; and quinolones such as moxifloxacin, gatifloxacin, and evofloxacin are playing an increasingly important role.[43-48] In addition, beta-lactamase inhibitors, including second and third generation cephalosporins, also are available.[41] A more detailed discussion of antibiotic therapy and the selection process are presented in subsequent sections of this review.

Antibiotic Outcome-Effectiveness and Total Cost of Therapy. Unfortunately, limited data exist to guide physicians in the cost-effective treatment of acute exacerbation of chronic bronchitis (ABE/COPD). One important study, however, attempted to determine the antimicrobial efficacy of various agents and compared total outcome costs for patients with ABE/COPD.[51] For the purpose of this analysis, a retrospective review was performed of 60 outpatient medical records of individuals with a diagnosis of COPD associated with acute episodes seen in the pulmonary clinic of a teaching institution.

The participating patients had a total of 224 episodes of ABE/COPD requiring antibiotic treatment. Before review, empirical antibiotic choices were divided into first-line (amoxicillin, co-trimoxazole, tetracyclines, erythromycin); second-line (cephradine, cefuroxime, cefaclor, cefprozil); and third-line (azithromycin, amoxicillin-clavulanate, ciprofloxacin) agents. The designations "first-line," "second-line," and "third-line" were based on a consensus of resident pulmonologists, and was not intended to indicate superiority of one group of drugs vs. another. The residents were asked, "What antibiotic would you choose to treat a patient with ABE/COPD on their initial presentation, on their second presentation, and on a subsequent presentation, if each episode was separated by 2-4 weeks?"[52]

The results have potentially interesting implications for antibiotic selection in the outpatient environment. In this study, patients receiving first-line agents (amoxicillin, co-trimoxazole, tetracyclines, erythromycin) failed significantly more frequently (19% vs 7%; $p < 0.05$) than those treated with third-line agents (azithromycin, amoxicillin-clavulanate, ciprofloxacin). Moreover, patients prescribed first-line agents were hospitalized significantly more often for ABE/COPD within two weeks of outpatient treatment as compared with patients prescribed third-line agents (18.0% vs 5.3% for third-line agents; p < 0.02). Time between subsequent ABE/COPD episodes requiring treatment was significantly longer for patients receiving third-line agents compared with first-line and second-line agents (p < 0.005).[51] The high failure rate with such older agents as amoxicillin, tetracycline, and erythromycin correlates well with recent reports of increasing antibiotic resistance.[52-54]

As might be expected, initial pharmacy acquisition costs were lowest with first-line agents (first-line, U.S. $10.30 ± 8.76; second-line, U.S. $24.45 ± 25.65; third-line, U.S. $45.40 ± 11.11; p < 0.0001), but third-line agents showed a trend toward lower mean total costs of ABE/COPD treatment (first-line, U.S. $942 ± 2173; second-line, U.S. $563 ± 2296; third-line, U.S. $542 ± 1946). The use of so-called third-line antimicrobials, azithromycin, amoxicillin-clavulanate, or ciprofloxacin, significantly reduced the failure rate and need for hospitalization, prolonged the time between ABE/COPD episodes, and were associated with a lower total cost of management for ABE/COPD. Well-designed, prospective studies are needed to confirm these findings and determine how critical pathways should be constructed to maximize outcome-effectiveness of antibiotics used for ABE/COPD.

Based on these results, the authors of this retrospective analysis suggest that these trends should be of interest to the following groups: 1) managed care decision-makers involved in the formulary selection process; 2) physicians whose objective is to optimize outcome-effectiveness of antibiotic therapy; and 3) patients with ABE/COPD, since definitive treatment of the initial presentation is necessary to minimize work disability, permit continuance of normal activities, reduce hospitalizations requiring more intensive therapy, and prevent further clinical deterioration from bronchitis to pneumonia.[52]

In addition, the reduction in hospitalization rate observed with second-line and third-line agents, when compared with first-line agents, may have potential impact on the mortality of patients with COPD. In a recent study of 458 patients with COPD who required admission to hospital for AECB, mortality was 13% after a median length of stay of 10 days; mortality at 180 days was 35%.[55] The severity of ventilator-related impairment of lung function in patients with COPD is strongly related to death both from obstructive lung disease and from all causes.[55,56] Moreover, patients who experience frequent episodes of ABE/COPD are at risk for accelerated loss of lung function, and effective antibiotic therapy may slow this decline. The use of third-line antibiotics in the outpatient setting could decrease the number of hospitalizations and the degenerative disease process, and thus prolong the survival of patients with COPD. Further evaluation of this hypothesis is required.[52,54-57]

Based on the data collected in this study, the use of azithromycin, amoxicillin-clavulanate, or ciprofloxacin for the treatment of ABE/COPD resulted in significantly fewer physician office visits and appeared to prevent hospitalizations when compared with first- or second-line antimicrobial therapy.[52] Whether there is any difference among these agents remains to be evaluated longitudinally. Additionally, the repetitive nature of return visits to the emergency department or outpatient clinic for ABE/COPD may assist in identifying patients who require initial treatment with more effective agents to prevent ABE/COPD-related hospital admissions and progression of the disease.

PHARMACOTHERAPY FOR PATIENT STABILIZATION: A MULTI-MODAL APPROACH FOR OPTIMIZING CLINICAL OUTCOMES

Optimizing outcomes in patients with ABE/COPD requires prudent but prompt administration of pharmacological agents directed at relieving bronchoconstriction and improving oxygenation. A multi-modal approach to initial stabilization is the rule rather than the exception. As might be expected, pharmacological approaches for chronic maintenance therapy differ somewhat from those used for acute management. In both cases, it should be stressed that the response to various pharmacotherapeutic modalities may vary from one patient to another; hence, sequencing and combining therapy (using such agents as oxygen, beta-agonists, anticholinergics, and/or corticosteroids) according to previously documented patterns of clinical response may represent the most logical approach in the majority of patients. The role of antibiotic therapy is discussed in a separate section.

Table 6. Characteristics of Bronchodilators Delivered by Metered-Dose Inhaler

Medication	Dose (mg)/Puff	Beta-1-Agonist*	Beta-2-Agonist*
Ipatropium bromide/ albuterol sulfate (Combivent®)-Preferred	0.18/ 0.10	+	+ + + +
Isoproterenol	0.08	+ + +	+ + +
Isoetharine	0.34	+ +	+ +
Metaproterenol	0.65	+	+ + +
Terbutaline	0.20	+	+ + + +
Albuterol	0.09	+	+ + + +
Bitolterol	0.37	+	+ + + +
Pirbuterol	0.20	+	+ + +
Salmeterol	0.04	+	+ + + +

* The number of plus signs denotes the relative level of activity.

HOME-BASED TREATMENT PLANS FOR PRIMARY CARE PRACTICE

After evaluation and initial treatment in the office or clinic setting, several adjustments to the patient's outpatient medical regimen may be considered.

Oxygen. First, patients with severe COPD may be eligible for home oxygen therapy. Although this generally is not initiated as part of the emergency department treatment, patients may benefit from a referral for subsequent consideration for home oxygen therapy. Patients with a PaO_2 of less than 55 mmHg at rest or a PaO_2 between 55 and 60 mmHg with evidence of cor pulmonale may meet Medicare criteria for reimbursable oxygen supplementation. It has been shown that home oxygen therapy prolongs survival, reduces polycythemia, decreases the risk of pulmonary hypertension, and reduces the risk of right ventricular failure. Accordingly, patients who meet these criteria should be referred to appropriate providers who can arrange for home oxygen supplementation.

Bronchodilators. Long-term management of the patient with COPD

Anticholinergic*	Onset (Min)	Peak (Min)	Duration (Min)
+ + + +	5-15	60-120	240-480
-	3-5	5-10	60-90
-	3-5	5-20	60-150
-	5-15	10-60	60-180
-	5-30	60-120	180-360
-	5-15	60-90	240-360
-	5-10	60-90	300-480
-	5-10	30-60	180-240
-	10-20	180	720

*The number of plus signs denotes the relative level of activity.

almost always requires use of various bronchodilating agents. Studies have shown that most patients with COPD respond to bronchodilators.[58,59] (*Please see Table 6.*) Significant improvements in pulmonary function may occur in response to inhaled beta-agonists, inhaled anticholinergic agents, and oral methylxanthines. Accordingly, appropriate patients should be discharged on bronchodilators, beginning with either inhaled beta-agonists or inhaled anticholinergics. Although the older, non-selective beta-agonists are effective in COPD, when used for long-term therapy, patients should be on one of the newer, longer acting, beta-2 selective agonists such as metaproterenol, albuterol, terbutaline, or bitolterol. For long-term maintenance, these agents are typically used in a dose of two puffs up to four times a day by metered-dose inhaler. (*Please see Table 7.*) Some patients, however, may require larger doses, and studies in patients with chronic disease have found dose-related improvements at up to 1600 mcg.[60]

In large studies, albuterol has been found to improve pulmonary function for stable patients with COPD.[60] The effectiveness, however, decreases over time. Albuterol is safe for the long-term management of COPD, as the incidence of drug-related adverse events is low. Patients with COPD tend to be older, and as such, have decreased sensitivity to adrenergic compounds. Some authors have found that the response to anticholinergic compounds in chronic therapy may be superior to beta-agonists for routine use.

Anticholinergic Agents. Anticholinergics probably should be used for routine maintenance in most patients with COPD. Inhaled quaternary ammonium anticholinergic agents have been found in some studies to lead to greater bronchodilation than beta-agonists or theophylline. Since older patients have a decrease in responsiveness to the adrenergic receptors, the cholinergic receptors become even more important in the older patients with COPD. Ipratropium is the primary agent used by metered-dose inhaler in this country. It is relatively safe, with side effects generally limited to dry mouth or the sensation of a "metallic" taste in the mouth. Again, this agent leads to increasing bronchodilation as the dose increases up to 600 mcg. Ipratropium is available in 500 mcg doses by metered-dose inhaler.

A meta-analysis of seven long-term studies comparing ipratropium with beta-agonists demonstrated that ipratropium leads to greater improvement in FEV_1 and even greater improvements in force vital capacity over the course of 90 days. Ipratropium leads to greater improvements in quality-of-life measurements. The improvements in pulmonary function are greatest in patients who have stopped smoking compared to current smokers. Furthermore, patients using ipratropium are less likely than patients using beta-agonists to develop a decreased response over time.[61] Ipratropium has minimal side effects that primarily are related to dry mouth or leaving a bad taste in the mouth.

Inhalers. Prior to discharge from the primary care clinic or office, patients should be instructed in the proper means of using metered-dose inhalers. Many patients will benefit from the use of a spacer device. A typical discharge regimen will include albuterol by metered-dose inhaler either on an as needed basis for rescue therapy or for chronic maintenance therapy.[62,63] In addition, most patients with COPD should be using ipratropium by metered-dose inhaler for chronic maintenance therapy. These drugs are available as

Table 7. Beta-Agonist Dosages

Albuterol (Proventil, Ventolin)	2-4 puffs q4h	0.5 cc (2.5 mg) in 2.5 cc NS
Bitolterol (Tornalate)	2 puffs q8h	0.5 cc (0.2% [1mg]) in 2 cc NS
Isoetharine (Bronkosol)	4 puffs q4h	0.5 cc (0.25%) in 3 cc NS
Isoproterenol (Isuprel)	5-15 puffs (1:200) q4h	0.5 cc (0.5%) in 3 cc NS
Metaproterenol (Alupent, Metaprel)	2-3 puffs q3-4h	0.3 cc (1.5 mg) in 2.5 cc NS
Pirbuterol (Maxair)	2 puffs q4-6h	
Terbutaline (Brethine)	2 puffs q4-6h	
Salmeterol (Serevent)	2 puffs q12h	

combination therapy in metered-dose inhalers. Patients who have prominent nighttime symptoms may benefit from a long-acting beta-agonist such as salmeterol. Patients should be counseled, however, that salmeterol should not be used for rescue therapy.

Theophylline. Theophylline does have dose-related effects on pulmonary function in patients with stable COPD. This drug may be used for patients who cannot or will not use metered-dose inhalers, patients who are not responding to otherwise maximal therapy, or patients who have prominent nighttime symptoms. Therapy is usually initiated at a dose of 300 mg twice a day with monitoring of the theophylline level. Therapeutic theophylline levels are considered to be between 10 and 20 micrograms per cc, although the FDA has changed labeling requirements for these drugs to suggest that consideration be given to maintain the level between 10 and 15 micrograms per cc.

Theophylline metabolism is affected by a number of factors and patients should be cautioned not to increase their dose without seeking medical advice.

Corticosteroids. About 25% of patients with COPD will respond to oral steroids. Patients with a significant degree of reversibility of pulmonary function on baseline testing are most likely to respond to steroids.[64] It seems reasonable to initiate a two-week trial of oral steroids for patients with COPD. Studies indicate that there may be a role for inhaled corticosteroids in patients with COPD. In this regard, one study found that the addition of inhaled corticosteroids over the course of two years decreased morbidity and improved airway obstruction when used in conjunction with an inhaled beta-2 agonist.[65] A more recent study found a short-term improvement in lung function in smokers with COPD treated with inhaled steroids, but this then was followed by continued deterioration in lung function.[66]

ANTIBIOTICS: SUMMARY

While many episodes of acute exacerbation of COPD are caused by viral infection, the weight of evidence seems to indicate that patients respond to oral antibiotics—especially when the exacerbation is associated with signs and symptoms of acute, bacterial bronchitis that is superimposed on COPD with a presentation characterized by fever, dyspnea, increase in sputum production, or change in the color of sputum.[61] Available antibiotics with evidence-based support for their efficacy and which have indications for ABE/COPD have been discussed in detail.

Patients with ABE/COPD who are deemed suitable for oral, outpatient therapy and who do not have signficant IOTT criteria in the SERF pathway (*please see Table 4*) that suggest the specific need for more extensive gram-negative coverage, should be discharged with a compliance-sensitive antibiotic that provides adequate coverage of *S. pneumoniae, H. influenzae*, and *M. catarrhalis*.

Macrolides/Azithromycin. Based on evidence-based trials and pharmatectural criteria (duration of therapy, reduced dosing frequency, drug interaction profile, cost, and spectrum of coverage), macrolides such as azithromycin should be considered a first-line agent in patients with ABE/COPD who, on the basis of clinical judgement, are likely to be infected with *S. pneumoniae, H. influenzae,* or *M. catarrhalis.*[6,7,15-18,68-70]

It should be stressed that one of the advanced macrolides, azithromycin, has the advantage of a simplified dosing schedule; the most convenient dosing schedule is 500 mg PO once daily for only three days. Azithromycin (500 mg on day 1 and 250 mg on days 2-5) did not affect the plasma levels or pharmacokinetics of theophylline administered as a single intravenous dose. However, because the effect of azithromycin on plasma levels or pharmacokinetics of theophylline is not known, until further data are available, prudent medical practice dictates careful monitoring of plasma levels of theophylline in COPD patients receiving azithromycin and theophylline concomitantly. The same precaution should be applied to patients receiving warfarin and azithromycin concomitantly. Other macrolides generally require a similar monitoring strategy.

Clarithromycin, another advanced generation macrolide, requires a much longer course of therapy and, as a seven-day course, is more expensive ($58-$68 for a 7-day course) than a five-day course of azithromycin ($43-$46). In general, the decision to use a macrolide such as azithromycin is based on consideration of its generally acceptable cost ($43-$46 for a 5-day treatment regimen), as well as its real-world advantages, which include convenient, once-daily dosing; a correct spectrum of coverage; favorable drug interaction profile; and toleration data (gastrointestinal side effects occur in about 3-5% of patients taking a 5-day, multiple-dose regimen). The oral tablet formulation permits consumption of the antibiotic without regard to food ingestion.

Fluoroquinolones. Patients who are macrolide treatment failures, are suspected of gram-negative infection with enterobacteria, and/or present with multiple IOTT points on the SERF pathway may be effectively served by a fluoroquinolone such as levofloxacin, moxifloxacin, gatifloxacin, or ciprofloxacin, the latter of which is not recommended when *S. pneumoniae* is the presumed causative agent. Levofloxacin is well-tolerated, with the most common side effects including nausea, diarrhea, headache, and constipation. Food does not affect the absorption of the drug, but it should be taken at least two hours before or two hours after antacids containing magnesium or aluminum, as well as sucralfate, metal cations such as iron, and multivitamin preparations with zinc. Dosage adjustment for levofloxacin is recommended in patients with impaired renal function (clearance < 50 mL/min).

Although no significant effect of levofloxacin on plasma concentration of theophylline was detected in 14 health volunteers studied, because other quinolones have produced increases in patients taking concomitant theophylline, theophylline levels should be closely monitored in patients on levofloxacin and dosage adjustments made as necessary. Monitoring patients on warfarin also is recommended in patients on quinolones. All quinolones have been associated with cartilage damage in animal studies; therefore, they are not recommended for use in children, adolescents, and pregnant and nursing women. Cephalosporins also are available and effective for treatment of ABE/COPD.

Moxifloxacin is the only fluoroquinolone antibiotic indicated in the United States for a five-day treatment of ABE/COPD. Other fluoroquinolones are indicated for seven, 7-10, or 7-14 days for the treatment of ABE/COPD. Moxifloxacin is generally well tolerated. In clinical trials, the most common adverse events were nausea (8%), diarrhea (6%), dizziness (3%), headache (2%), abdominal pain (2%), and vomiting (2%). The agent is contraindicated in persons with a history of hypersensitivity to moxifloxacin or any quinolone antibiotic. The safety and effectiveness of moxifloxacin in pediatric patients, adolescents (> age 18), pregnant women, and lactating women have not been established.

Moxifloxacin has been shown to prolong the QT interval of the electrocardiogram in some patients. The drug should be avoided in patients with known prolongation of the QT interval, patients with uncorrected hypokalemia, and patients receiving Class lA (e.g., quinidine, procainamide) or Class lll (e.g., amiodarone, sotalol) antiarrhythmic agents, due to the lack of clinical experience with the drug in these patient populations. Pharmacokinetic studies between moxifloxacin and other drugs that prolong the QT interval such as cisapride, erythromycin, antipsychotics, and tricyclic antidepressants have not been performed. An additive effect of moxifloxacin and these drugs cannot be excluded; therefore, moxifloxacin should be used with caution when given concurrently with these drugs.

The effect of moxifloxacin on patients with congenital prolongation of the QT interval has not been studied; however, it is expected that these individuals may be more susceptible to drug-induced QT prolongation. Because of limited clinical experience, moxifloxacin should be used with caution in patients with ongoing proarrhythmic conditions, such as clinically significant bradycardia or acute myocardial ischemia. As with all quinolones, moxifloxacin should be used with caution in patients with known or suspected central nervous system (CNS) disorders or in the presence of other risk factors that may predispose to seizures or lower the seizure threshold.

Gatifloxacin, a broad-spectrum 8-methoxy fluoroquinolone antibiotic, has been approved for the safe and effective treatment of approved indications, including community-acquired respiratory tract infections, such as bacterial exacerbation of chronic bronchitis (ABE/COPD); acute sinusitis; and CAP caused by indicated, susceptible strains of gram-positive and gram-negative bacteria. The recommended dose for gatifloxacin is 400 mg once daily, for all individuals with normal renal function. Dosage adjustment is required in patients with impaired renal function (creatinine clearance < 40 mL/min).

Gatifloxacin is primarily excreted through the kidneys and less than 1% is metabolized by the liver. In clinical trials, gatifloxacin has been found to be a well-tolerated treatment in 15 international clinical trials at 500 study sites. Gatifloxacin may have the potential to prolong the QTc interval of the electrocardiogram in some patients; due to limited clinical experience, gatifloxacin should be avoided in patients with known prolongation of the QTc interval, in patients with uncorrected hypokalemia, and in those receiving Class IA (e.g., quinidine, procainamide) or Class III (e.g., amiodarone, sotalol) antiarrhythmic agents. Gatifloxacin should be used with caution when given together with drugs that may prolong the QTc interval (e.g., cisapride, erythromycin, antipsychotics, tricyclic antidepressants), and in patients with ongoing proarrhythmic conditions (e.g., clinically significant bradycardia or acute myocardial ischemia).

Gatifloxacin should be used with caution in patients with known or suspected CNS disorders or patients who have a predisposition to seizures. The most common side effects associated with gatifloxacin in clinical trials were gastrointestinal. Adverse reactions considered to be drug related and occurring in greater than 3% of patients were: nausea (8%), vaginitis (6%), diarrhea (4%), headache (3%), and dizziness (3%).

Oral doses of gatifloxacin should be administered at least four hours before the administration of ferrous sulfate; dietary supplements containing zinc, magnesium, or iron (such as multivitamins); aluminum/magnesium-containing antacids; or Videx (didanosine, or ddI). Concomitant administration of gatifloxacin and probenecid significantly increases systemic exposure to gatifloxacin. Concomitant administration of gatifloxacin and digoxin did not produce significant alteration of the pharmacokinetics of gatifloxacin; however, patients taking digoxin should be monitored for signs and/or symptoms of digoxin toxicity.

Patients with a greater risk of respiratory failure are more likely to benefit from antibiotic therapy. This would include patients of advanced age and patients with significant lung impairment, impairment due to other co-morbid conditions, frequent exacerbations, or steroid use. Accordingly, a small percentage of these patients may require intensification and amplification of antibiotic therapy (i.e., the movement from azithromycin to a fluoroquinolone) to cover gram-negative organisms in addition to the three common offenders cited above.

Less expensive and still widely used in certain institutions and health plans, many of the older agents (sulfa-derivatives, tetracyclines, and amoxicillin) are becoming resistant to *S. pneumoniae* or do not cover beta-lactamase-producing organisms and, as a result, may no longer represent the best choice for empiric therapy of ABE/COPD.[71-77] The finding in one retrospective study that such antimicrobials as azithromycin, amoxicillin-clavulanate, or ciprofloxacin significantly reduced the failure rate and need for hospitalization, prolonged the time between ABE/COPD episodes, and were associated with a lower total cost of management for ABE/COPD compared to the older agents is extremely provocative and requires further investigation.[76]

Even until clarification of outcome-effectiveness is forthcoming, clinicians should be aware that a number of newer antibiotic agents are available, including advanced generation macrolides and quinolones, which have the advantage of a broader spectrum of activity, simplified dosing regimens, and lower resistance rates.[78]

Pneumonia in Patients with COPD. The development of pneumonia in a patient with COPD frequently will provide an indication for admission. However, there are younger patients with very mild COPD who have good ventilatory status; do not have other concomitant medical diseases; and on the basis of clinical judgment, may be given a trial of outpatient antibiotic therapy. Protocols for treatment of CAP are widely published. (*Please see Table 8.*) However, most patients with COPD complicated by pneumonia will require admission.

The small percentage of patients who are discharged, and therefore judged appropriate for outpatient treatment, should be treated for the most common causative agents, which include *S. pneumoniae, H. influenzae, M. catarrhalis, M. pneumoniae*, and *C. pneumoniae*. Given the spectrum of organisms encountered, it is probably preferable to initiate therapy with either a macrolide/azalide such as azithromycin or, as an alternative, an advanced generation fluorquinolone.

COMMUNITY-ACQUIRED PNEUMONIA (CAP)—OMBIRT PANEL OVERVIEW AND RECOMMENDATIONS FOR OUTPATIENT MANAGEMENT

Despite a general consensus that empiric, outpatient treatment of CAP requires, at the least, mandatory coverage of such organisms as *S. pneumoniae, H. influenzae*, and *M. catarrhalis*, as well as atypical organisms (*M. pneumoniae, C. pneumoniae*, and *L. pneumophila*), antibiotic selection strategies for achieving this spectrum of coverage vary widely. New treatment guidelines for CAP have been issued by such national associations as the Infectious Disease Society of America (IDSA, 2000), the American Thoracic Society (ATS, 2001), and the Centers for Disease Control and Prevention (CDC) Drug-Resistant *Streptococcus pneumoniae* Therapeutic Working Group (CDCDR-SP-WG, 2000).

Deciphering the strengths, subtleties, and differences among recommendations issued by different authoritative sources can be problematic and confusing. Because patient disposition practices and treatment pathways vary among institutions and from region to region, management guidelines for CAP in the geriatric patient must be "customized" for the local practice environment. Unfortunately, no single set of guidelines is applicable to every patient or practice environment; therefore, clinical judgment must prevail. This means taking into account local antibiotic resistance patterns, epidemiological and infection incidence data, and patient demographic features.

Patient Management Recommendations. The OMBIRT Panel concurs that appropriate use of antibiotics requires radiographic confirmation of the diagnosis of CAP. In this regard, physicians should use clinical judgment when ordering chest x-rays, with the understanding that the diagnostic yield of this radiographic modality in CAP is increased in patients with fever greater than 38.5°C; presence of new cough; and abnormal pulmonary findings suggestive of consolidation, localized bronchoconstriction, or pleural effusion.

Accordingly, a chest x-ray is recommended and encouraged by the OMBIRT Panel, as well as by such national associations as the IDSA, ATS, and American College of Emergency Physicians (ACEP), to confirm the diagnosis of outpatient CAP; however, the panel acknowledges that, on occasion, logistical issues may prevent radiographic confirmation at the time of diagnosis and treatment.

The approach to antibiotic therapy usually will be empiric, and must account for a number of clinical, epidemiological, and unpredictable factors related to antibiotic resistance patterns and respiratory tract pathogens. As a general rule, appropriate antibiotic choice for the patient with CAP requires consideration of strategies that will yield clinical cure in the patient "today," combined with antibiotic selection strategies that prevent accelerated emergence of drug-resistant organisms that will infect the community "tomorrow."

Based on the most current clinical studies, the principal six respiratory tract pathogens that must be covered on an empiric basis in individuals with outpatient CAP include: *S. pneumoniae, H. influenzae, M. catarrhalis, C. pneumoniae, M. pneumoniae*, and *L. pneumophilia*. In addition, the OMBIRT Panel emphasized that there may be a "disconnect," i.e., an incompletely understood and not entirely predictable relationship between an antibiotic's MIC level and its association with positive clinical outcomes in CAP. This disconnect may be explained by the unique qualities of an antimicrobial, such as tissue penetration and/or pharmacokinetics, patient medication compliance, and other factors.

Double-blinded, prospective clinical trials comparing new generation macrolides vs. new generation fluoroquinolones demonstrate similar outcomes in terms of clinical cure and bacteriologic eradication rates in outpatients with CAP.[79] However, emergence of resistance among *S. pneumoniae* species to new generation fluoroquinolones has been reported in a number of geographic regions, including the United States, Hong Kong, and Canada, and this may have implications for treatment.

The frequency of DRSP (drug-resistant *S. pneumoniae*) causing outpatient CAP, as estimated by the CDC, is very low (i.e., in the range of 0.14-1.9%). The CDC working group panel on drug-resistant Streptococcus pneumoniae (CDCDRSP-WG) cautions against overuse of new generation fluoroquinolones in outpatient CAP, and recommends their use as alternative agents when: 1) first-line therapy with advanced generation macrolides such as azithromycin fail; 2) patients are allergic to first-line agents; or 3) the case is a documented infection with DRSP.[80]

Given concerns about antibiotic overuse, the potential for emerging resistance among DRSP to fluoroquinolones, and the increasing recognition of atypical pathogens as causative agents in patients with outpatient CAP, the OMBIRT Panel concurs with the CDCDRSP-WG recommendation advocating macrolides as initial agents of choice in outpatient CAP. The OMBIRT Panel also noted that the Canadian Consensus Guidelines for CAP Management and the 2001 ATS (American Thoracic Society) Consensus Guideline Recommendations also include advanced generation macrolides as initial therapy for outpatient CAP.

In this regard, two safe and effective advanced generation macrolides, azithromycin and clarithromycin, currently are available for outpatient, oral-based treatment of CAP (IV azithromycin also is indicated for in-hospital management of patients who are risk-stratified as having more serious disease). Based on outcome-sensitive criteria and pharmatectural considerations such as cost, daily dose frequency, duration of therapy, side effects, and drug interactions, the OMBIRT Panel recommends as first-line, preferred initial therapy in CAP, azithromycin, with clarithromycin or doxycycline as alternative agents; and as second-line therapy, moxifloxacin, gatifloxacin, or levofloxacin when appropriate, according to CDC guidelines and other association-based protocols.

Physicians are urged to prescribe antibiotics in CAP at the time of diagnosis and to encourage patients to fill and begin taking their prescriptions for CAP on the day of diagnosis. Ideally, patients should initiate their first course of oral therapy within eight hours of diagnosis, a time frame that appears reasonable based on studies in hospitalized patients indicating improved survival in patients who received their first IV dose within eight hours of diagnosis. Primary care practitioners also are urged to instruct patients in medication compliance, and in the case of short (5-day) courses of therapy, educate their patients that although they are only consuming medications for a five-day period, the antibiotic remains at the tissue site of infection for about 7-10 days and continues to deliver therapeutic effects during that period.

Either verbal or on-site re-evaluation of patients is recommended within a three-day period following diagnosis and initiation of antibiotic therapy. Follow-up in the office or clinic within three days is recommended in certain risk-stratified patients, especially the elderly, those with co-morbid illness, and those in whom medication compliance may be compromised. More urgent follow-up may be required in patients with increasing symptoms, including dyspnea, fever, and other systemic signs or symptoms. Follow-up chest x-rays generally are not recommended in patients with outpatient CAP, except in certain high-risk groups, such as those with right middle lobe syndrome, and in individuals in whom the diagnosis may have been uncertain.

RISK STRATIFICATION AND PATIENT DISPOSITION: OUTPATIENT VS. INPATIENT MANAGEMENT

Overview. The OMBIRT Panel concurred that determining whether to admit or discharge a patient with pneumonia is one of the most important decisions made by a primary care physician when managing patients suspected of having CAP. For this reason, there have been increasing efforts to identify patients with CAP who can appropriately be treated as outpatients.[73-75,81] The disposition decision for patients with pneumonia should take into account the severity of the pneumonia, as well as other medical and psychosocial factors that may affect the treatment plan and clinical outcome.[82-84]

In the absence of respiratory distress or other complicating factors, many young adults can be adequately treated with appropriate oral antibiotic therapy. This is less often the case for the elderly patient with CAP, because comorbid conditions and other risk factors may complicate the course of the illness. Even when following appropriate treatment and dispositon, patients may have symptoms, including cough, fatigue, dyspnea, sputum production, and chest pain that can last for several months. To address this issue of patient disposition and treatment setting, a variety of investigators have proposed criteria to identify patients requiring hospitalization. Patients felt to be at low risk have a median length of stay of seven days, while those at medium risk have a median length of stay of 12-13 days.

Among the factors most physicians use to make admission decisions for pneumonia are the presence of hypoxemia, overall clinical status, the ability to maintain oral intake, hemodynamic status, and the patient's home environment. Using clinical judgment, however, physicians tend to overestimate the likelihood of death from pneumonia.[82] These findings have led some investigators to employ more stringent prediction rules. For example, the chest radiograph may help identify patients who are at high risk for mortality. The presence of bilateral effusions, moderate-size pleural effusions, multi-lobar involvement, and bilateral infiltrates are associated with a higher risk of mortality.

A landmark study presented a prediction rule (Pneumonia Severity Index [PSI]) to identify low-risk patients with CAP.[73] Using such objective criteria as patient age, coexistent medical conditions, and vital signs, patients are assigned either to a low-risk class, which has a mortality rate of about 0.1% in outpatients, or to higher risk categories. Patients with any risk factors are then evaluated with a second scoring system that assigns individuals to one of three higher risk categories, which have mortality rates ranging from 0.7% to 31%.[82] In addition to the factors noted in this prediction rule, patients who are immunocompromised as a result of AIDS or chronic alcohol use frequently require hospitalization.

Once the clinician has determined hospitalization is required, the need for intensive care unit (ICU) admission also must be evaluated. A variety of factors are associated with an increased risk for mortality, including increasing age (> age 65), alcoholism, chronic lung disease, immunodeficiency, and specific laboratory abnormalities, including azotemia and hypoxemia. These patients may require admission to the ICU.

Prognostic Scoring. There have been many efforts to assess severity and risk of death in patients with pneumonia.[83,85-88] The study by Fine and colleagues has received considerable attention and is used as a benchmark by many clinicians.[82] This study developed a prediction rule, the PSI, to assess 30-day mortality in patients with CAP. The rule was derived and validated with data from more than 52,000 inpatients, and then validated with a second cohort of 2287 inpatients and outpatients as part of the Pneumonia PORT study. Subsequent evaluation and validation has been performed with other cohorts, including geriatric patients and nursing home residents.[89,90]

In this risk-stratification scheme, patients are assigned to one of five risk classes (1 is lowest risk, 5 is highest risk) based upon a point system that considers age, co-existing disease, abnormal physical findings, and abnormal laboratory findings. Elderly patients cannot be assigned to Class 1, as a requirement is age younger than 50 years.[82]

In older patients, age contributes the most points to the overall score. For example, it should be noted that males older than age 70 and females older than age 80 would be assigned to Class 3 on the basis of age alone, without any other risk factor. In the Fine study, patients assigned to Class 1 and 2 were typically younger patients (median age, 35-59 years) and patients in Class 3-5 were older (median age, 72-75 years).[82]

Outpatient management is recommended for Classes 1 and 2, brief inpatient observation for Class 3, and traditional hospitalization for Classes 4 and 5.[83,91] For a geriatric patient to qualify for outpatient treatment based on these recommendations, he or she would have to be younger than 70 years of age if male or younger than 80 years of age if female, and have no additional risk factors. Inpatient observation or traditional hospitalization would be recommended for all other patients based on this rule. Other studies have suggested outpatient management for Class 3 patients.[73,92]

Patients considered eligible for management as outpatients must be able to take oral fluids and antibiotics, comply with outpatient care, and be able to carry out activities of daily living (ADLs) or have adequate home support to assist with ADLs.[82-84] Other factors cited in previous studies but not included in the PSI also have been found to increase the risk of morbidity or mortality from pneumonia. These include: other comorbid illnesses (diabetes mellitus, COPD, post-splenectomy state), altered mental status, suspicion of aspiration, chronic alcohol abuse or malnutrition, and evidence of extrapulmonary disease.[93] Additional laboratory studies that may suggest increased severity of illness include white blood cell count less than 4 or greater than 30, absolute neutrophil count less than 1, elevated protime or partial thromboplastin time, decreased platelet count, or radiographic evidence of multilobar involvement, cavitation, and rapid speeding.[93]

Severe pneumonia may require ICU admission. In the Fine study, 6% of patients in Class 3, 11% of patients in Class 4, and 17% of patients in Class 5 required ICU admission.[82] The ATS guidelines define severe pneumonia as the presence of at least one of the following: respiratory rate greater than 30, severe respiratory failure ($PaO_2/FIO_2 < 250$), mechanical ventilation, bilateral infiltrates or multilobar infiltrates, shock, vasopressor requirement, or oliguria (urine output < 20 cc per hour). The presence of at least one of these is highly sensitive (98%) but only 32% specific for the need for ICU management.[94] It is emphasized that the above guidelines for admission should not supercede clinical judgment when assessing the need to hospitalize patients.[82,83,91,93]

ANTIBIOTIC SELECTION IN THE PATIENT WITH PNEUMONIA

Introduction. Antibiotic therapy is the mainstay of management for outpatients with CAP. As previously emphaszied, antibiotic therapy should be initiated promptly, as soon as the diagnosis is strongly suspected or confirmed, and after appropriate microbiological studies or samples have been obtained. Chest x-rays should be performed to confirm the diagnosis.

It should be stressed that there is no absolute or consistent consensus on precisely which drug, or combination of drugs, constitutes the most outcome-effective choice for managing CAP in outpatients. However, virtually all panels and guideline documents, including the OMBIRT Panel, agree that antimicrobial coverage, as a baseline spectrum of coverage, must include sufficient activity against the following bacterial pathogens: *S. pneumoniae, H. influenzae*, and *M. catarrhalis*, as well as against the atypical pathogens *Mycoplasma, Legionella*, and *C. pneumoniae*. Therefore, such macrolides as azithromycin and advanced generation fluoroquinolones which, because of their activity against both bacterial and atypical pathogens commonly encountered in CAP, have supplanted cephalosporins and amoxicillin-clavulanate as preferred monotherapeutic options for treatment of outpatients with CAP.

Beyond this non-negotiable caveat mandating coverage for the six afore-mentioned pathogens, there are important differences among recommendations and expert panels for empiric treatment of pneumonia. Variations among the guidelines usually depend upon: 1) their emphasis or focus on the need to empirically cover drug-resistant *S. pneumoniae* (DRSP) species as part of the initial antimicrobial regimen; 2) their concern about using antimicrobials (fluoroquinolones) with an over-extended (too broad) spectrum of coverage; 3) their concern about the potential of growing resistance to a class (fluoroquinolones) which has agents that currently are active against DRSP species; 4) their preference for monotherapeutic vs. combination therapy; 5) the date when the guidelines were released (recent vs several years old); and 6) their emphasis on drug costs, patient convenience, and options for step-down (IV to oral) therapeutic approaches. Clearly, these factors and the relative emphasis placed on each of them will influence antimicrobial selection for the patient with pneumonia.

With these issues and drug selection factors in mind, the most recent guidelines issued by the IDSA, CDCDRSP-WG, and ATS attempt to both risk-stratify and "drug-stratify" patients according to their eligibility for receiving agents as initial empiric therapy that have activity against DRSP. Before presenting the OMBIRT Panel's detailed analysis of the current treatment landscape for CAP, a number of points should be emphasized. First, the relative importance of *S. pneumoniae* as a cause of outpatient CAP is difficult to determine. Nevertheless, a review of the literature by the CDCDRSP-WG suggests that *S. pneumoniae* accounts for about 2-27% of all cases of CAP treated on an outpatient basis.[95-97] In addition, surveillance studies have suggested that about 7% of invasive *S. pneumoniae* species in the United States showed a significant degree of penicillin resistance.[98] Hence, this group estimates that only 0.14% (7% of 2%) to 1.9% (7% of 27%) of outpatients with bacterial pneumonia have pneumococcal infections with levels of resistance high enough to warrant consideration of alternative treatment.

This analysis has made the CDC panel conclude that because CAP in outpatients who are appropriately triaged and risk-stratified is generally not immediately life-threatening and because *S. pneumoniae* isolates with penicillin MICs of no less than 4 mcg/mL are uncommon, antibiotics with predictable activity against highly penicillin-resistance pneuomococci are not necessary as part of the initial regimen. From a practical, drug-selection perspective, the working group, therefore, suggests that oral fluoroquinolones are not first-line treatment in outpatients with CAP because of concerns about emerging resistance. Consequently, oral macrolide or beta-lactam monotherapy is recommended by the CDC working group as initial therapy in patients with pneumonia considered to be amenable to outpatient management.

COMMUNITY-ACQUIRED PNEUMONIA (CAP) OUTPATIENT MANAGEMENT

Appropriate and Adequate Intensity of Antimicrobial Coverage. Because macrolides and extended spectrum quinolones are effective, appropriate agents for treatment of CAP, they frequently get equal billing as initial-choice agents for management of CAP. Despite their excellent track record and proven efficacy, however, the macrolides and extended spectrum quinolones have clinically significant differences that should be considered in the antibiotic treatment equation for CAP. Accordingly, a careful analysis of the benefits and potential pitfalls of these agents should include a full accounting of the relevant similarities and differences. It will help emergency physicians and intensivists develop criteria that suggest the appropriateness and suitability that each of these classes may have in specific patient subgroups.

Although the previously cited six organisms (S. pneumoniae, H. influenzae, and M. catarrhalis, and atypical pathogens Mycoplasma, Legionella, and C. pneumoniae) are the most commonly implicated pathogens in patients with CAP, there are patients who are susceptible to infection with gram-negative enteric organisms such as Klebsiella, E. coli, and Pseudomonas. In other cases, the likelihood of infection with DRSP is high. When infection with these pathogens is likely, intensification of empiric coverage should include antibiotics with activity against these gram-negative species and/or DRSP. However, it should be noted that patients with infections caused by the aforementioned respiratory pathogens usually are managed on an inpatient basis.

Clinical features or risk factors that may suggest the need for intensification and expansion of bacterial and/or gram-negative pathogen coverage include the following: 1) increasing fragility (> age 85, comorbid conditions, previous infection, etc.) of the patient; 2) acquisition of the pneumonia in a skilled nursing facility; 3) the presence of an aspiration pneumonia, suggesting involvement with gram-negative or anaerobic organisms; 4) chronic alcoholism, increasing the likelihood of infection with Klebsiella pneumoniae; 5) pneumococcal pneumonia in an underlying disease-compromised individual who has not been vaccinated with pneumococcal polysaccharide antigen (Pneumovax); 6) history of infection with gram-negative, anaerobic, or resistant species of S. pneumoniae; 7) history of treatment failure; 8) previous hospitalizations for pneumonia; 9) patient requires or has had previous ICU hospitalization for pneumonia; 10) acquisition of pneumonia in a community with high and increasing resistance among S. pneumoniae species; and 11) immunodeficiency and/or severe underlying disease.

As emphasized earlier in this review, most consensus panels, infectious disease experts, textbooks, and peer-reviewed antimicrobial prescribing guides recommend, as the initial or preferred choice, those antibiotics that, within the framework of monotherapy or combination therapy, address current etiologic and mortality trends in CAP. As a general rule, for empiric initial therapy in patients without modifying host factors that predispose to enteric gram-negative or pseudomonal infection, they recommend those antibiotics that provide coverage against the bacterial pathogens *S. pneumoniae, H. influenzae*, and *M. catarrhalis*, as well as against atypical pathogens *Mycoplasma, Legionella,* and *C. pneumoniae*.[99]

Correct Spectrum Coverage. When antimicrobial monotherapy is desirable, cost-effective, and/or clinically indicated, extended spectrum quinolones and advanced generation macrolides best satisfy the empiric coverage requirements for patients with CAP. These antimicrobial agents are among the therapeutic classes of choice for management of CAP in the outpatient setting. (*Please see Table 8.*)

Although third generation cephalosporins, beta-lactam antibiotics, and TMP/SMX (trimethoprim-sulfamethoxazole) are still deemed valuable by many authorities and practitioners (in particular, in combination with other agents for in-hospital management of CAP), these agents, for the most part, have been given alternative status for oral therapy. This is because they are not, as a rule, clinically indicated for treatment of atypical organisms, including *Mycoplasma, Legionella*, and *C. pneumoniae*, whose increasing importance now mandates initial empiric coverage of atypical organisms.

Because advanced generation macrolides and extended spectrum quinolones constitute the principal oral treatment options for CAP, the following sections will discuss indications, clinical trials, side effects, and strategies for their use in CAP. The focus of the discussion will be on newer antibiotics that: 1) provide coverage of bacterial and atypical organisms causing CAP; and 2) are able, when indicated, to provide compliance-enhancing and cost-effective treatment within the context of antimicrobial monotherapy. It should be stressed that these agents also may be used as part of combination therapy for CAP.

Table 8. OMBIRT Panel Guidelines—Empiric Antimicrobial Therapy of Choice for Outpatient and in-Hospital Management of Patients with CAP

PATIENT PROFILE/ETIOLOGIC AGENTS
Outpatients
Patients deemed to be suitable for outpatient/oral therapy, i.e., no systemic toxicity, high likelihood of compliance, and supportive home environment[*]
In-Hospital management of mild severity CAP
(excludes nursing home patients, immunosuppressed patients, patients with sepsis, renal failure, aspiration, the elderly and other serious co-morbid conditions)
In-Hospital CAP (not in intensive care unit) with underlying risk factors or comorbid conditions:
In-Hospital management (COPD, history of pneumonia, diabetes, etc.)
CAP acquired in the nursing home environment
(increased likelihood of gram-negative, *E. coli*, *Klebsiella pneumoniae*)
CAP in the elderly individual with chronic alcoholism
(increased likelihood of *Klebsiella pneumoniae* infection)

* Oral therapy/outpatient treatment recommendations are appropriate only for those otherwise healthy patients with CAP of mild enough severity that they are judged to be suitable candidates for outpatient management with oral antibiotics.

§ Quinolones are restricted for use in patients > 18 years of age.

¶ If *S. pneumoniae* demonstrates complete resistance to extended spectrum quinolones (very rare), third-generation cephalosporins, and macrolides, then vancomycin may be required as part of initial therapy, although this would be necessary only in rare circumstances.

FIRST-LINE ANTIBIOTIC THERAPY[†]	ALTERNATIVE FIRST-LINE THERAPY
Azithromycin PO	Moxifloxacin PO (preferred) OR Levofloxacin PO OR Gatifloxacin PO OR Clarithromycin PO
Azithromycin IV plus ceftriaxone IV	Azithromycin IV[††]
Azithromycin IV plus ceftriaxone IV	Levofloxacin IV OR Gatifloxacin IV OR Cefotaxime[**] plus azithromycin IV
Azithromycin IV plus ceftriaxone IV	Levofloxacin IV OR Gatifloxacin IV OR Cefotaxime plus azithromycin IV
Azithromycin IV plus ceftriaxone IV	Cefepime IV plus azithromycin IV OR Levofloxacin IV OR Gatifloxacin IV

[†] First-line therapy recommendations take into consideration cost of the drug (which may vary from one institution to another), convenience of dosing, daily dose frequency, spectrum of coverage, side effects, and risk of drug-drug interactions.

[††] Identifying hospitalized patients with CAP that is mild enough to warrant azithromycin monotherapy is difficult; therefore combination therapy with ceftriaxone is preferred in almost all hospitalized patients.

[**] Cefotaxime requires q 8 hour dosing for treatment of CAP.

ADVANCED GENERATION MACROLIDES: CORRECT SPECTRUM, FIRST-LINE COVERAGE IN OUTPATIENT CAP

The established new generation macrolide antibiotics include the erythromycin analogues azithromycin and clarithromycin.[100,101] Compared to erythromycin, which is the least expensive macrolide, the major advantages of these newer antibiotics are significantly decreased gastrointestinal side effects, which produce enhanced tolerance, improved bioavailability, higher tissue levels, and pharmacokinetic features that permit less frequent dosing and better compliance, as well as enhanced activity against *H. influenzae*.[102,103] In particular, the long tissue half-life of azithromycin allows this antibiotic to be prescribed for a shorter duration (5 days) than comparable antibiotics given for the same indications.

Macrolides in CAP Therapy: An Overview. Given the cost differences between azithromycin and clarithromycin, as well as the improved compliance patterns associated with short-duration therapy, any rational approach to distinguishing between these agents must consider prescription, patient, and drug resistance barriers. From the outset, it is fair to say that these macrolides, to a great degree, have supplanted the use of erythromycin (as well as cephalosporins and tetracyclines) in community-acquired infections of the lower respiratory tract.

In some institutions, this is not the case. Although erythromycin, in particular, has been considered by some to be the antibiotic of choice for CAP, its lack of efficacy against *H. influenzae*, as well as its adverse gastrointestinal side effects, potential for drug-drug interactions, and poor compliance profile, are now recognized as clinically important liabilities in emergency practice.[104,105] It is, however, effective against pneumococcal pneumonia, Mycoplasma pneumonia, and many atypical infections, including Legionella. Food decreases the absorption of erythromycin, which interferes with drug metabolism; therefore, many experts caution this drug should not be considered for use in elderly patients on theophylline or warfarin.[90,99]

From the perspective of providing definitive, cost-effective, and compliance-promoting therapy, the newer macrolide antibiotics, which include both azithromycin and clarithromycin, have recently emerged as some of the drugs of choice—along with the new, extended spectrum quinolones—for outpatient management of CAP.[106] When used as oral agents, they play a central role in management of pneumonia in otherwise healthy elderly individuals who do not require hospitalization.

Macrolides have the advantage of a simplified dosing schedule, especially azithromycin, which is given once daily for only three days (500 mg PO qd x 3 days). Clarithromycin requires a longer (1000 mg/d for 7 days) course of therapy and costs more. In general, the decision to use a macrolide such as azithromycin rather than erythromycin is based on weighing the increased cost of a course of therapy with azithromycin against its real-world advantages, which include a more convenient dosing schedule, its broader spectrum of coverage, its favorable drug interaction profile, and its decreased incidence of gastrointestinal side effects, which occur in 3-5% of patients taking a five-day, multiple-dose regimen.[107] The introduction of a tablet formulation permits consumption of the antibiotic without regard to food ingestion.

Comparative Studies. Although advanced generation fluoroquinolones have enhanced coverage against DRSP as compared to macrolides, most studies suggest comparable outcomes. One prospective, double-blind, multicenter trial reviewed the safety and efficacy of moxifloxacin and clarithromycin in adult patients with radiographically documented CAP.[79] Patients were treated for 10 days with either oral moxifloxacin 400 mg qd, or clarithromycin 500 mg bid. Among 382 patients, both drugs were highly effective, with a 95% clinical resolution rate and 96% bacterial resolution. Drug-related adverse events occurred at comparable rates with the two antibiotics, although nausea and/or vomiting was a more frequent cause of premature discontinuation in the clarithromycin group than in the moxifloxacin group. Taste perversion was almost twice as common in those given clarithromycin (7%) as in those given moxifloxacin (4%).[79]

EXTENDED SPECTRUM FLUOROQUINOLONES, INDICATION FOR INITIAL EMPIRIC USE, INTENSIFICATION OF COVERAGE, AND PATIENT SELECTION

The extended spectrum quinolones—moxifloxacin, levofloxacin, and gatifloxacin—are indicated for treatment of CAP because they are active against many gram-positive organisms that may infect the lower respiratory tract, including *S. pneumoniae* and S. *aureus*, as well as covering atypical pathogens, including *C. pneumoniae, L. pneumophila*, and *M. pneumoniae*. Levofloxacin also is active against gram-negative organisms, including *E. coli, H. influenzae, H. parainfluenzae, Klebsiella pneumoniae*, and *M. catarrhalis*.

Several studies and surveillance data suggest that some newly available, expanded spectrum fluoroquinolones, including levofloxacin (which is approved for PRSP), are efficacious for the treatment of *S. pneumoniae*, including penicillin-resistant strains.[76,80,108] In one study, microbiologic eradication from sputum was reported among all 300 patients with pneumococcal pneumonia treated with oral levofloxacin.[108] In a study of in vitro susceptibility of *S. pneumoniae* clinical isolates to levofloxacin, none of the 180 isolates (including 60 isolates with intermediate susceptibility to penicillin and 60 penicillin-resistant isolates) was resistant to this agent.[76] In addition, a surveillance study of antimicrobial resistance in respiratory tract pathogens found levofloxacin was active against 97% of 9190 pneumococcal isolates and found no cross-resistance with penicillin, amoxicillin-clavulanate, ceftriaxone, cefuroxime, or clarithromycin.

Despite high level activity against pneumococcal isolates and a formal FDA approval/indication for levofloxacin use in suspected DRSP lower respiratory tract infection, the CDCDRSP-WG recent guidelines do not advocate the use of expanded spectrum fluoroquinolones for first-line, empiric treatment of pneumonia. This is because: 1) of their broad, perhaps, over-extended spectrum of coverage that includes a wide range of gram-negative organisms; 2) of concern that resistance among pneumococci will emerge if there is widespread use of this class of antibiotics; 3) their activity against pneumococci with high penicillin resistance (MIC = 4 mcg/mL) makes it important that they be reserved for selected patients with CAP; 4) use of fluoroquinolones has been shown to result in increased resistance to *S. pneumoniae* in vitro; and 5) population-based surveillance in the United States has shown a statistically significant increase in ofloxacin resistance among pneumococcal isolates between Jan. 1, 1995, and Dec. 31, 1997 (unpublished data, Active Bacterial Core Surveillance, CDC).[80]

From a practical, drug selection perspective, the CDCDRSP-WG has recommended that fluoroquinolones be reserved for selected patients with CAP, and these experts have identified specific patient subgroups that are eligible for initial treatment with extended-spectrum fluoroquinolones. However, outpatients with CAP, according to the CDCDRSP-WG and OMBIRT Panel recommendations, are managed preferentially with an oral macrolide (or doxycycline).

For hospitalized patients, advanced generation fluoroquinolones are recommended for adults and elderly patients in whom one of the first-line regimens (cephalosporin plus a macrolide) has failed, those who are allergic to the first-line agents, or those who have a documented infection with highly drug-resistant pneumococci (i.e., penicillin MIC = 4 mcg/mL).[109] Other guideline panels and recommendations, such as those issued by the IDSA (2000) and the ATS (2001), do not prioritize between two-drug, combination (cephalosporin plus macrolide) vs. advanced generation fluoroquinolone monotherapy.

OMBIRT PANEL SUMMARY FOR EMPIRIC ANTIBIOTIC SELECTION IN OUTPATIENTS WITH ABE/COPD AND CAP—MATCHING BUGS WITH DRUGS

A variety of antibiotics are available for outpatient management of pulmonary infections. Although the selection process can be daunting, as mentioned, a sensible approach, accompanied by specific recommendations for antibiotic selection in patients with outpatient bacterial infections of the respiratory tract has been generated by the OMBIRT Panel. Regardless of the specific antimicrobial selected, one of the most important issues for the primary care practitioner is to ensure that the appropriate intensity and spectrum of coverage are provided, according to patient and community/epidemiological risk factors and patterns. The significant majority of cases of both ABE/COPD and CAP are appropriately managed with a macrolide. In the minority of cases (i.e, those in which infection with gram-negative organisms is suspected or if there is structural lung disease), the practitioner, based on clinical judgment, may consider shifting to and intensifying therapy with an extended spectrum quinolone.

ABE/COPD. As a rule, the clinical criteria for initiating antibiotic therapy in patients with a documented history of chronic obstructive pulmonary disease (COPD), and who are suspected of having ABE/COPD, include the presence of at least two of the following three symptoms: increasing purulence of sputum, increasing volume of sputum production, and increasing cough and/or dyspnea. In contrast, patients with symptoms of acute tracheobronchitis who have no previous history of COPD initially should not be treated with antibiotics, since antibiotics have not been shown to improve outcomes in this patient population.

Given concerns about antibiotic overuse and the potential for emerging resistance among DRSP to fluoroquinolones, the panel concurs with other national guidelines specifying advanced generation macrolides such as azithromycin (or clarithromycin) as initial therapy for outpatient ABE/COPD and the use of fluoroquinolones or amoxicillin-clavulanate as alternative agents in patients who fail therapy or who have risk factors predictive of gram-negative infection. Patients who do not respond to oral therapy with one class of antibiotics (relapse) may be treated with a course of antibiotics with different gaps in coverage. Reinfections should be treated with antibiotics that have been shown to be effective in previous exacerbations.

A number of relatively inexpensive, well-tolerated antibiotics also are available, including amoxicillin, trimethoprim-sulfamethoxazole, doxycycline, and tetracycline. Antimicrobial resistance, particularly involving *H. influenzae, M. catarrhalis,* and *S. pneumoniae,* has become increasingly problematic with many of these agents, specifically with older members of each of these drug classes. There is a growth of amoxicillin-resistant, beta-lactamase-producing *H. influenzae.* New agents are providing solutions to these difficulties. The azalide antibiotic azithromycin has the advantage of an appropriate spectrum of coverage, an acceptable safety profile, reasonable cost, and a unique patient-dosing schedule that improves patient compliance.

The newer fluoroquinolones, moxifloxacin, gatifloxacin, and levofloxacin are advantageous when gram-negative bacteria predominate;

ciprofloxacin is another appropriate choice in this subgroup, especially those with structural lung disease such as bronchiectasis and documented infection with gram-negative species such as *Pseudomonas*. When there is documented infection with DRSP, levofloxacin or moxifloxacin are prudent choices. Amoxicillin-clavulanate also has in vitro activity against beta-lactamase-producing *H. influenzae* and *M. catarrhalis*, as well as *S. pneumoniae*; moreover, the agent's clinical efficacy in lower respiratory tract infection attributable to enzyme-producing strains has been demonstrated.

CAP. The overwhelming majority of well-designed, double-blinded, prospective clinical trials comparing new generation macrolides (azithromycin and clarithromycin) vs. new generation fluoroquinolones (moxifloxacin, gatifloxacin, and levofloxacin) demonstrate comparable outcomes in terms of clinical cure and bacteriologic eradication rates in outpatients with CAP. However, emergence of resistance among *S. pneumoniae* species to new generation fluoroquinolones has been reported in a number of geographic regions, including the United States, Hong Kong, and Canada, and this may have implications for treatment.

Although not precisely known, the frequency of DRSP causing outpatient CAP, as estimated by the CDC, is very low (i.e., in the range of 0.14-1.9%). Accordingly, the CDCDRSP-WG cautions against overuse of new generation fluoroquinolones in outpatient CAP, and recommends their use as alternative agents when: 1) first-line therapy with advanced generation macrolides such as azithromycin fails; 2) patients are allergic to first-line agents; or 3) the cases are documented infection with DRSP.

Given concerns about antibiotic overuse, the potential for emerging resistance among DRSP to fluoroquinolones, and the increasing recognition of atypical pathogens as causative agents in patients with outpatient CAP, the OMBIRT Panel concurs with the CDCDRSP-WG recommendation advocating macrolides as initial agents of choice in outpatient CAP. The OMBIRT Panel also noted that the Canadian Consensus Guidelines for CAP Management and the 2001 ATS (American Thoracic Society) Consensus Guideline Recommendations also specify advanced generation macrolides as initial therapy for outpatient CAP.

In this regard, two safe and effective advanced generation macrolides, azithromycin and clarithromycin, currently are available for outpatient, oral-based treatment of CAP (IV azithromycin also is indicated for in-hospital management of patients who are risk-stratified as having more serious disease). Based on outcome-sensitive criteria and pharmatectural considerations such as cost, daily dose frequency, duration of therapy, side effects, and drug interactions, the OMBIRT Panel recommends as first-line, preferred initial therapy in CAP, azithromycin, with clarithromycin or doxycycline as alternative agents; and, as second-line therapy, moxifloxacin, gatifloxacin, or levofloxacin when appropriate, according to CDCDRSP-WG guidelines, epidemiological patterns in the local community, and other association-based protocols issued by the IDSA and ATS.

REFERENCES

1. Statistics VaH. Current Estimates from the National Health Interview Survey. NHS Publication. 1990:1643.

2. Cydulka R, McFadden E, Emerman C, et al. Patterns of hospitalization in elderly

The OMBIRT Consensus Panel and Scientific Roundtable†: **Gideon Bosker, MD, FACEP**, Panel Chairman and Moderator, Yale University School of Medicine; **Bill Billica, MD FAAFP**, Department of Family Practice, Banner Health System, Phoenix, AZ; **Phillip Bonanni, MD**, Primary Care and Internal Medicine, University of Rochester School of Medicine; **Susan I. Fesmire, MD,** Assistant Professor, Department of Internal Medicine, Aston Ambulatory Care Center, The University of Texas Southwestern Medical Center; **Robert Haddon, MD**, Urgency Care Clinics, Cleveland Clinic, Cleveland, OH; **Gary Merlino, DO**, Department of Family Medicine, Mt. Sinai Hospital, Miami, FL; **Sam Sandowski, MD**, Department of Family Practice, SUNY Medical College; **Ethel Smith, MD**, Department of Family Practice, MetroWest Health Center, Cleveland Clinic, Cleveland, OH; **Paul Stander, MD, FACP,** Regional Medical Director, Banner Health System, Phoenix, AZ; **Gregory Volturo, MD, FACEP**, University of Massachusetts Medical School.

* OMBIRT - Outpatient Management of Bacterial Infections in the Respiratory Tract

patients with asthma and chronic obstructive pulmonary disease. *Am J Respir Crit Care Med* 1997;156:1807-1812.

3. Kanner RE, Renzetti AD, Jr., Stanish WM, et al. Predictors of survival in subjects with chronic airflow limitation. *Am J Med* 1983;74:249-255.

4. Salit IE, Mederski B, Morisset R, et al. Azithromycin for the treatment of acute LRTIs: A multicenter, open-label study of infections in medicine. *Infect Med* 1998;15:773-777.

5. Wilson R. The role of infection in COPD. *Chest* 1998;113: 242S-248S.

6. Shu D, et al. A Controlled randomized multicenter trial comparing 5 days of azithromycin to 10-14 days of clarithromycin for the treatment of acute bacterial exacerbations of chronic bronchitis. In: *American Society for Microbiology*. 37th Interscience Conference on Antimicrobial Agents and Chemotherapy; Sept. 28-Oct. 1, 1997; Toronto, Ont. Washington, D.C.; pg. 372.

7. Rosen MJ. Treatment of exacerbations of COPD. *Am Fam Phys* 1992;45:693-697.

8. Cydulka R, McFadden E, Emerman C, et al. Patterns of hospitalization in elderly patients with asthma and chronic obstructive pulmonary disease. *Am J Respir Crit Care Med* 1997;156:1807-1812.

9. Celli BR, Snider GL, Heffner J. Standards for the diagnosis and care of patients with chronic obstructive pulmonary disease. *Am J Respir Crit Care Med* 1995;152:S77-S120.

10. Kanner RE, Renzetti AD, Jr., Stanish WM, et al. Predictors of survival in subjects with chronic airflow limitation. *Am J Med* 1983;74:249-255.

11. Gump DW, Philips CA, Forsyth BR. Role of infection in chronic bronchitis. *Am Rev Respir Dis* 1976;113:465-474.

12. Blasi F, Legnani D, Lombardo VM, et al. *Chlamydia pneumoniae* infection in acute exacerbations of COPD. *Eur Respir J* 1993;6:19-22.

13. Beaty CD, Grayston JT, Wang SPP, et al. *Chlamydia pneumoniae,* strain TWAR, infection in patients with chronic obstructive pulmonary disease. *Am Rev Respir Dis* 1991;144:1408-1410.

14. Rodnick JE, Gude JK. The use of antibiotics in acute bronchitis and acute exacerbations of chronic bronchitis. *West J Med* 1988;149:347-351.

15. Wallace RJ Jr. Newer oral antimicrobials and newer etiologic agents of acute bronchitis and acute exacerbations of chronic bronchitis. *Semin Respir Infect* 1988;3:49-54.

16. Wallace RF Jr, Steele LC, Brooks DL, et al. Amoxicillin/clavulanic acid in the treatment

of lower respiratory tract infections caused by beta-lactamase-positive *Haemophilus influenzae* and *Branhamella catarrhalis. Antimicrob Agents Chemother* 1985;27:912-915.

17. Hopkins SJ. Clinical toleration and safety of azithromycin in adults and children. *Rev Contemp Pharmacother* 1994;5:383-389.

18. Nightingale CH, Belliveau PP, Quintiliani R. Cost issues and considerations when choosing antimicrobial agents. *Infect Dis Clin Pract* 1994;3:8-11.

19. Eller J, Ede A, Schaberg T, et al. Infective exacerbations of chronic bronchitis: Relation between bacteriologic etiology and lung function. *Chest* 1998;113:1542-1548.

20. Knaus WA, Harrell FEJ, Lynn J, et al. The SUPPORT Program prognostic model. Objective estimates of survival for seriously ill hospitalized adults. Study to understand prognosis and preferences for outcomes and risks of treatments. *Ann Intern Med* 1995;122:191-203.

21. Lange P, Nyboe J, Appleyard M, et al. Relationship of ventilatory impairment and of chronic mucous secretion to mortality from chronic obstructive lung disease and from all causes. *Thorax* 1990;45:579-585.

22. Sherman CB, Zu X, et al. Longitudinal lung function decline in subjects with respiratory symptoms. *Am Rev of Resp Dis* 1992;146:855-859.

23. Warren Whitlock on behalf of the Multicenter Chronic Obstructive Pulmonary Disease Study Group. Multicenter comparison of azithromycin and amoxicillin/clavulanate in the treatment of patients with chronic obstructive pulmonary disease. *Curr Therapeutic Res* 1995;56:10.

24. Grossman RF. The value of antibiotics and the outcomes of antibiotic therapy in exacerbations of COPD. *Chest* 1998;113:249S-255S.

25. DebAbate CA, Mathew CP, Warner JH, et al. The safety and efficacy of a short course (5-day) moxifloxacin vs. azithromycin in the treatment of patients with acute exacerbation of chronic bronchitis. *Respir Med* 2000;94:1029-1037.

26. Kreis S, Herrera N, Golzar N, et al. A comparison of moxifloxacin and azithromycin in the treatment of acute exacerbations of chronic bronchitis. *JCOM* 2000;7:33-37.

27. Bauernfreind A, Jungwirth R., Eberlein E. Comparative pharmacodynamics of clarithromycin and azithromycin against respiratory pathogens. *Infection* 1995;23:316-321.

28. Guggenbichler JP, Kastner H. The influence of macrolide antibiotics on the fecal and oral flora. *Infect Medicate* 1998;15(Suppl D):17-25.

29. Adam D, Grimm H, Lode H, et al. Comparative pharmacodynamics of clarithromycin and azithromycin against respiratory pathogens. *Infection* 1996;24:270.

30. Retsema JA. Susceptibility and resistance emergence studies with macrolides. *Int J Antimicrob Agents* 1999;11:S15-S21.

31. Girard AE, Cimochowski CR, Faiella JA. Correlation of increased azithromycin concentrations with phagocyte infiltration into sites of localized infection. *J Antimicrob Chemother* 1996;37(Suppl. C):9-19.

32. Chodosh S, Schreurs A, Siami G, et al. Efficacy of oral ciprofloxacin vs. clarithromycin for treatment of acute bacterial exacerbations of chronic bronchitis. The Bronchitis Study Group. *Clin Infect Dis* 1998;27:730-738.

33 Fagon JY, Chastre J. Severe exacerbations of COPD patients: The role of pulmonary infections. *Semin Respir Infect* 1996;11:109-118.

34. Gump DW, Philips CA, Forsyth BR. Role of infection in chronic bronchitis. *Am Rev Respir Dis* 1976;113:465-474.

35. Blasi F, Legnani D, Lombardo VM, et al. *Chlamydia pneumoniae* infection in acute exacerbations of COPD. *Eur Respir J* 1993;6:19-22.

36. Beaty CD, Grayston JT, Wang SP, et al. Chlamydia pneumoniae, strain TWAR, infection in patients with chronic obstructive pulmonary disease. *Am Rev Respir Dis* 1991;144:1408-1410.

37. Eller J, Ede A, Schaberg T, et al. Infective exacerbations of chronic bronchitis: Relation between bacteriologic etiology and lung function. *Chest* 1998;113:1542-1548.

38. Saint S, Bent S, Vittinghoff E, et al. Antibiotics in chronic obstructive pulmonary disease exacerbations. A meta-analysis [see comments]. *JAMA* 1995;273:957-960.

39. Ball P, Harris JM, Lowson D, et al. Acute infective exacerbations of chronic bronchitis. *QJM* 1995;88:61-68.

40. Macfarlane JT, Colville A, Guion A, et al. Prospective study of etiology and outcome of adult lower-respiratory-tract infections in the community. *Lancet* 1993;341:511-514.

41. Wilson R. The role of infection in COPD. *Chest* 1998;113:242S-248S.

42. Shu D, et al. A controlled randomized multicenter trial comparing 5 days of azithromycin to 10-14 days of clarithromycin for the treatment of acute bacterial exacerbations of chronic bronchitis. In: American Society for Microbiology, ed. 37th Interscience Conference on Antimicrobial Agents and Chemotherapy; 1997 Sept.-Oct. 28-1; Toronto, Ont. Washington, D.C.; 1997:372

43. Rosen MJ. Treatment of exacerbations of COPD. *Am Fam Phys* 1992;45:693-697.

44. Rodnick JE, Gude JK. The use of antibiotics in acute bronchitis and acute exacerbations of chronic bronchitis. *West J Med* 1988;149:347-351.

45. Wallace RJ, Jr. Newer oral antimicrobials and newer etiologic agents of acute bronchitis and acute exacerbations of chronic bronchitis. *Semin Respir Infect* 1988;3:49-54.

46. Wallace RF Jr, Steele LC, Brooks DL, et al. Amoxicillin/clavulanic acid in the treatment of lower respiratory tract infections caused by beta-lactamase-positive *Haemophilus influenzae* and *Branhamella catarrhalis*. *Antimicrob Agents Chemother* 1985;27:912-915.

47. Hopkins SJ. Clinical toleration and safety of azithromycin in adults and children. *Rev Contemp Pharmacother* 1994;5:383-389.

48. Nightingale CH, Belliveau PP, Quintiliani R. Cost issues and considerations when choosing antimicrobial agents. *Infect Dis Clin Pract* 1994;3:8-11.

49. Chodosh S, DeAbate CA, et al. Short-course moxifloxacin therapy for treatment of acute bacterial excaerbations of chronic bronchitis. *Respir Med* 2000;94:18-27.

50. Wilson R, Kubin R, et al. Five-day moxifloxacin comparedd with 7 day clarithromycin for the treatment of acute exacerbations of chronic bronchitis. *J Anitimicrob Ther* 1999;44:501-513.

51. Destache CJ, Dewan N, O'Donohue WJ, et al Clinical and economic considerations in the treatment of acute exacerbations of chronic bronchitis. *J Antimicrob Chemother* 1999;43:A107-A113.

52. Davies. J. Inactivation of antibiotics and the dissemination of resistance genes. *Science* 1994;264:375-382.

53. Jorgensen JH, Doern GV, Maher LA, et al. Antimicrobial resistance among respiratory isolates of *Haemophilus influenzae, Moraxella catarrhalis,* and *Streptococcus pneumoniae* in the United States. *Antimicrob Agents Chemother* 1990;34:2075-2080.

54. Doern GV. Trends in antimicrobial susceptibility of bacterial pathogens of the respiratory tract. *Am J Med* 1995;99:3S-7S.

55. Knaus WA, Harrell FEJ, Lynn J, et al. The SUPPORT Program prognostic model. Objective estimates of survival for seriously ill hospitalized adults. Study to understand prognosis and preferences for outcomes and risks of treatments. *Ann Intern Med* 1995:122:191-203.

56. Lange P, Nyboe J, Appleyard M, et al. Relationship of ventilatory impairment and of

chronic mucous secretion to mortality from chronic obstructive lung disease and from all causes. *Thorax* 1990;45:579-585.

57. Sherman CB, Zu X, et al. Longitudinal lung function decline in subjects with respiratory symptoms. *Am Rev of Resp Dis* 1992;146:855-859.

58. Tashkin DP, Bleecker E, Braun S, et al. Results of a multicenter study of nebulized inhalant bronchodilator solutions. *Am J Med* 1996;100:62S-69S.

59. Cazzola M, Di Perna F, Noschese P, et al. Effects of formoterol, salmeterol or oxitropium bromide on airway responses to salbutamol in COPD. *Eur Respir J* 1998;11:1337-1341.

60. Corris PA, Neville E, Nariman S, et al. Dose-response study of inhaled salbutamol powder in chronic airflow obstruction. *Thorax* 1983;38:292-296.

61. Colice GL. Nebulized bronchodilators for outpatient management of stable chronic obstructive pulmonary disease. *Am J Med* 1996;100:11S-18S.

62. Rennard Sa, Serby Ca, Ghafouri Ma, et al. Extended therapy with ipratropium is associated with improved lung function in patients with COPD. *Chest* 1996;110:62-70.

63. Friedman M. A multicenter study of nebulized bronchodilator solutions in chronic obstructive pulmonary disease. *Am J Med* 1996;100:30S-39S.

64. Chanez P, Vignola AM, O'Shaugnessy T, et al. Corticosteroid reversibility in COPD is related to features of asthma. *Am J Respir Crit Care Med* 1997;155:1529-1534.

65. Kerstjens Ha, Brand Pa, Hughes Ma, et al. A comparison of bronchodilator therapy with or without inhaled corticosteroid therapy for obstructive airways disease. *N Engl J Med* 1992;327:1413-1419.

66. Pauwels R, Claes-Goran L, Laitinen L, et al. Long-term treatment with inhaled budesonide in persons with mild chronic obstructive pulmonary disease who continue smoking. *N Engl J Med* 1999;340:1948-1953.

67. Saint S, Bent S, Vittinghoff E, et al. Antibiotics in chronic obstructive pulmonary disease exacerbations. A meta-analysis [see comments]. *JAMA* 1995;273:957-960.

68. Bosker G. *Pharmatecture: Minimizing Medications To Maximize Results.* St. Louis: Facts and Comparisons; 1999.

69. Salit IE, Mederski B, Morisset R, et al. Azithromycin for the treatment of acute LRTIs: A multicenter, open-label study. *Infect Med* 1998;15:773-777.

70. Destache CJ, Dewan N, O'Donohue OJ, et al. Clinical and economic considerations in the treatment of acute exacerbations of chronic bronchitis. *J Antimicrob Chemother*

1999;43:107-113.

71.   Bartlett JG, Mundy M. Community-acquired pneuominia. *N Engl J Med* 1995;333:1618-1624.

72.   Fine MD, Smith MA, et al. Prognosis and outcomes of patients with community acquired pneumonia. A meta-analysis. *JAMA* 1996;275:134-141.

73.   Marrie TJ, Lau CY, Wheeler SL, et al. A controlled trial of a critical pathway for treatment of community-acquired pneumonia. *JAMA* 2000;283:749-755.

74.   Dean NC, Suchyta MR, Bateman KA. Implementation of admission decision support for community-acquired pneumonia. A pilot study. *Chest* 2000;117:1368-1377.

75.   Flanders WD, Tucker G, Krishnadasan A, et al. Validation of the pneumonia severity index: Importance of study-specific recalibration. *J Gen Intern Med* 1999;14:333-340.

76.   Kulgman KP, Capper T, et al In vitro susceptibility of penicillin-resistant S. pneumoniae to levofloxacin, selection of resistant mutants, and time-kill synergy studies of levofloxacin combined with vancomycin, telcoplanin, fusidic acid, and rifampin. *Antimicrob Agents Chemother* 1996;40:2802-2804.

77.   Levaquin Product Information. Ortho-McNeil Pharmaceuticals. January 1997.

78.   Vincent J, et al. Pharmacokinetics and safety of trovafloxacin in healthy male volunteers following administration of single intravenous doses of the prodrug, alatrofloxacin. *J Antimicrob Chemother* 1997;39(supp B):75-80.

79.   Fogarty C, Grossman C, et al. Efficacy and safety of moxifloxacin vs clarithromycin in community-acquired pneumonia. *Infect Med* 1999;16:11.

80.   Heffelfinger JD, Dowell SF, et al. A report from the Drug-resistant Streptococcus pneumoniae Therapeutic Working Group. Management of community-acquired pneumonia in the era of pneumococcal resistance. *Arch Int Med* 2000;160:1399.

81.   Hoe LK, Keang LT. Hospitalized low-risk community-acquired pneumonia: Outcome and potential for cost-savings. *Respirology* 1999;4:307-309.

82.   Fine MJ, Auble TE, Yealy DM, et al. A prediction rule to identify low-risk patients with community-acquired pneumonia. *N Engl J Med* 1997;336:243-250.

83.   Auble TE, Yealy DM, Fine MJ. Assessing prognosis and selecting an initial site of care for adults with community-acquired pneumonia. *Infect Dis Clin North Am* 1998;2:741-759.

84.   Dean NC. Use of prognostic scoring and outcome assessment tools in the admission decision for community-acquired pneumonia. *Clin Chest Med* 1999;20:521-529.

85. Farr BM, Sloman AJ, Fisch MJ. Predicting death in patients hospitalized for community-acquired pneumonia. *Ann Intern Med* 1991;115:428-436.

86. Fine JM, Smith MA, Carson CA, et al. Prognosis and outcomes of patients with community-acquired pneumonia. *JAMA* 1996;275:134-141.

87. Houston MS, Silverstein MD, Suman VJ. Risk factors for 30-Day mortality in elderly patients with lower respiratory tract infection. *Arch Intern Med* 1997;157:2190-2195.

88. Conte HA, Chen YT, Mehal W, et al. A prognostic rule for elderly patients admitted with community-acquired pneumonia. *Am J Med* 1999;106:20-28.

89. Ewig S, Kleinfeld T, Bauer T, et al. Comparative validation of prognostic rules for community-acquired pneumonia in an elderly population. *Eur Respir J* 1999;14:370-375.

90. Mylotte JM, Naughton B, Saludades C, et al. Validation and application of the pneumonia prognosis index to nursing home residents with pneumonia. *JAGS* 1998;46:1538-1544.

91. Marston BJ, Plouffe JF, et al. Incidence of community-acquired pneumonia requiring hospitalization. Results of a population-based active surveillance study in Ohio. The Community-Based Pneumonia Incidence Study Group. *Arch Int Med* 1997;157:1709-1718.

92. Atlas SJ, Benzer TI, Borowsky LH, et al. Safely increasing the proportion of patients with community-acquired pneumonia treated as outpatients. An interventional trial. *Arch Intern Med* 1998;158:1350-1356.

93. American Thoracic Society: Guidelines for the Initial Management of adults with Community-Acquired Pneumonia: Diagnosis, Assessment of Severity, and Initial Antimicrobial Therapy. *Am Rev Respir Dis* 1993;148:1418-1426.

94. Ewig S, Ruiz M, Mensa J, et al. Severe community-acquired pneumonia. Assessment of severity criteria. *Am J Respir Crit Care Med* 1998;158:1102-1108.

95. Marrie TJ. Community-acquired pneumonia: Epidemiology, etiology, treatment. *Infect Dis Clinic North Am* 1998;12:723-740.

96. Brentsson E, Lagergard T. Etiology of community-acquired pneumonia in outpatients. *Eur J Clin Microbiol* 1986;5:446-447.

97. Langille DB, Yates L, Marrie TJ. Serological investigation of pneumonia as it presents to the physician's office. *Can J Infect Dis* 1993;4:328.

98. Whitney CG, Barrett N, et al. Increasing prevalence of drug-resistant Streptococcus pneumoniae (DRSP): Implications for therapy for pneumonia. In: Programs and

Abstracts of the 36th Annual Meeting of the Infectious Disease Society of America, November 12-15, 1998. IDSA, Abstract 51.

99.   Antibiotic Update 1998: Outcome-effective treatment for bacterial infections managed in the primary care and emergency department setting. *Emerg Med Rep* 1997;18:1-24.

100.   Enoxacin-A new fluoroquinolone. *Med Lett Drugs Ther* 1992;34:103-105.

101.   Cooper B, Lawer M. Pneumococcal bacteremia during ciprofloxacin therapy for pneumococcal pneumonia. *Am J Med* 1989;87:475.

102.   Flynn CM, et al. In vitro efficacy of levofloxacin alone or in combination tested against multi-resistant *Pseudomonas aeruginosa* strains. *J Chemother* 1996;8:411-415.

103.   Dholakia N, et al. Susceptibilities of bacterial isolates from patients with cancer to levofloxacin and other quinolones. *Antimicrob Agents Chemother* 1994;38:848-852.

104.   Garibaldi RA. Epidemiology of community-acquired respiratory tract infections in adults. Incidence, etiology, and impact. *Am J Med* 1985;78:32-37.

105.   Fang GD, Fine M, Orloff J, et al. New and emerging etiologies for community-acquired pneumonia with implications for therapy. *Medicine* 1990;69:307-316.

106.   Habib MP, et al. Intersci Conf Antimicrob Agents Chemother 1996;36. Abstract L002. 36th Interscience Conference on Antimicrobial Agents and Chemotherapy. New Orleans, LA. Sept. 15-18, 1996.

107.   File TM, et al. Abstr Intersci Conf Antimicrob Agents Chemother 1996;36. Abstract L001 (LM1). 36th Interscience Conference on Antimicrobial Agents and Chemotherapy. New Orleans, LA. Sept. 15-18, 1996.

108.   File TM, Dunbar L, et al. A multicenter, randomized study comparing the efficacy and safety of intravenous and/or oral levofloxacin versus ceftriaxone and/or cefuroxime in treatment of adults with community-acquired pneumonia. *Antimicrob Agents Chemother* 1997;41:1965-1972.

109.   Cleeland R, Squires E. Antimicrobial activity of ceftriaxone: A review. *Am J Med* 1984;77:3.

KEY, SELECTED REFERENCES

1.   Sethi S. Infectious exacerbations of chronic bronchitis: Diagnosis and management. *J Antimicrob Chemother* 1999;43(Suppl A): 97-105. Review.

2.   Sachs FL. Chronic bronchitis. *Clin Chest Med* 1981;2:79-89. Review.

3. Ball P, Tillotson G, Wilson R. Chemotherapy for chronic bronchitis. Controversies. *Presse Med* 1995;24:189-194. Review.

4. Grossman RF. Acute exacerbations of chronic bronchitis. *Hosp Pract* 1997;32:85-89, 92-94.

5. Sethi S. Infectious etiology of acute exacerbations of chronic bronchitis. *Chest* 2000;117(5 Suppl 2):380S-3855S. Review.

6. Zuck P, Rio Y. [Antibiotic therapy in exacerbations of chronic bronchitis]. *Presse Med* 1997;26:1492-1494. French.

7. Read RC. Infection in acute exacerbations of chronic bronchitis: A clinical perspective. *Respir Med* 1999;93:845-850. Review.

8. Niederman MS. [Clinical contribution of the newer fluoroquinolones in acute bacterial exacerbation of chronic bronchitis]. *Medicina* (B Aires). 1999;59(Suppl 1):23-30. Spanish.

9. Nicotra MB, Kronenberg RS. Con: antibiotic use in exacerbations of chronic bronchitis. *Semin Respir Infect* 1993;8:254-258. Review.

10. Verghese A, Ismail HM. Acute exacerbations of chronic bronchitis. Preventing treatment failures and early reinfection. *Postgrad Med* 1994;96:75-76, 79-82, 87-89. Review.

11. Isada CM. Pro: Antibiotics for chronic bronchitis with exacerbations. *Semin Respir Infect* 1993;8:243-253. Review.

12. Adams SG, Anzueto A. Antibiotic therapy in acute exacerbations of chronic bronchitis. *Semin Respir Infect* 2000;15:234-247. Review.

13. Carbon C. Acute and chronic bronchitis. *Microb Drug Resist* 1995;1:159-162. Review.

14. Buchenroth M. [Antibiotic therapy in bronchial infections. 1: Acute and chronic bronchitis]. *MMW Fortschr Med* 1999;141:49-50. German.

15. Grossman RF. Management of acute exacerbation of chronic bronchitis. *Can Respir J* 1999;6(Suppl A):40A-45A. Review.

16. Wilson R. Ten years of ciprofloxacin: the past, present and future. Acute exacerbations of chronic bronchitis. Introduction. *J Antimicrob Chemother* 1999;43(Suppl A):95-6.

17. Wilson R, Wilson CB. Defining subsets of patients with chronic bronchitis. *Chest* 1997;112(6 Suppl):303S-309S. Review.

18. McHardy VU, Inglis JM, Calder MA, et al. A study of infective and other factors in exacerbations of chronic bronchitis. *Br J Dis Chest* 1980;74:228-238.

19.   Grossman RF. How do we achieve cost-effective options in lower respiratory tract infection therapy? *Chest* 1998;113(3 Suppl): 205S-210S.

20.   Wilson R, Grossman R. Introduction: The role of bacterial infection in chronic bronchitis. *Semin Respir Infect* 2000;15:1-6. Review.

21.   Niroumand M, Grossman RF. Airway infection. *Infect Dis Clin North Am* 1998;12:671-688. Review.

22.   Adams SG, Anzueto A. Treating acute exacerbations of chronic bronchitis in the face of antibiotic resistance. *Cleve Clin J Med* 2000;67:625-628, 631-633. Review.

23.   Ayoub A, Rekik WK. [Chronic bronchitis exacerbations: justifications and indications of antibiotic therapy]. *Tunis Med* 1996;74:271-276. Review. French.

24.   Ball P, Make B. Acute exacerbations of chronic bronchitis: An international comparison. *Chest* 1998;113(3 Suppl):199S-204S.

25.   Riise GC, Larsson S, Larsson P, et al. The intrabronchial microbial flora in chronic bronchitis patients: A target for N-acetylcysteine therapy? *Eur Respir J* 1994;7:94-101.

26.   Donner CF. Infectious exacerbations of chronic bronchitis. ORIONE Board. Monaldi *Arch Chest Dis* 1999;54:43-48. Review.

27.   Allegra L, Catena E, Pozzi E, et al. [Effectiveness of and tolerance to ceftibuten in the treatment of chronic bacterial bronchitis exacerbations in an elderly population]. *Minerva Med* 1996;87: 479-485. Italian.

28.   Niederman MS. Antibiotic therapy of exacerbations of chronic bronchitis. *Semin Respir Infect* 2000;15:59-70. Review.

29.   Ball P, Harris JM, Lowson D, et al. Acute infective exacerbations of chronic bronchitis. *QJM* 1995;88:61-68.

30.   Ball P. Infective pathogenesis and outcomes in chronic bronchitis. *Curr Opin Pulm Med* 1996;2:181-185. Review.

31.   Paster RZ, McAdoo MA, Keyserling CH, et al. A comparison of a five-day regimen of cefdinir with a seven-day regimen of loracarbef for the treatment of acute exacerbations of chronic bronchitis. *Int J Clin Pract* 2000;54:293-299.

32.   San Pedro G, George R. Treating acute exacerbations of chronic bronchitis. *Hosp Pract* (Off Ed). 2000;35:43-50. Review.

33.   Grossman RF. Guidelines for the treatment of acute exacerbations of chronic bronchitis. *Chest* 1997;112(6 Suppl):310S-313S. Review.

34.   Finch RG. A review of worldwide experience with sparfloxacin in the treatment of com-

munity-acquired pneumonia and acute bacterial exacerbations of chronic bronchitis. *Int J Antimicrob Agents* 1999;12:5-17. Review.

35.   Shteingardt IN, Bukreeva EB, Khristoliubova EI, et al. [Etiologic structure of exacerbations in chronic bronchitis]. *Ter Arkh* 1988;60:93-95. Russian.

36.   Gonzales R, Sande MA. Acute bronchitis in the healthy adult. *Curr Clin Top Infect Dis* 2000;20:158-173. Review.

37.   Melbye H, Berdal BP. [Acute bronchitis in adults. Clinical findings, microorganisms and use of antibiotics]. *Tidsskr Nor Laegeforen* 1994;114:814-817. Norwegian.

38.   Robertson CE, Ford MJ, Munro JF, et al. The efficacy of a new formulation of trimethoprim and sulphadiazine in acute exacerbations of chronic bronchitis. *Methods Find Exp Clin Pharmacol* 1983;5:127-129.

39.   Staley H, McDade HB, Paes D. Is an objective assessment of antibiotic therapy in exacerbations of chronic bronchitis possible? *J Antimicrob Chemother* 1993;31:193-197. Review.

40.   Hamacher J, Vogel F, Lichey J, et al. Treatment of acute bacterial exacerbations of chronic obstructive pulmonary disease in hospitalised patients-a comparison of meropenem and imipenem/cilastatin. COPD Study Group. *J Antimicrob Chemother* 1995;36(Suppl A):121-133.

41.   Zithromax® Package Insert. Pfizer, Inc. Revised, May 2002

CME QUESTIONS

16.   Antimicrobial coverage in patients with ABE/COPD typically requires using an antibiotic that covers which of the following organism(s)?

A.   *S. pneumoniae*

B.   *M. catarrhalis*

C.   *H. influenzae*

D.   All of the above

E.   None of the above

17.   Antimicrobial coverage in patients with CAP typically requires using an antibiotic that covers the following organism(s):

A.   *S. pneumoniae* and *C. pneumoniae.*

B.   *M. catarrhalis* and *Legionella.*

C.   *H. influenzae* and *Mycoplasma pneumoniae.*

D.   All of the above

E.   None of the above

18. As a rule, antimicrobial therapy is indicated in patients who have at least two of the following three symptoms:

A.   increased wheezing, fever, or rhinorrhea.

B.   increased purulence, malaise, and rhinorrhea.

C.   increasing purulence of sputum, increasing sputum volume, or increasing cough/dyspnea.

D.   All of the above

E.   None of the above

19. Use of antibiotics for "chronic prophylaxis" against ABE/COPD should be:

A.   encouraged in older patients with emphysema.

B.   encouraged in younger patients with recurrent acute bronchitis.

C.   encouraged in patients on oxygen therapy.

D.   discouraged.

20. Which of the following fluoroquinolone antibiotics are approved as a five-day course for the treatment of ABE/COPD?

A.   TMP/SMX and clarithromycin

B.   Clarithromycin and levofloxacin

C.   Clarithromycin and azithromycin

D.   Moxifloxacin

E.   None of the above

21. According to the CDC Drug-Resistant Streptococcus pneumoniae Working Group (CDCDRSP-WG), the frequency of DRSP causing out-patient CAP is estimated to be about:

A.   0.14-1.9%.

B.   14%-19%.

    C.   1.4-9%.

    D.   19%-41%.

    E.   None of the above

22.   Which of the following is *not* encouraged for outpatient management of patients with CAP?

    A.   Initiating therapy within the first eight hours of diagnosis

    B.   Instructing patients in medication compliance

    C.   Verbal or on-site re-evaluation withing three days or sooner

    D.   Follow-up CXR

    E.   All of the above

For instructions on how to participate in this CME activity, please see the back of this book (page 717).

Outcome-Effective Management of Acute Coronary Syndromes: Guidelines, Protocols, and Recommendations for Treatment

INTRODUCTION

Over the past decade, impressive reductions in mortality, reinfarction, and length of hospital stay have been reported in large-scale studies of patients with acute myocardial infarction (AMI). Despite these advances, substantial challenges remain in identifying the optimal combination of therapeutic agents (e.g., fibrinolytics, low-molecular weight heparins [LMWHs] or unfractionated heparin [UFH], and glycoprotein [GP] IIb/IIIa inhibitors) that will maximize outcomes while minimizing drug-related adverse events in patients with ST-elevation myocardial infarction (STEMI).

When one considers percutaneous interventional approaches (angioplasty and stenting), in addition to these various pharmacologic options available for establishing coronary reperfusion, the decision-making process for providers at all levels becomes even more difficult. Regardless of the modality used to establish reperfusion, there are a number of pathophysiological and clinical issues that must be factored into the efficacy and safety equation evaluating optimal medical approaches to AMI management. These include, among other considerations, suboptimal macroperfusion and

Authors: **Charles V. Pollack, Jr., MA, MD, FACEP**, Chairman, Department of Emergency Medicine Pennsylvania Hospital, Associate Professor of Emergency Medicine, University of Pennsylvania School of Medicine, Philadelphia, PA, and **Marc Cohen, MD,** Director of Clinical Research, Hahnemann University Hospital, Professor of Medicine, MCP-Hahnemann University School of Medicine, Philadelphia, PA.

microperfusion, recurrent ischemia, reinfarction, and the risk of intracranial hemorrhage.

It also is clear that anticoagulant agents, especially LMWHs, have continued to play a central—and based on the results of recent clinical trials, an increasingly important—role in pharmacological reperfusion therapy for AMI. Until recently, UFH and aspirin, along with a fibrinolytic agent, routinely were administered to most patients with acute coronary ischemia. However, recent trials (ASSENT-3, HART II, and ENTIRE) support a pivotal role for the LMWH enoxaparin in the setting of fibrinolysis.[1-3] Compared to UFH, enoxaparin has more predictable kinetics, is less protein-bound, has less potential for inducing platelet activation, and requires no monitoring; this is a combination of benefits that provides a strong foundation for achieving potentially better outcomes when this LMWH is given in combination with fibrinolytic agents.

The track record of enoxaparin's success—and its superiority to UFH—in unstable angina (UA) and non-ST elevation MI (NSTEMI) has been impressive; therefore, the rapidly evolving story of its outcome-enhancing role in STEMI should come as no surprise to clinicians who follow the evolution of reperfusion strategies. Most previous studies comparing enoxaparin to UFH in unstable angina have demonstrated less reocclusion, enhanced late patency of the infarct-related vessel, and/or a reduction in reinfarction rate when compared with UFH. The superior outcomes with enoxaparin vs. UFH across the entire spectrum of acute coronary syndromes (ACS), including its most recent value in STEMI as reported in ASSENT-3, have lifted this antithrombin agent to a prominent and unique position among pharmacological modalities used to manage acute coronary ischemia.

As would be expected, GP IIb/IIIa inhibitors also have undergone intense scrutiny for their role in the management of STEMI, and the results of adding this class of agents to fibrinolytic therapy have been mixed. Pilot studies with platelet GP IIb/IIIa inhibitors and reduced-dose fibrinolytic agents have shown enhanced patency of the epicardial infarct-related artery, and signs of improved tissue reperfusion.

The phase III Global Use of Strategies to Open Occluded Coronary Arteries (GUSTO)-V trial of 16,588 patients demonstrated a reduction in ischemic complications of STEMI with half-dose reteplase and abciximab, as compared to full-dose reteplase alone. The incidence of any ischemic or bleeding complication was 31.7% in the reteplase group and 28.6% in the combination group (p < 0.0001). GUSTO-V, however, failed to show a significant reduction in 30-day mortality, and there was a significant increase in non-cerebral bleeding complications with combination therapy at seven days. Particularly concerning was that the incidence of intracranial hemorrhage was twice as high in the combination arm as in the reteplase arm, although the difference did not quite reach significance (p = 0.069).[4] These considerations were seen as offsetting potential benefits and dampening enthusiasm for an imminent paradigm shift that would routinely include abciximab as a preferred agent in fibrinolytic protocols in the absence of percutaneous coronary intervention (PCI).

Although fibrinolysis is widely available and has demonstrated its ability to improve coronary flow, limit infarct size, and improve survival in AMI patients, many individuals with STEMI are not considered suitable candidates for such treatment. Patients with absolute or relative contraindications to fibrinolytic therapy and cardiogenic shock, for example, must receive prompt reperfusion therapy via some alternative means. The prevalence of such limitations has led many clinicians to advocate PCI as the primary therapy and treatment of choice for AMI.

PCI, which may include percutaneous transluminal coronary angioplasty (PTCA) and coronary stenting, has many theoretical and practical advantages over fibrinolysis and is becoming the preferred strategy for most patients with AMI. First, there is a larger patient eligibility pool for PCI, a lower risk of intracranial bleeding, and a significantly higher initial reperfusion rate. This strategy always affords earlier definition of coronary artery anatomy and the ability to risk stratify patients invasively, thereby permitting rapid triage to surgical intervention when indicated. On the other hand, many patients with STEMI present to centers at which PCI is not readily available.

Several trials of varying sizes comparing primary PCI with fibrinolysis have been reported in the past 10 years. Interventions in the early trials were performed using PTCA, prior to the current widespread use of coronary stents. Despite a clear and consistent benefit of primary PTCA in restoring patency of the infarct-related artery, differences in mortality in the individual trials have been difficult to evaluate due to small sample sizes and differences in study design, patient selection, and medical therapy. However, recent trials comparing coronary stenting to fibrinolysis have been more definitive in clarifying the superiority of invasive techniques in the management of appropriately risk-stratified patients with ACS.

With these clinical controversies and treatment options in clear focus, the authors of this review and its accompanying protocols critically evaluate recent clinical trials and outline an evidence-based strategy that employs pharmacological and/or invasive interventions based on risk-group stratification for maximizing outcomes in patients with STEMI.

Likewise, the optimal evaluation and management of patients with suspected ACS who do not manifest the electrocardiographic features of STEMI have been a recent focus of intense study, updated guidelines, and controversy. In non-ST-segment elevation (NSTE) ACS, debate has centered on optimal means of risk stratification, aggressiveness of medical therapy tied to assigned risk, and the overall need and urgency of interventional management and revascularization. Updated guidelines published by the American College of Cardiology (ACC) and American Heart Association (AHA) provide evidence-based recommendations to address these issues. As in STEMI, the LMWH enoxaparin is specifically cited as a preferred therapeutic agent. The authors will address issues specific to NSTEMI and also provide CEVAT-endorsed pathways for these patients.

OVERVIEW OF GUIDELINES

A wide range of mechanical and pharmacological options are available for restoring perfusion in coronary arteries that have been occluded by thrombosis in AMI. These include: 1) PCI (intracoronary stenting and/or angioplasty); 2) fibrinolysis, which may include some combination of a fibrinolytic agent, an anticoagulant, and aspirin; or 3) fibrinolysis-facilitated mechanical reperfusion (i.e., pretreatment with a fibrinolytic agent or some combination of a fibrinolytic agent and GP IIb/IIIa platelet antagonist followed by PCI).

Determining which of these approaches is optimal for a patient can be difficult, and requires a multi-factorial assessment. In this regard, the best approach for establishing coronary reperfusion after STEMI depends on a number of clinical factors, among them: patient eligibility for specific interventions (medical vs invasive) based on risk stratification; adherence to risk-stratification protocols; availability of institutional resources for performing interventional techniques; availability of cardiologists with sufficient experience in percutaneous coronary reperfusion techniques; the ability to provide prompt transfer to another hospital for patients who may require PCI; and the presence of exclusion and inclusion factors that determine patient eligibility for fibrinolysis.

The key point is that selection of a reperfusion strategy is a fluid process that must account for myriad patient, institutional, and risk factors to yield optimal outcomes. *(Please see Figures, in which protocols for evaluating and managing acute coronary syndromes are presented.)*

Although the guidelines presented in this review prioritize some strategies and agents over others, the dominant approach for a particular patient type identified in the guidelines may not always be the most suitable strategy for the individual patient if institutional, timing, or physician factors are not synchronized with the implementation of a specific intervention. Accordingly, sound clinical judgment should prevail when applying guidelines articulated in this review.

CANDIDATES FOR FIBRINOLYSIS

Optimizing outcomes in patients with ACS requires matching patients with strategies that will produce the best results in specific clinical subgroups. Identifying those patients who represent ideal candidates for fibrinolysis, and who are likely to have outcomes that are at least as favorable as they would have with percutaneous interventions, has become an area of intense focus among cardiologists and emergency physicians. A number of factors that should be considered when assessing patients with AMI for either percutaneous or fibrinolytic therapy are discussed in the following sections.

Patient Age. In general, published trials do not provide evidence to support withholding fibrinolytic therapy on the basis of a patient's age alone. In fact, the Fibrinolytic Therapy Trialists' (FTT) Collaborative Group concluded that, "clearly, age alone should no longer be considered a contraindication to fibrinolytic therapy."[5] At the same time, it must be recognized that patients older than age 75 do have a higher incidence of hemorrhagic stroke than younger patients. Moreover, the recent GUSTO-V trial suggested a greater incidence of adverse outcomes when abciximab was combined with UFH and tenecteplase in patients older than age 75.[4] This must be balanced in the individual patient against the consideration that older patients are more likely to die with STEMI if treated conservatively.

Time from Chest Pain Onset—The Therapeutic Window. The generally accepted therapeutic time window for administration of a fibrinolytic agent after the onset of ST segment elevation AMI is 6-12 hours. Considerable data support this time period.[5-13] Without question, the earlier treatment is initiated, the greater the likelihood that the patient will experience a good outcome. This is the case in patients who present within the first six hours of AMI. Delayed administration (i.e., those occurring between 6 and 12 hours after AMI onset) also confers benefit, although of a lesser magnitude.[14]

The Late Assessment of Fibrinolytic Efficiency (LATE) trial, which compared fibrinolytic therapy with placebo, found a significant 26% decrease in 35-day mortality in patients treated with alteplase, heparin, and aspirin 6-12 hours after the onset of symptoms.[15] There is no significant decrease in mortality among patients treated 12-24 hours after symptom onset. These studies, then, clearly establish benefit from treatment at 0 to 12 hours in patients who are otherwise appropriate candidates for fibrinolytic therapy. Treatment beyond that time is not supported by results of currently available trials. The exception may be a patient with a "stuttering" pattern of chest pain between 12 and 24 hours after symptom onset, emphasizing the importance of an adequate history. If there is evidence of marked ST segment elevation on a 12-lead ECG, the patient should be considered at least a potential fibrinolytic candidate.

Previous Myocardial Infarction or Coronary Artery Bypass Grafting. In the setting of AMI, a previous myocardial infarction (MI) should not preclude consideration for treatment with fibrinolytic agents, although there is evidence that PCI may be preferable.[5] Without treatment, there is a potential for greater loss of function in the newly infarcting region of the myocardium. Although the GISSI-1 trial showed no treatment benefits with fibrinolytic therapy in patients with previous MI,[16] the ISIS-2 trial demonstrated a 26% relative mortality rate reduction for patients with previous MIs treated with fibrinolytic therapy.[7] The FTT (Fibrinolytic Therapy Trialists') Collaborative Group meta-analysis further demonstrates that patients with a history of past MI who receive fibrinolytic therapy for recurrent AMI have a mortality rate of 12.5%, compared with 14.1% among control patients.[5]

Many studies have reported successful fibrinolysis in AMI patients with prior coronary artery bypass graft (CABG). Complete thrombotic occlusion of the bypass graft is the cause of AMI in approximately 75% of cases, as opposed to native vessel occlusion. It has been suggested that because of the large mass of thrombus and absent flow in the graft, conventional fibrinolytic therapy may be inadequate to restore flow. Because patients who have undergone CABG may be relatively resistant to fibrinolytic therapy, they should be considered for direct angioplasty or combined fibrinolysis and angioplasty; fibrinolysis is appropriate if PCI is not available.[17]

Stroke. A history of previous stroke or transient ischemic attack (TIA) is a major risk factor for hemorrhagic stroke after treatment with fibrinolytic therapy. A history of previous ischemic stroke should remain a strong relative contraindication to fibrinolytic therapy. A history of previous hemorrhagic stroke within one year should remain an absolute contraindication. American College of Cardiology (ACC) Guidelines should be consulted for additional information and specific exclusion criteria.[18,19]

Recent Surgery and Trauma. Recent surgery or trauma is considered a relative contraindication to fibrinolytic therapy. The term "recent" has been variably interpreted, however, in fibrinolytic therapy trials. In the GISSI-1 trial, patients were excluded if they had surgery or trauma within the previous 10 days.[16] In the ASSET trial, patients were excluded for surgery or trauma within the previous six weeks.[20] Other fibrinolytic therapy trials have not defined "recent surgery or trauma." It is prudent to consider alternative inter-

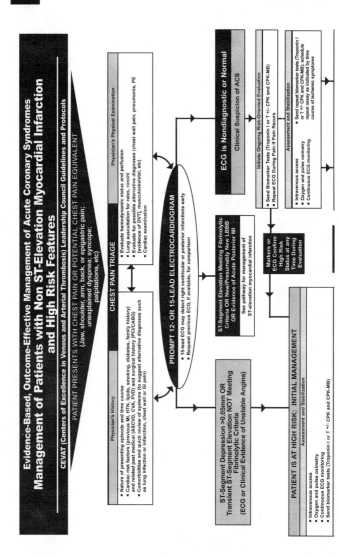

Evidence-Based, Outcome-Effective Management of Acute Coronary Syndromes
Management of Patients with Non ST-Elevation Myocardial Infarction
and High Risk Features

CEVAT (Centers of Excellence in Venous and Arterial Thrombosis) Leadership Council Guidelines and Protocols

PATIENT PRESENTS WITH CHEST PAIN OR POTENTIAL CHEST PAIN EQUIVALENT
(Jaw, shoulder, arm, back, or epigastric pain; unexplained dyspnea; syncope; palpitations, etc)

CHEST PAIN TRIAGE

Physician's History
- Nature of presenting episode and time course
- Cardiac risk factors (previous MI, HTN, lipids, smoking, diabetes, family history) and related past medical (ASCVD, CVA, PVD) and surgical history (PCI/CABG)
- Comorbidities and quick review of systems (to suggest alternative diagnoses such as lung infection or infarction, chest wall or GI pain)

Physician's Physical Examination
- Evaluate hemodynamic status and perfusion
- Lung auscultation for rales, ronchi
- Evaluate for possible alternative diagnoses (chest wall pain, pneumonia, PE evidence of DVT), musculoskeletal, etc)
- Cardiac examination

PROMPT 12- OR 15-LEAD ELECTROCARDIOGRAM
- 15-lead ECG may detect right ventricular or posterior infarctions early
- Request previous ECG, if available, for comparison

ST-Segment Elevation Meeting Fibrinolytic
Criteria OR New/Presumably New LBBB
OR Evidence of Acute Posterior MI

See pathway for management of
ST-elevation myocardial infarction

ST-Segment Depression >0.05mm OR
Transient ST-Segment Elevation NOT Meeting
Fibrinolytic Criteria
(ECG or Clinical Evidence of Unstable Angina)

Markers or
ECG Confirm
High Risk
Status at any
Time During
Evaluation

ECG Is Nondiagnostic or Normal

Clinical Suspicion of ACS

Initiate Ongoing Risk-Oriented Evaluation
- Send Biomarker Tests (Troponin I or T +/- CPK and CPK-MB)
- Repeat ECG During Pain If Pain Recurs

Assessment and Stabilization
- Intravenous access
- Oxygen and pulse oximetry
- Continuous ECG monitoring
- Send repeat biomarker tests (Troponin I or T +/- CPK and CPK-MB); schedule repeat assay as indicated by time course of ischemic symptoms

PATIENT IS AT HIGH RISK: INITIAL MANAGEMENT
Assessment and Stabilization
- Intravenous access
- Oxygen and pulse oximetry
- Continuous ECG monitoring
- Send biomarker tests (Troponin I or T +/- CPK and CPK-MB)

Pharmacologic Intervention

- Aspirin 160-325mg PO
- Nitroglycerin SL/TC/IV ischemic chest for pain, morphine sulfate for immediate relief of pain
- Anticoagulate with enoxaparin (preferred) or UFH
- Consider β-blocker therapy
- Consider initiating eptifibatide or tirofiban infusion

TIMI Risk Score
= 5-7:
Patient is at
HIGH RISK

Calculate TIMI Risk Score: 1 point Each for Presence of
- Age > 65 years
- Prior stenosis > 50 %
- > 3 CAD risk factors
- ASA in last 7 days
- > 2 anginal events in last 24 hours
- ST deviation
- Elevated biomarkers

TIMI Risk Score = 3-4: Patient is at INTERMEDIATE RISK:
INITIAL MANAGEMENT:
Pharmacologic Intervention
- Aspirin 160-325mg PO
- Nitroglycerin SL/TC/IV for ischemic pain. Morphine sulfate as needed
- Anticoagulate with enoxaparin 1mg/kg SQ q 12h
- Consider β-blocker if patient on maintenance β-blocker, if hypertensive, or if tachycardic

TIMI Risk Score = 0-2: Patient is at LOW RISK:
INITIAL MANAGEMENT:
Pharmacologic Intervention
- Aspirin 160-325mg PO
- Nitroglycerin SL/TC/IV for ischemic pain. Morphine sulfate as needed
- Consider anticoagulation with enoxaparin 1mg/kg SQ q 12h or UFH
- Consider expedited R/O protocol including early provocative testing

Continue Risk-Oriented Evaluation

According to agreements and protocols among departments of emergency medicine, cardiology, radiology, and catheterization lab
- Lower Risk Patients may not Require an Extended Observation Period
- Serial ECGs, Serial Biomarker Assays, and Consider Rest or Provocative Testing to Evaluate for the Appearance of High-Risk Features (see below)

High Risk Features
- Persistent Ischemic Chest Pain
- > 20 min Ischemic Chest Pain at Rest or More Than 2 Episodes of Pain in 24h
- Positive Biomarker
- ST-Segment Deviation > 0.05mm
- Positive Objective Ischemia Test or LVEF Less Than 40%
- Sustained Ventricular Tachycardia or Hemodynamic Instability
- Signs of Pump Failure (Rales, New MR Murmur, New S3 Gallop)

High-Risk Feature Manifests During Risk-Oriented Evaluation

High-Risk Feature Not Present During Risk-Oriented Evaluation

Consider Referral for Provocative Testing

If TIMI Risk Score was 3-4:
- Cardiology follow-up as outpatient
- Discharge on aspirin 81-162 mg PO qd
- Consider discharge on clopidogrel 75 mg PO qd

If TIMI Risk Score was 0-2:
- Primary care physician vs cardiology follow-up as outpatient
- Consider discharge on aspirin 81-162 mg PO qd

Catheterization Lab Available In-House or by Transfer Within 24-36 Hours?

YES / **NO**

Dominant Strategy: Acute Intervention
- Administer eptifibatide (preferred) or tirofiban
- Expedite transfer to cath lab
- Continue anticoagulation
- Administer clopidogrel (300mg PO then 75mg PO qd) in catheterization lab if CABG not necessary once coronary anatomy is defined

Alternative Strategy: Medical Management
- Administer clopidogrel (300mg PO then 75mg PO qd)
- Continue anticoagulation with enoxaparin (preferred) or UFH
- Consider initiating eptifibatide (preferred) or tirofiban infusion
- Consider transfer for elective catheterization
- Cardiology admission
- Transfer for catheterization if other high risk features (see below) manifest or if patient deteriorates

High Risk Features
- Persistent ischemic chest pain
- > 20 min chest pain at rest or more than 2 episodes of pain in 24h
- Positive biomarker
- Worsening or persistent ST-segment deviation despite therapy
- Sustained ventricular tachycardia
- Age > 75
- Hemodynamic instability
- Signs of pump failure (rales, new MR murmur, new S3 gallop)

YES

CE/VAT PANEL REPORTS
Charles Pollack, Jr., MA, MD, FACEP
Editor-in-Chief

THOMSON
★
AMERICAN HEALTH
CONSULTANTS

ventions such as PCI, if available, in patients with AMI with a history of any surgical procedures within 2-4 weeks, and within three weeks for major surgery—or significant trauma within the preceding 2-4 weeks.

Elevated Blood Pressure. Current evidence indicates that a patient with a history of chronic hypertension should not be excluded from fibrinolytic therapy if his/her blood pressure is under control at the time of presentation or if it can be predictably lowered to acceptable levels using standard therapy for ischemic chest pain. In this regard, the patient's blood pressure at admission also is an important indicator of risk of intracerebral hemorrhage.

The FTT meta-analysis[5] demonstrates that the risk of cerebral hemorrhage increases with a systolic blood pressure of greater than 150 mmHg on admission, and further increases when systolic blood pressure is 175 mmHg or greater. Despite an increased mortality rate during days 0 and 1, the FTT meta-analysis demonstrated an overall, long-term benefit of 15 lives saved per 1000 for patients with systolic blood pressures of greater than 150 mmHg and 11 lives saved per 100 for patients with systolic blood pressures of 175 mmHg or greater.[5] Although these results appear to indicate an acceptable risk-benefit ratio for patients with substantially increased systolic blood pressure, a persistent blood pressure of greater than 180/110 mmHg generally is considered an absolute contraindication to fibrinolytic therapy. The American Heart Association (AHA)/ACC guidelines' recommendation that a blood pressure of greater than 180/110 mmHg is a relative contraindication is derived from the TIMI-II trial, in which intracranial hemorrhage occurred in 9.1% (n = 22) of patients with a systolic blood pressure of greater than 180 or diastolic blood pressure of greater than 110 before receiving thrombolytic therapy, compared with 1.4% (n = 9) of patients without an elevated blood pressure.[18,19]

Hypotension. The benefit of fibrinolytic therapy in patients with hypotension remains controversial. The FTT meta-analysis, however, supports this approach.[5] Patients with an initial systolic blood pressure of less than 100 mmHg who were not treated with fibrinolytic therapy had a very high risk of death (35.1%), and those who were treated with fibrinolytic therapy had the largest absolute benefit (60 lives saved per 1000 patients).[5] Based on this evidence, the FTT Collaborative Group suggests that hypotension, heart failure, and perhaps even shock should not be contraindications to fibrinolytic therapy.[5] The value of PCI in these patients also has been established. Overall, the data support immediate treatment directed toward myocardial reperfusion, regardless of the method (PCI or fibrinolysis) as indicated by clinical judgment and availability.

Menstrual Bleeding. Experts have debated whether actively menstruating women with AMI are candidates for fibrinolysis. Because natural estrogen is cardioprotective, there has been little experience with fibrinolysis among premenopausal women. Significant adverse effects, however, have not been reported by clinicians who administer fibrinolytic therapy to such patients. Gynecologists indicate that any excessive vaginal bleeding that may occur after receiving fibrinolytic therapy should be readily controllable by vaginal packing; therefore, this can be considered bleeding from a compressible site.

The Electrocardiogram. Combined with the patient's history and physical examination, the 12-lead ECG is the key determinant of eligibility for fibrinolysis. Electrocardiographic eligibility can be established by either: 1) ST segment elevation of 1 mm or more in two or more anatomically contiguous standard limb leads and 2 mm or more elevation in two or more contiguous precordial leads; or 2) new or presumed new left bundle branch block (LBBB). No evidence of benefit from fibrinolytic therapy is found in patients with ischemic chest pain who lack either of these criteria.

Patients with LBBB and AMI are at an increased risk of experiencing a poor outcome; accordingly, these patients should be rapidly and aggressively managed in the emergency department (ED) with appropriate reperfusion therapies.[5,21] This observation was noted prior to the introduction of fibrinolytic agents and continues to be true today. In patients with AMI, new-onset LBBB is a marker for a significantly worse prognosis in terms of higher mortality, lower left ventricular ejection fraction, and increased incidence of cardiovascular complications.[5,21] The development of new LBBB in the setting of AMI suggests proximal occlusion of the left anterior descending artery; such an obstruction places a significant portion of the left ventricle in ischemic jeopardy. Despite this increased risk of a poor outcome, patients with LBBB are less likely to receive fibrinolytic agents than are patients with ST-elevation without LBBB. It should be stressed that patients with new onset LBBB show significant benefit when treated with fibrinolytic therapy.[5]

Patients with AMI in the anterior, inferior, or lateral anatomic locations benefit from administration of fibrinolytic therapy. The relatively favorable prognosis associated with inferior infarction without fibrinolytic therapy requires larger sample sizes to detect a significant survival benefit. The large ISIS-2 trial[7] demonstrated a statistically significant mortality benefit for fibrinolytic therapy in patients with inferior AMI: the mortality at five weeks was 6.5% for streptokinase plus aspirin vs. 10.2% for placebo. Patients with inferior AMI and coexisting right ventricular infarctions as detected by additional-lead ECGs are likely to benefit because a larger portion of myocardium is involved. Acute, isolated posterior wall MI, frequently diagnosed only by placement of posterior leads, may represent yet another electrocardiographic indication for fibrinolysis. Although improved outcomes are unproven in large fibrinolytic trials, patients with isolated posterior AMI may be considered as possible candidates for reperfusion therapy.

In general, the larger the size of the myocardial infarct, the greater the potential mortality reduction with fibrinolytic therapy. The size of an AMI—and therefore the associated risk of cardiovascular complications and death—is reflected by either the absolute number of leads showing ST segment elevation on the ECG or a summation of the total ST segment deviation from the baseline (i.e., both ST segment depressions and elevations).

The current evidence strongly indicates that fibrinolytic therapy should not be used routinely in patients with ST segment depression only on the 12-lead ECG. Mortality rates actually may be increased by administration of fibrinolytics in this patient population. The TIMI-3 trial[22] demonstrated a significant difference in outcome in fibrinolytic-treated patients with only ST segment depression: 7.4% incidence of death compared with 4.9% in the placebo group. These findings also are supported in the FTT meta-analysis, which demonstrated that the mortality rate among patients with ST segment depression who received fibrinolytic therapy was 15.2%, compared with 13.8% among controls.[5]

Recent Cardiopulmonary Resuscitation (CPR). CPR is not a contraindication to fibrinolytic therapy unless CPR has been prolonged (i.e., greater than 10 minutes) or extensive chest trauma from manual compression is evident.[23] Although the in-hospital mortality rate is higher in AMI patients who experience cardiac arrest and then receive ED-based fibrinolytic agents, no difference is found in the rates of bleeding complications. No hemothorax or cardiac tamponade occurred in cardiac arrest patients receiving fibrinolytics.[23] One study reported that up to 25 minutes of CPR did not place patients at increased risk for complications of fibrinolysis. Although prolonged CPR that is performed for greater than 20 minutes is not an absolute contraindication to thrombolysis, it should, perhaps, be considered a relative contraindication; primary PCI may be preferred in this subgroup when it is available.[24,25]

STEMI FIBRINOLYTIC STRATEGIES: NEW CONSIDERATIONS FOR LOW MOLECULAR WEIGHT HEPARINS

An important advance in fibrinolytic management of AMI is the emerging evidence defining a pivotal role for enoxaparin. Although the largest body of published literature evaluating LMWH in the setting of acute coronary ischemia has focused on enoxaparin, other LMWHs, including dalteparin, also have been evaluated.[26-28] Because the most recent, significant data to emerge from large, well-designed, prospective trials involve enoxaparin, its role in pharmacological strategies for reperfusion will be discussed in detail.

In this regard, the recently published ASSENT-3 trial was designed to compare the effectiveness and safety of enoxaparin vs. UFH as part of a full-dose tenecteplase regimen.[1] This trial enrolled 6095 patients with AMI marked by pain of less than six hours duration, and randomly assigned patients to one of three regimens: 1) full-dose tenecteplase plus enoxaparin (30 mg IV bolus followed immediately by 1 mg/kg SC q12 hr) for a maximum of seven days (enoxaparin group, n = 2040); 2) half-dose tenecteplase with weight-adjusted, low-dose UFH and a 12-hour infusion of abciximab (abciximab group, 2017); and 3) full-dose tenecteplase with weight-adjusted UFH for 48 hours (UFH group, n = 2038). The primary end points were the composites of 30-day mortality, in-hospital reinfarction, or in-hospital refractory ischemia (efficacy end point); and the above end point plus in-hospital intracranial hemorrhage or in-hospital major bleeding complications (efficacy plus safety end point).

Although ASSENT-3 was not powered to show a difference in mortality alone, it should be noted that the combination of full-dose tenecteplase plus enoxaparin produced the lowest 30-day mortality rates (5.4%) in patients with AMI reported in large clinical trials evaluating fibrinolytic strategies in similar patient populations. Consistent with this finding is the fact that there were significantly fewer adverse efficacy end points in the enoxaparin and abciximab groups than in the UFH group: 233/2037 (11.4%) vs. 315/2038 (15.4%; RR 0.74 [95% CI, 0.63-0.87], p = 0.0002) for enoxaparin, and 223/2017 (11.1%) vs. 315/2038 (15.4%; RR 0.72 [0.61-0.84], p < 0.0001) for abciximab. The same was true for the efficacy plus safety end point: 280/2037 (13.7%) vs. 347/2036 (17.0%; RR 0.81 [0.70-0.93], p = 0.0037) for enoxaparin, and 287/2016 (14.2%) vs. 347/2036 (17.0%; RR 0.84 [0.72-0.96], p = 0.01416) for abciximab.[1]

The investigators concluded that the tenecteplase plus enoxaparin or abciximab regimens reduced the frequency of ischemic complications in AMI, producing an overall relative reduction in primary adverse end points of about 26% in the enoxaparin-tenecteplase and abciximab groups as compared to the UFH group. From a practical, time-to-treat myocardial salvage perspective, the convenience factor of the enoxaparin regimen must not be under-emphasized. The abciximab arm required initiation of two infusions (abciximab plus UFH) and administration of three IV boluses (tenecteplase, abciximab, and heparin). In contrast, the enoxaparin arm was much more convenient, requiring two simple bolus infusions, one of tenecteplase and one of enoxaparin. Its ease of administration, acceptable safety profile, and relatively lower cost make the tenecteplase plus enoxaparin arm the optimal reperfusion regimen studied in this trial.

These practical advantages, combined with a lower bleeding rate and maintenance of overall effectiveness in terms of safety and efficacy across the full-spectrum of high risk patient subgroups with AMI (i.e., including the elderly and diabetic subsets) supports a paradigm shift to enoxaparin/tenecteplase or enoxaparin in combination with other fibrin-specific thrombolytics, as the preferred pharmacotherapeutic approach to fibrinolysis-mediated therapy of AMI. Although the ASSENT-3 trial evaluated a fibrinolytic regimen consisting of tenecteplase, it is reasonable to suggest that enoxaparin also should be the preferred anticoagulant agent, over UFH, when used in combination with other fibrinolytic agents such as alteplase and reteplase. In fact, in the second trial of Heparin and Aspirin Reperfusion Therapy (HART II), 400 patients with STEMI were randomized to receive either enoxaparin (30 mg intravenous bolus then 1 mg/kg subcutaneously every 12 hours) or UFH intravenous infusion as adjunct to aspirin and a 90-minute infusion regimen of alteplase. The primary end points were infarct-related patency at 90 minutes after initiation of fibrinolytic therapy, reocclusion at 5-7 days, and safety. The TIMI grade 2 or 3 flow was comparable between groups, 80.1% with enoxaparin and 75.1% with heparin.[2]

Reocclusion within one week occurred in 9.1% of the patients who received heparin and in only 3.1% of those who received enoxaparin (p = 0.1). Bleeding complications were comparable between groups. This study showed that enoxaparin was effective and safe in patients with AMI and that it may be a convenient, safe, and effective substitute for UFH in conjunction with alteplase in this indication.[2]

Baird and others assessed the efficacy and safety of enoxaparin vs. heparin in 300 patients with AMI who received fibrinolytic therapy. The enoxaparin group received a 40 mg intravenous bolus followed by subcutaneous injections, while the heparin group received a 5000 unit bolus plus 30,000 units per 24 hours with adjustment to maintain an appropriate aPTT. The triple end point of death, AMI, or readmission with unstable angina at three months occurred in 36% of those who received heparin and in 26% of those who received enoxaparin (p = 0.04). Major bleeding was comparable between groups.[29]

There are several considerations that support the important role of enoxaparin in combination with tenecteplase and other fibrinolytics as the optimal regimen for appropriately selected patients with AMI. First, the results obtained in ASSENT-3[1] with half-dose tenecteplase plus abciximab are very similar to those with half-dose reteplase and abciximab seen in GUSTO-V;[4] this supports the hypothesis that a more potent antiplatelet agent increases flow in the infarct-related coronary artery. However, in both trials, the benefits of abciximab in a fibrinolytic regimen were obtained at the cost of a higher rate of thrombocytopenia, major bleeding complications, and blood transfusions, thereby mitigating its attractiveness. Moreover, as is the case in GUSTO-V, no benefit, and perhaps even harm, was observed in ASSENT-3 patients treated with the abciximab/half-dose fibrinolytic regimen who were older than age 75;[1] this reinforces the need for caution regarding the use of this combination in elderly patients. Although these observations are made on the basis of sub-group analysis (and its inherent limitations), in contrast to GUSTO-V, ASSENT-3 also suggested an inferior result, compared to heparin, for the abciximab regimen in diabetic patients, a finding that should prompt addition-al investigation.

The ENTIRE-TIMI 23 evaluated enoxaparin with full-dose tenecteplase (TNK) and half-dose TNK plus abciximab.[3] Patients (n = 483) with STEMI presenting less than six hours from symptom onset were randomized to full-dose TNK and either UFH (bolus 60 U/kg; infusion 12 U/kg per hour) or enoxaparin (1.0 mg/kg subcutaneously every 12 hours after an initial 30 mg intravenous bolus), or half-dose TNK plus abciximab and either UFH (bolus 40 U/kg; infusion 7 U/kg per hour) or enoxaparin (0.3 to 0.75 mg/kg subcuta-neously every 12 hours after an initial intravenous bolus of 30 mg). With full-dose TNK and UFH, the rate of TIMI 3 flow at 60 minutes was 52% and was 48-51% with enoxaparin. Using combination therapy, the rate of TIMI 3 flow was 48% with UFH and 47-58% with enoxaparin. The rate of TIMI 3 flow among all UFH patients was 50%, and was 51% among enoxaparin patients.

Through a period extending for 30 days, death/recurrent MI occurred in the full-dose TNK group in 15.9% of patients with UFH and in 4.4% with enoxa-parin (p = 0.005). In the combination therapy group, the rates were 6.5% with UFH and 5.5% with enoxaparin; with combination therapy, it was 5.2% using UFH and 8.5% with enoxaparin.[3] Based on these results, the investigators con-cluded that enoxaparin is associated with similar TIMI 3 flow rates to UFH at an early time point, while exhibiting advantages over UFH with respect to ischemic events through 30 days. These findings with enoxaparin are achieved with a similar risk of major hemorrhage.

There are some interesting aspects of this study that should be noted.

Through 30 days, the composite end point of death/MI in patients in the full-dose TNK group was 15.9% with UFH and 4.4% with enoxaparin (p = 0.005). This was mediated largely by a reduction in the rate of nonfatal reinfarction: 12.2% with UFH and 1.9% with enoxaparin (p = 0.003). In the combination therapy group, death/MI occurred in 6.5% of UFH patients and 5.5% of enoxaparin patients. The pooled rate among all UFH patients was 11.3% and was 4.9% in enoxaparin patients (p = 0.01).

Of the 224 patients who underwent PCI, 13 (5.8%) experienced a major hemorrhage that was at an instrumented site in 10 patients. When PCI was performed in patients who had been assigned to full-dose TNK, the rate of major hemorrhage with UFH was 4.9% and was 1.8% with enoxaparin. When PCI was performed in patients assigned to combination therapy, the rates of major hemorrhage were 7.7% with UFH and 8.0% with enoxaparin. Across both forms of pharmacological reperfusion, the rate of major hemorrhage in the PCI cohort was 6.3% in patients receiving UFH and 5.6% in patients receiving enoxaparin.[3]

The findings of ENTIRE-TIMI 23[3] and ASSENT-3[1] suggest that large phase III trials are now needed to evaluate enoxaparin as a replacement for UFH in a variety of pharmacological reperfusion regimens including different lytics in full-dose and as part of combination therapy regimens with different GP IIb/IIIa inhibitors. The convenient mode of administration and lack of need for anticoagulation monitoring with enoxaparin also make it an attractive agent for testing as part of a prehospital treatment strategy for STEMI, as is being explored in the ASSENT-3 Plus study.

STEMI—PRIMARY PERCUTANEOUS CORONARY INTERVENTIONS (PCI)

The mandate to implement prompt reperfusion therapy in fibrinolytic-ineligible patients, as well as the other limitations of fibrinolytic therapy, have encouraged many clinicians to advocate PTCA, and more recently PCI with coronary artery stenting, as the primary treatment modality for the majority of patients with AMI.

Recent studies suggest the introduction of coronary artery stenting likely will favorably alter the outcomes of AMI patients, making stent placement a superior method of management for appropriately selected patients at institutions where physicians are experienced in this procedure.

Stenting represents a significant advance in the management of patients with AMI by PCI. In the recent past, early use of stenting in the AMI patient was considered problematic due to the real possibility of prompt stent thrombosis or subsequent unexpected stent restenosis. With the introduction of aggressive antiplatelet therapy using aspirin and antagonists of platelet ADP and GP IIb/IIIa receptors, the rates of stent thrombosis have significantly decreased. Exploring early stent placement in the AMI patient, the PAMI-stent trial compared urgent treatment with PTCA with or without stenting in 900 patients.[30] Stenting significantly reduced both stenosis and reocclusion at six months. No differences in death, reinfarction, or stroke at six months, however, were noted. Thus, it appears that in selected patients with AMI, primary stenting can be applied safely and effectively, resulting in a lower incidence of recurrent infarction and a significant reduction in the need for subsequent target-vessel revascularization compared with balloon angioplasty.

The purpose of the Stent versus Thrombolysis for Occluded Coronary Arteries in Patients with Acute Myocardial Infarction (STOPAMI) study was to assess whether coronary stenting combined with blockade of platelet GP IIb/IIIa receptors produces a greater degree of myocardial salvage than fibrinolysis with an accelerated infusion of alteplase.[31] In this study, a total of 140 patients with STEMI were enrolled in a randomized trial, with 71 assigned to receive a stent plus abciximab, and 69 to receive intravenous alteplase. The primary end point was the degree of myocardial salvage, determined by means of serial scintigraphic studies, and the secondary end point was a composite of death, reinfarction, and stroke within six months after randomization. In the group that received a stent plus abciximab, the median size of the final infarct was 14.3% of the left ventricle, as compared with a median of 19.4% in the alteplase group. The cumulative incidence of death, reinfarction, or stroke at six months was lower in the stent group than in the alteplase group (8.5 vs 23.2%, p = 0.02; RR, 0.34; 95% CI, 0.13-0.88).[31] The investigators concluded that in patients with AMI, coronary stenting plus abciximab produces a greater degree of myocardial salvage and a better clinical outcome than does fibrinolysis without aggressive antiplatelet therapy.

Recent research has evaluated the use of therapeutic combinations, including GP IIb/IIIa receptor inhibition with both PCI and fibrinolysis, low-dose fibrinolysis followed by primary angioplasty, and intracoronary stent placement during PCI. As emphasized, reperfusion with primary PCI may be improved with the use of GP IIb/IIIa inhibitors, although there are conflicting results regarding their use in non-PCI patients. Abciximab with intracoronary stenting in AMI has been studied in the RAPPORT,[32] ADMIRAL,[33] and CADILLAC trials.[34] In the RAPPORT trial,[32] a significant reduction in the combined end point of death, MI, and urgent need for revascularization with the use of abciximab was noted at 30 days; no significant differences, however, were seen at six months. An increase in major bleeding episodes and the need for transfusions was encountered in the abciximab group, but may have been due to high-dose heparin therapy.

The ADMIRAL trial[33] reported a significantly lower rate of occurrence of the combined end point of death, recurrent MI, and target vessel revascularization at 30 days in the treatment (abciximab) group. In addition, lower doses of heparin were given to patients in the abciximab group, and no increase in major bleeding was observed. The CADILLAC trial[34] randomized primary PCI patients with AMI to PTCA or stenting and also evaluated the potentially additive effects of abciximab vs. placebo to both approaches. CADILLAC randomized 2082 patients from 76 centers in 9 countries to one of four treatment groups: angioplasty alone; angioplasty plus abciximab; stenting alone (using the MultiLink or MultiLink Duet stent); or stenting plus abciximab. The primary end point was major adverse clinical events (MACE) at six months, which included a composite incidence of death, reinfarction, disabling stroke, or the need for repeat revascularization. At six months, patients who received a stent plus abciximab had the lowest rates of combined death, reinfarction, disabling stroke, or the need for repeat revascularization compared to patients who received primary PTCA alone or PTCA plus abciximab. Ultimate outcome with stenting, however, was found to be independent of the use of abciximab.[34]

The use of GP IIb/IIIa inhibitors in the setting of AMI treated with PCI is still being intensively studied, and the consistency of benefit vs. the increased risk of bleeding with these agents has not yet been clearly defined.

Even though PCI may be the optimal management approach to AMI, PCI may not always be readily available, necessitating rapid transfer to another facility. Indications for transfer of a patient with AMI to a regional, tertiary care facility with PCI and cardiovascular surgery capabilities include patients with contraindications to fibrinolytic therapy who may benefit from PCI or CABG, persistent hemodynamic instability, persistent ventricular dysrhythmias, or postinfarction or post-reperfusion ischemia. Hospital transfer for primary PCI is strongly suggested in patients with fibrinolytic agent contraindications. The urgent transfer of a fibrinolytic-eligible AMI patient for primary PCI to another institution is not recommended until fibrinolytic therapy is initiated; the delay in restoring perfusion in such a patient is not acceptable in most instances. If the patient is an acceptable candidate for fibrinolysis, the fibrinolytic agent should be started before or during transport to the receiving hospital.

Prior agreement between the ED and the inpatient physicians at institutions both with and without PCI capability must be obtained so that PCI consideration will not introduce further delays in fibrinolytic drug administration; such cooperation has been shown to limit additional delays in the administration of fibrinolytic agents in patients who are considered for PCI in AMI.[35] If performed without a time delay by experienced hands, PCI appears to produce improved outcomes in the urgent management of AMI. It must be stressed that while PCI is felt to be superior in the treatment of AMI, benefit is largely limited to patients whose interventional management is initiated within 90-120 minutes of arrival to the hospital ED.[18,36,37]

If the time required to mobilize staff and arrange for PCI is prolonged (i.e., greater than approximately 2 hours to balloon catheter inflation or stenting across the culprit coronary lesion), then fibrinolysis is preferred.[36] Delays beyond this time period are unacceptable if the patient originally was a fibrinolytic candidate. These various time periods are suggestions; individual patient and system issues must be considered in the treatment decisions.

NON-ST-SEGMENT-ELEVATION ACUTE CORONARY SYNDROMES: CURRENT MANAGEMENT OPTIONS

Perhaps one of the most important aspects of managing patients with acute coronary ischemic syndromes is the ability to risk-stratify patients into those individuals who will benefit most from either pharmacological or percutaneous strategy-mediated reperfusion. It is difficult to generate a reliable and user-friendly patient selection process that will guarantee an optimal outcome for each individual case. Although a number of risk-stratification tools have been suggested by clinical experts and associations, the TIMI risk factor analysis has emerged as one of the most widely accepted approaches to date for identifying patients who are most likely to benefit from specific strategies.[38]

TIMI Risk Factor Stratification. The following factors are assessed in the TIMI risk-stratification scheme: 1) presence of chest pain; 2) significant elevation of cardiac markers; 3) history of three or more conventional cardiac risk factors (e.g., diabetes, smoking, elevated LDL-cholesterol, etc.); 4) age 65 years or older; 5) known coronary artery disease (CAD), defined as documented 50% or greater stenosis in at least one major coronary artery; 6) ASA use within one week of presentation; 7) two or more episodes of resting angina during the previous 24 hours prior to presentation; and 8) new ST-segment deviation (persistent depression or transient elevation not meeting fibrinolytic criteria) of 0.5 mm or greater in limb and/or precordial leads.[38]

As the number of risk factors increases from 0/1 to 6-7/7, the risk of death, MI, or urgent revascularization within 14 days increases from 4.7% to 40.9% in a stepwise fashion. Many institutions are utilizing the risk score, which is available on-line at www.clinicaltrialresults.org, in early diagnostic and therapeutic decision making for the patient presenting with a non-ST-elevation acute coronary syndrome. It also is utilized as an example of systematic risk stratification in the attached CEVAT guidelines for ACS.

LMWH in NSTEMI. The optimal management approach to patients with unstable angina (UA) and NSTEMI continues to undergo refinement. New studies, however, increasingly support a paradigm shift toward enoxaparin playing a central role in patients with ACS, whether treated with medical or percutaneous interventions. An institutional analysis from a single center was

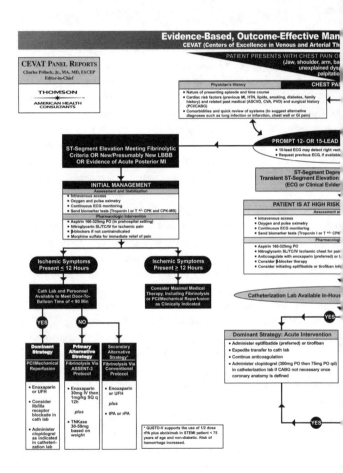

Evidence-Based, Outcome-Effective Man
CEVAT (Centers of Excellence in Venous and Arterial Th

PATIENT PRESENTS WITH CHEST PAIN O
(Jaw, shoulder, arm, ba
unexplained dys
palpitatio

CEVAT PANEL REPORTS

Charles Pollack, Jr., MA, MD, FACEP
Editor-in-Chief

THOMSON
—★—
AMERICAN HEALTH
CONSULTANTS

Physician's History

- Nature of presenting episode and time course
- Cardiac risk factors (previous MI, HTN, lipids, smoking, diabetes, family history) and related past medical (ASCVD, CVA, PVD) and surgical history (PCI/CABG)
- Comorbidities and quick review of systems (to suggest alternative diagnoses such as lung infection or infarction, chest wall or GI pain)

CHEST PAI

PROMPT 12- OR 15-LEAD

- 15-lead ECG may detect right vent
- Request previous ECG, if available

ST-Segment Elevation Meeting Fibrinolytic Criteria OR New/Presumably New LBBB OR Evidence of Acute Posterior MI

ST-Segment Depre
Transient ST-Segment Elevation
(ECG or Clinical Eviden

INITIAL MANAGEMENT

Assessment and Stabilization

- Intravenous access
- Oxygen and pulse oximetry
- Continuous ECG monitoring
- Send biomarker tests (Troponin I or T +/- CPK and CPK-MB)

Pharmacologic Intervention

- Aspirin 160-325mg PO (in prehospital setting)
- Nitroglycerin SL/TC/IV for ischemic pain
- β-blockers if not contraindicated
- Morphine sulfate for immediate relief of pain

PATIENT IS AT HIGH RISK

Assessment an

- Intravenous access
- Oxygen and pulse oximetry
- Continuous ECG monitoring
- Send biomarker tests (Troponin I or T +/- CPK

Pharmacologi

- Aspirin 160-325mg PO
- Nitroglycerin SL/TC/IV ischemic chest for pair
- Anticoagulate with enoxaparin (preferred) or U
- Consider β-blocker therapy
- Consider initiating eptifibatide or tirofiban infe

Ischemic Symptoms Present ≤ 12 Hours

Ischemic Symptoms Present ≥ 12 Hours

Cath Lab and Personnel Available to Meet Door-To-Balloon Time of < 90 Min

Consider Maximal Medical Therapy, Including Fibrinolysis or PCI/Mechanical Reperfusion as Clinically Indicated

Catheterization Lab Available In-Hous

YES

Dominant Strategy: Acute Intervention

- Administer eptifibatide (preferred) or tirofiban
- Expedite transfer to cath lab
- Continue anticoagulation
- Administer clopidogrel (300mg PO then 75mg PO qd) in catheterization lab if CABG not necessary once coronary anatomy is defined

YES   **NO**

Dominant Strategy

PCI/Mechanical Reperfusion

- Enoxaparin or UFH
- Consider IIb/IIIa receptor blockade in cath lab
- Administer clopidogrel as indicated in catheterization lab

Primary Alternative Strategy

Fibrinolysis Via ASSENT-3 Protocol

- Enoxaparin 30mg IV then 1mg/kg SQ q 12h

  plus

- TNKase 30-50mg based on weight

Secondary Alternative Strategy*

Fibrinolysis Via Conventional Protocol

- Enoxaparin or UFH

  plus

- tPA or rPA

* GUSTO-V supports the use of 1/2 dose rPA plus abciximab in STEMI patient < 75 years of age and non-diabetic. Risk of hemorrhage increased.

YES

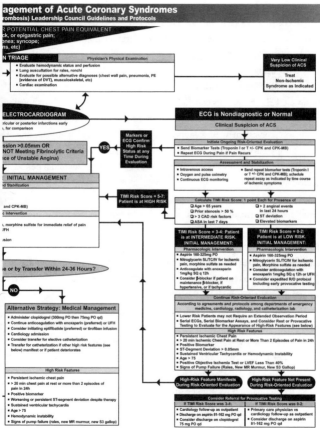

reported at the American College of Cardiology Scientific Assembly in March 2001. Conducted by investigators at the Royal Infirmary of Edinburgh, the study demonstrated that enoxaparin is superior to UFH in patients with UA/NSTEMI: 7.1% vs. 8.6% (p = 0.02) death/MI at 43 days. Decisions to proceed to revascularization were independent of trial randomization.[39]

The group analyzed a population comprising 6098 patients for death or MI at 43 days using chi-squared tests; 983 patients undergoing coronary artery bypass grafting were excluded. Clinicians were blinded to the use of enoxaparin vs. UFH. The authors concluded that patients undergoing PCI (compared with those who were not) sustained more events, including events prior to PCI, which was consistent with a higher risk population. Enoxaparin treatment, when compared with UFH treatment, benefited both patients treated solely medically and those patients who underwent PCI following an initial period of medical stabilization.[39]

Another investigative cardiology group from Greece reported the results of a trial comparing enoxaparin vs. tinzaparin in the management of unstable coronary artery disease (EVET Study).[40] The researchers noted that LMWHs are rapidly emerging as an alternative form of antithrombotic therapy to the standard UFH. Despite similarities in origin, synthesis, and structure, the LMWHs have different pharmacokinetic and pharmacodynamic characteristics and may elicit different efficacies.

The aim of EVET was to compare head-to-head the efficacy of enoxaparin vs. tinzaparin in the management of ACS. In a prospective study, 438 patients with UA or non-Q wave MI were randomized to receive either subcutaneous injections of 1 mg/kg enoxaparin twice daily (n = 220) or 175 IU/kg tinzaparin once daily (n = 218) for seven days. The primary end points were death, MI, refractory angina, and recurrence of UA. Secondary end points were rehospitalization due to UA or MI, death, and the need for revascularization at 30 days.[40]

At seven days, recurrence of UA occurred significantly less frequently in the enoxaparin than in the tinzaparin group (24/220 vs 41/218, p = 0.029). No statistically significant differences were observed between these two groups with respect to death, MI, or refractory angina at seven days. At 30 days there were no differences between the two groups regarding rehospitalization and death, but the need for revascularization occurred significantly less frequently in the patients assigned to enoxaparin (36/220 vs 57/218, p = 0.019). Bleeding complication rates were similar in the two groups. These investigators concluded that antithrombotic treatment with enoxaparin for seven days was more effective than with tinzaparin for reducing the incidence of recurrent angina in patients with UA or non-Q wave MI in the early phase.[40]

Invasive vs. Medical Therapy. The syndrome of UA and MI without ST-elevation accounts for about 1.4 million hospital admissions annually in the United States. As discussed in previous sections, until recently, therapy has focused primarily on medical management using a combination of antianginal agents and anti-thrombotic agents, including aspirin and LMWH. The most current studies have attempted to evaluate and compare early invasive and conservative strategies in patients with unstable coronary syndromes treated with GP IIb/IIIa inhibitors such as tirofiban.[41]

The TACTICS (Thrombolysis in Myocardial Infarction 18 [TACTICS TIMI 18]) investigators enrolled 2220 patients with UA and MI without ST-segment elevation who had electrocardiographic evidence of changes in the ST segment or T wave, elevated levels of cardiac markers, a history of coronary artery disease, or all three findings.[41] All patients were treated with aspirin, heparin, and tirofiban. Patients were randomly assigned to an early invasive strategy, in which routine catheterization was performed no later than 48 hours after presentation and revascularization was performed as appropriate; or to a more conservative (selectively invasive) strategy, in which catheterization was performed only if the patient had objective evidence of recurrent ischemia or an abnormal stress test. The primary end point was a composite of death, non-fatal MI, and rehospitalization for an ACS at six months.

At six months, the rate of the primary end point was 15.9% with the use of the early invasive strategy and 19.4% with the use of the conservative strategy (OR 0.78; 95% CI, 0.62-0.97; p = 0.025). The rate of death or non-fatal MI at six months was similarly reduced (7.3% vs 9.5%; OR, 0.74; 95% CI, 0.54-1.00; p < 0.05). The economic analysis suggested a neutral cost for this added benefit.[41]

Based on these results, the investigators concluded that in patients with UA and MI without ST-segment elevation who were treated with the GP IIb/IIIa inhibitor tirofiban, the use of an early invasive strategy significantly reduced the risk of major cardiac events.

The economic analysis from TACTICS TIMI 18 was presented at the AHA 2000 Scientific Assembly. The results were as follows: Mean hospital costs for the invasive arm were $14,660 and $12,667 for the conservative arm, with a difference in groups of $1994 (CI $6888-3329). However, mean six-month follow-up costs were $6063 in the invasive patients and $7203 in the conservative patients; a difference of -1140 (CI -2165- -50). The primary end point was total cost, which was $629 more in the conservative group with a CI of -1273-2465; therefore, the two arms were considered equivalent.[19]

LMWH in PCI. Recent trials also have assessed the safety of enoxaparin in the setting of PCI not associated with STEMI. The NICE-3 registry experience evaluated the incidence of bleeding while performing catheterization in 661 patients with ACS, all of whom received enoxaparin plus a GP IIb/IIIa inhibitor (abciximab, eptifibatide, or tirofiban, at clinician's discretion).[42] At the time of catheterization, enoxaparin (0.3 mg/kg IV) was administered if more than eight hours had elapsed since the last subcutaneous dose. The combination of enoxaparin with different GP IIb/IIIa inhibitors resulted in similar clinical outcomes and bleeding frequency in comparison to those seen in the large GP IIb/IIIa inhibitor trials, which were conducted with UFH.[42]

The NICE-4 registry experience studied the combination of enoxaparin with abciximab during PCI.[43] Enoxaparin was given as a 0.75 mg/kg intravenous bolus, while abciximab was administered in its usual fashion. Data from the first 310 patients who received enoxaparin and abciximab revealed that the incidence of major non-CABG bleeding and transfusion in this group was 0.6%, which compared favorably with an incidence of 2.7% occurring in patients receiving abciximab and low-dose heparin in the EPILOG trial.[44] Another group assessed the safety and outcomes in patients with UA or NSTE-MI. Of the 451 patients, a non-randomized 293 underwent catheterization within eight hours of the morning enoxaparin injection, which was followed by immediate PCI in 132 patients (28%). The procedures were done without additional heparin or enoxaparin. Major bleeding occurred in 0.8% of those who received catheterization, comparable to the 1.2% in those who were not studied.[45]

In 200 patients receiving elective PCI after three days of aspirin and tirofiban, another group performed a randomized comparison of peri-procedural heparin vs. enoxaparin. Clinical outcomes and major bleeding were comparable between the groups at 30 days.[46] While not a study in the setting of PCI, the pharmacokinetics, pharmacodynamics, and safety of the combination of tirofiban with enoxaparin vs. heparin in non-Q wave MI was addressed in a 55-patient series. As with most studies, more minor bleeding occurred with the enoxaparin combination, while major bleeding was comparable. The combination of tirofiban and enoxaparin resulted in a more consistent inhibition of platelet aggregation and lower adjusted bleeding time than did the combination with heparin. One study measured anti-Xa levels in patients undergoing angiography with or without PCI using the NICE-3 enoxaparin regimen and found stable levels. This investigation evaluated anti-Xa levels with enoxaparin in patients undergoing coronary angiography with or without PCI. The levels averaged 0.99 + 0.02 IU/mL in patients undergoing coronary angiography (n = 293) and 0.98 + 0.03 IU/mL in PCI patients, demonstrating remarkable reproducibility with little (< 3%) variation in a large population of patients.[47]

The FRISC II (Fragmin during instability in coronary artery disease) trial assessed the role of three months of dalteparin therapy after the use of PCI in patients with UA or NSTEMI or after the use of fibrinolysis in AMI.[48] While the initial randomization compared three months of dalteparin vs. placebo, a second randomization, in a 2-by-2 design, compared the use of early PCI with its more conservative use. At six months, the composite of death or AMI was decreased by early PCI from 12.1% to 9.4% in those with less aggressive use (p = 0.031).[48] Dalteparin decreased adverse coronary events during the three-month administration primarily in patients who received conservative use of PCI. It was further observed that there was no benefit from the three-month dalteparin administration in patients who were in the non-invasive segment of the study.

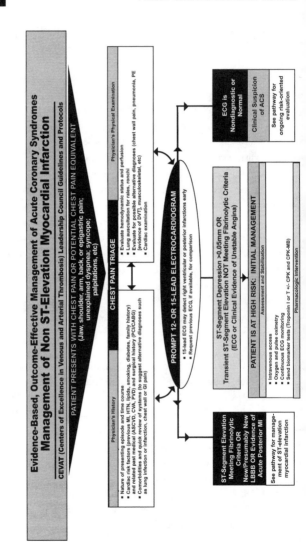

Evidence-Based, Outcome-Effective Management of Acute Coronary Syndromes Management of Non ST-Elevation Myocardial Infarction

CEVAT (Centers of Excellence in Venous and Arterial Thrombosis) Leadership Council Guidelines and Protocols

PATIENT PRESENTS WITH CHEST PAIN OR POTENTIAL CHEST PAIN EQUIVALENT
(Jaw, shoulder, arm, back, or epigastric pain; unexplained dyspnea; syncope; palpitations, etc)

CHEST PAIN TRIAGE

Physician's History

- Nature of presenting episode and time course
- Cardiac risk factors (previous MI, HTN, lipids, smoking, diabetes, family history) and related past medical (ASCVD, CVA, PVD) and surgical history (PCI/CABG)
- Comorbidities and quick review of systems (to suggest alternative diagnoses such as lung infection or infarction, chest wall or GI pain)

Physician's Physical Examination

- Evaluate hemodynamic status and perfusion
- Lung auscultation for rales, ronchi
- Evaluate for possible alternative diagnoses (chest wall pain, pneumonia, PE [evidence of DVT], musculoskeletal, etc)
- Cardiac examination

PROMPT 12- OR 15-LEAD ELECTROCARDIOGRAM

- 15-lead ECG may detect right ventricular or posterior infarctions early
- Request previous ECG, if available, for comparison

ST-Segment Elevation Fibrinolytic Criteria OR New/Presumably New LBBB OR Evidence of Acute Posterior MI

See pathway for management of ST-elevation myocardial infarction

ST-Segment Depression >0.05mm OR Transient ST-Segment Elevation NOT Meeting Fibrinolytic Criteria (ECG or Clinical Evidence of Unstable Angina)

PATIENT IS AT HIGH RISK: INITIAL MANAGEMENT

Assessment and Stabilization

- Intravenous access
- Oxygen and pulse oximetry
- Continuous ECG monitoring
- Send biomarker tests (Troponin I or T +/- CPK and CPK-MB)

Pharmacologic Intervention

ECG is Nondiagnostic or Normal

Clinical Suspicion of ACS

See pathway for ongoing risk-oriented evaluation

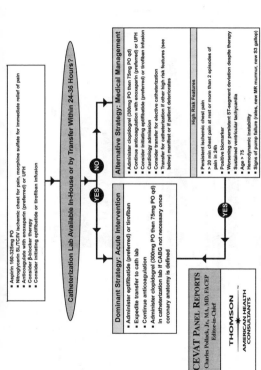

- Aspirin 160-325mg PO
- Nitroglycerin SL/TC/IV ischemic chest for pain, morphine sulfate for immediate relief of pain
- Anticoagulate with enoxaparin (preferred) or UFH
- Consider β-blocker therapy
- Consider initiating eptifibatide or tirofiban infusion

Catheterization Lab Available In-House or by Transfer Within 24-36 Hours?

NO

YES

Dominant Strategy: Acute Intervention

- Administer eptifibatide (preferred) or tirofiban
- Expedite transfer to cath lab
- Continue anticoagulation
- Administer clopidogrel (300mg PO then 75mg PO qd) in catheterization lab if CABG not necessary once coronary anatomy is defined

YES

Alternative Strategy: Medical Management

- Administer clopidogrel (300mg PO then 75mg PO qd)
- Continue anticoagulation with enoxaparin (preferred) or UFH
- Consider initiating eptifibatide (preferred) or tirofiban infusion
- Cardiology admission
- Consider transfer for elective catheterization
- Transfer for catheterization if other high risk features (see below) manifest or if patient deteriorates

High Risk Features

- Persistent ischemic chest pain
- > 20 min chest pain at rest or more than 2 episodes of pain in 24h
- Positive biomarker
- Worsening or persistent ST-segment deviation despite therapy
- Sustained ventricular tachycardia
- Age > 75
- Hemodynamic instability
- Signs of pump failure (rales, new MR murmur, new S3 gallop)

CEVAT PANEL REPORTS
Charles Pollack, Jr., MA, MD, FACEP
Editor-in-Chief

THOMSON

AMERICAN HEALTH
CONSULTANTS

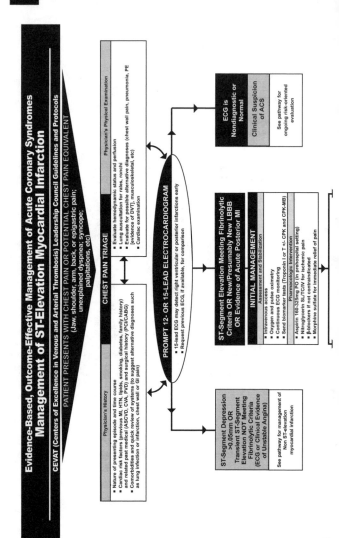

Evidence-Based, Outcome-Effective Management of Acute Coronary Syndromes
Management of ST-Elevation Myocardial Infarction

CEVAT (Centers of Excellence in Venous and Arterial Thrombosis) Leadership Council Guidelines and Protocols

PATIENT PRESENTS WITH CHEST PAIN OR POTENTIAL CHEST PAIN EQUIVALENT
(Jaw, shoulder, arm, back, or epigastric pain;
unexplained dyspnea; syncope; palpitations, etc)

Physician's History

- Nature of presenting episode and time course
- Cardiac risk factors (previous MI, HTN, lipids, smoking, diabetes, family history) and related past medical (ASCVD, CVA, PVD) and surgical history (PCI-CABG)
- Comorbidities and quick review of systems (to suggest alternative diagnoses such as lung infection or infarction, chest wall or GI pain)

CHEST PAIN TRIAGE

Physician's Physical Examination

- Evaluate hemodynamic status and perfusion
- Lung auscultation for rales, ronchi
- Evaluate for possible alternative diagnoses (chest wall pain, pneumonia, PE [evidence of DVT], musculoskeletal, etc)
- Cardiac examination

PROMPT 12- OR 15-LEAD ELECTROCARDIOGRAM

- 15-lead ECG may detect right ventricular or posterior infarctions early
- Request previous ECG, if available, for comparison

ST-Segment Depression >0.05mm OR Transient ST-Segment Elevation NOT Meeting Fibrinolytic Criteria (ECG or Clinical Evidence of Unstable Angina)

See pathway for management of Non ST-elevation myocardial infarction

ST-Segment Elevation Meeting Fibrinolytic Criteria OR New/Presumably New LBBB OR Evidence of Acute Posterior MI

INITIAL MANAGEMENT

Assessment and Stabilization

- Intravenous access
- Oxygen and pulse oximetry
- Continuous ECG monitoring
- Send biomarker tests (Troponin I or T +/- CPK and CPK-MB)

Pharmacologic Intervention

- Aspirin 160-325mg PO (in prehospital setting)
- Nitroglycerin SL/TC/IV for ischemic pain
- β-blockers if not contraindicated
- Morphine sulfate for immediate relief of pain

ECG is Nondiagnostic or Normal

Clinical Suspicion of ACS

See pathway for ongoing risk-oriented evaluation

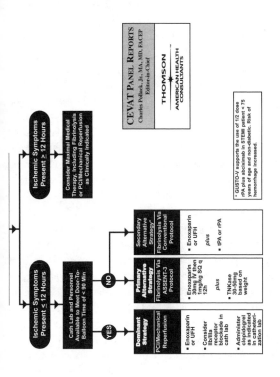

Ischemic Symptoms Present ≥ 12 Hours

Consider Maximal Medical Therapy, Including Fibrinolysis or PCI/Mechanical Reperfusion as Clinically Indicated

Ischemic Symptoms Present ≤ 12 Hours

Cath Lab and Personnel Available to Meet Door-To-Balloon Time of < 90 Min

YES

Dominant Strategy

PCI/Mechanical Reperfusion

- Enoxaparin or UFH
- Consider IIb/IIIa receptor blockade in cath lab
- Administer clopidogrel as indicated in catheterization lab

NO

Primary Alternative Strategy*

Fibrinolysis Via ASSENT-3 Protocol

- Enoxaparin 30mg IV then 1mg/kg SQ q 12h

  plus

- TNKase 30-50mg based on weight

Secondary Alternative Strategy*

Fibrinolysis Via Conventional Protocol

- Enoxaparin or UFH
- tPA or rPA

CEVAT PANEL REPORTS

Charles Pollack, Jr., MA, MD, FACEP
Editor-in-Chief

THOMSON
★
AMERICAN HEALTH
CONSULTANTS™

* GUSTO-V supports the use of 1/2 dose rPA plus abciximab in STEMI patient < 75 years of age and non-diabetic. Risk of hemorrhage increased.

In the Integrilin and Enoxaparin Randomized assessment of Acute Coronary Syndromes Treatment (INTERACT) trial, presented at the American College of Cardiology's 51st Annual Scientific Session, 746 patients who met high-risk criteria with non-ST elevation ACS all were given full-dose eptifibatide.[49] Patients were then randomized to receive either enoxaparin (1 mg/kg SQ q 12 for > 4 doses) or weight-adjusted UFH by infusion. Sixty percent of patients underwent cardiac catheterization, 30% underwent PCI, and 12% underwent CABG. The risk of bleeding at 48 and 96 hours for enoxaparin- and UFH-treated patients, respectively, was 1.1% vs. 3.8% (p = 0.014) and 1.8% vs. 4.6% (p = 0.03). Much more striking was the finding that ECG-determined ischemic events were much less common in enoxaparin- (14.1% and 12.7% at 0-48 and 48-96 hours, respectively) than UFH-treated patients (25.1% and 25.9%, both p-values less than 0.002). This is the largest randomized study of the combination of a LMWH and a GP IIb/IIIa agent to date.[49]

The Role of Enoxaparin in ACS. The use of enoxaparin in non-STEMI ACS is supported by data from the ESSENCE and TIMI 11B clinical studies.[50,51] In the ESSENCE study, the need for revascularization procedures at 30 days was significantly less frequent with enoxaparin compared with UFH (27.0% compared with 32.2%; p = 0.001). In the TIMI 11B study, urgent revascularization was required in 10.7% of patients who received enoxaparin and 12.6% of patients who received UFH at 43 days (p = 0.05). The incidence of cardiac and hemorrhagic events in patients undergoing PCI in the ESSENCE and TIMI 11B clinical studies was similar, irrespective of the initial type of anticoagulation (enoxaparin or UFH) and the timing of the intervention (PCI on treatment/within 12 hours of the final dose or at any time during initial hospitalization).[50,51]

Antithrombin therapy is considered an integral component of the management of non-ST elevation ACS. In the 2000 ACC/AHA non-ST elevation ACS Guidelines,[19] anticoagulation with UFH or LMWH was recommended as Class I, Level B. Although anticoagulation is clearly considered "standard of care" in the management of these patients, a level A recommendation was withheld because of the paucity of randomized, controlled data supporting the use of UFH and uncertainty about the use of LMWH in the catheterization lab and in combination with GP IIb/IIIa agents. In the 2002 update (www.acc.org or www.americanheart.org), these recommendations are issued regarding the use of anticoagulants:[52]

- Anticoagulation with subcutaneous LMWH or intravenous UFH should be added to antiplatelet therapy with ASA and/or clopidogrel (Class I, Level A).

- Enoxaparin is preferable to UFH as an anticoagulant in patients with UA/NSTEMI, unless CABG is planned within 24 hours (Class IIa, Level A).

The "upgrade" of the anticoagulation recommendation and the unusual step of singling out a specific agent among the LMWH class resulted from the inclusion of several recent studies of enoxaparin and perhaps a reconsideration of the strengths of the ESSENCE[50] and TIMI-11B[51] analyses.

The issue of performing PCI in patients anticoagulated with LMWH and therefore whose aPTT or activated clotting time (ACT) do not accurately reflect the extent of anticoagulation, was addressed by Collet et al, who showed in a study of 293 UA/NSTEMI patients that PCI can be performed safely with the usual dose of enoxaparin.[47] The NICE-1 data, in which the rate of bleeding (1.1% for major bleeding and 6.2% for minor bleeding in 30 days) was comparable to historical controls given UFH, has already been referenced.[53]

An alternative approach specifically recommended in the 2002 Guidelines is to use LMWH during the period of initial stabilization—that is, in the ED care of the non-ST elevation ACS patient. The dose can be withheld on the morning of the procedure, and if an intervention is required and more than eight hours has elapsed since the last dose of LMWH, UFH can be used for PCI according to usual practice patterns. Because the anticoagulant effect of UFH can be more readily reversed than that of LMWH, UFH is preferred in patients likely to undergo CABG within 24 hours, although the need for CABG cannot reliably be predicted in the ED.

Two LMWH compounds are approved by the U.S. FDA for the treatment of non-ST elevation ACS, enoxaparin and dalteparin. Dalteparin (Fragmin®) was shown in the FRIC study[54] to be noninferior in safety and efficacy to UFH, while in the ESSENCE[50] and TIMI-11B[51] studies, enoxaparin was shown to be clearly superior to UFH.

In summary, the most recent clinical trial data and specialty guidelines confirm enoxaparin as the LMWH of choice in patients with non-ST elevation ACS—and in most cases, as the preferable substitute for UFH. Moreover, they also provide increasing evidence that patients with PCI can be safely and effectively managed using a combination of enoxaparin and a GP IIb/IIIa antagonist. *(Please See Figures, in which protocols for evaluating and managing acute coronary syndromes are presented.)*

Pharmacoeconomic Implications of the Use of Enoxaparin in AMI. A number of studies support the observation that enoxaparin reduces the incidence of adverse cardiovascular end points, among them recurrent MI and the need for revascularization, without increasing major bleeding in patients with ACS, including UA and acute STEMI.[1,55-57] These clinical benefits are associated with economic benefits in terms of reduced expenditure on revascularization procedures, the requirement for additional drug therapies, and drug administration. Accordingly, several pharmacoeconomic analyses have been conducted on the use of enoxaparin in ACS.[58-61]

Enoxaparin has been shown to be associated with cost-saving compared with UFH in the management of UA and NSTEMI in health economic studies from Canada, the United States, the United Kingdom, South America, and France.[58-61] These cost savings accrue from reductions in administration costs (primarily associated with the subcutaneous dosing of enoxaparin compared with intravenous UFH); the amount of nursing time required (this also increases the availability of nurses for other duties); the need for revascularization procedures (and any complications arising from these procedures); and the duration of hospitalization.[60]

Oral Platelet Antagonists: The Role of Clopidogrel Pretreatment. The Clopidogrel in Unstable Angina to Prevent Recurrent Events (CURE) trial was designed to compare the efficacy and safety of the early and long-term use of clopidogrel plus aspirin with that of aspirin alone in patients with ACS and no ST-segment elevation.[62] In the CURE trial, 12,562 patients who had presented within 24 hours after the onset of symptoms were randomly assigned to receive either clopidogrel (300 mg immediately, followed by 75 mg once daily) or placebo, in addition to aspirin, for 3-12 months.

The first primary outcome (a composite of death from cardiovascular causes, nonfatal MI, or stroke) occurred in 9.3% of the patients in the clopidogrel group and 11.4% of the patients in the placebo group (RR with clopidogrel as compared with placebo, 0.80; 95% CI, 0.72-0.90; p < 0.001). The second primary outcome—the first primary outcome or refractory ischemia—occurred in 16.5% of the patients treated with clopidogrel and 18.8% of the patients in the placebo group (RR, 0.86; p < 0.001). The percentage of patients with major bleeding was greater in the clopidogrel group (RR, 1.38), although the percentage of patients with life-threatening bleeding was not greater.[62] Among 2568 patients receiving PCI in the CURE study, pretreatment with clopidogrel also was beneficial in those patients undergoing mechanical revascularization.[63] A clopidogrel loading dose for appropriately selected patients is recommended in the setting of ACS based on a study that demonstrates an onset of effect within two hours compared to greater than six hours without the loading dose.[64]

It should be emphasized that not all patients are appropriate candidates for clopidogrel. Transfusions are increased, and in PCI there was no benefit beyond 30 days. The benefit was limited to recurrent MI reduction only, and there was no concomitant use of GP IIb/IIIa blockers in this trial. The CURE study provides strong evidence for the addition of clopidogrel to aspirin in the ED as part of overall management of patients with UA/NSTEMI, in whom CABG is contraindicated or in whom a noninterventional approach is intended—an especially useful approach in hospitals that do not have a routine policy of early invasive procedures. One reasonable approach for hospitals in which patients with UA/NSTEMI undergo diagnostic catheterization within 24-36 hours of admission, is to withhold clopidogrel until it is clear that CABG will *not* be scheduled within the next several days; that is, it should not be initiated in the ED. A loading dose of clopidogrel can be given to a patient on the catheterization table if PCI is to be carried out immediately. If PCI is not performed, clopidogrel can be administered after the catheterization.

SUMMARY

Physicians' ability to intervene successfully in coronary ischemia emergencies continues to evolve and improve. It is clear that prompt revascularization ("time is muscle") is associated with the best possible outcomes in STEMI. A body of literature seems to be growing that indicates, when available, an interventional management strategy is to be preferred in these patients. Fibrinolytic therapy, however, if not contraindicated, still should be considered standard of care when an interventional approach is not possible or is not available within a very short period of time. The role of aggressive antiplatelet therapy in STEMI patients still is being evaluated. The importance of reliable and safe anticoagulation, regardless of management strategy, is clear.

Physicians also are coming to understand that "time is muscle" in non-ST elevation ACS as well; accordingly, management strategies are becoming increasingly aggressive. This is particularly true in the case of patients with high-risk features of NSTEMI, for whom the ACC and AHA now recommend GP IIb/IIIa receptor blockade and an urgent interventional management approach. Antiplatelet and anticoagulation therapies are essential in ACS patients without ST-segment elevation, as well. The new guidelines specifically cite enoxaparin as the agent of choice in this regard.

The guidelines presented here are intended to provide a user-friendly, evidence-based, clinical resource that assists the physician in the initial evaluation and management based entirely on data that should be available in an ED setting. The goals for management of ACS patients are rapid and accurate risk stratification, appropriate and institution-specific triage to interventional vs. medical strategies, and optimal pharmacologic therapy—all of which provide for a smooth and seamless transition of care between the ED and the cardiology service. These guidelines—and the CEVAT initiative that underlies them—are intended to assist skilled physicians in meeting those goals.

REFERENCES

1. Efficacy and safety of tenecteplase in combination with enoxaparin, abciximab, or unfractionated heparin: the ASSENT-3 randomised trial in acute myocardial infarction. *Lancet* 2001;358:605.

2. Ross AM, Molhoek GP, Knudtson ML, et al. A randomized comparison of low-

molecular-weight heparin and unfractionated heparin adjunctive to t-PA thrombolysis and aspirin (HART-II) [Abstract]. *Circulation* 2000;102(Suppl 18):II-600.

3. Antman EM, Louwerenburg HW, Baars HF, et al. Enoxaparin as adjunctive antithrombin therapy for ST-elevation myocardial infarction: results of the ENTIRE-Thrombolysis in Myocardial Infarction (TIMI) 23 Trial. *Circulation* 2002;105:1642.

4. Topol EJ. Reperfusion therapy for acute myocardial infarction with fibrinolytic therapy or combination reduced fibrinolytic therapy and platelet glycoprotein IIb/IIIa inhibition: the GUSTO V randomised trial. *Lancet* 2001;357:1905.

5. Indications for fibrinolytic therapy in suspected acute myocardial infarction: collaborative overview of early mortality and major morbidity results form all randomised trials of more than 1000 patients. Fibrinolytic Therapy Trialists' (FTT) Collaborative Group. *Lancet* 1994;343:311.

6. The effects of tissue plasminogen activator, streptokinase, or both on coronary-artery patency, ventricular function, and survival after acute myocardial infarction. The GUSTO Angiographic Investigators. *N Engl J Med* 1993;329:1615.

7. Randomized trial of intravenous streptokinase, oral aspirin, both, or neither among 17,187 cases of suspected acute myocardial infarction: ISIS-2. ISIS-2 (Second International Study of Infarct Survival) Collaborative Group. *Lancet* 1988;2:349.

8. Weaver WD, Cerqueira M, Hallstrom AP, et al. Prehospital-initiated vs hospital-initiated fibrinolytic therapy. The Myocardial Infarction Triage and Intervention Trial. *JAMA* 1993;270:1211.

9. GISSI-2: a factorial randomised trial of alteplase versus streptokinase and heparin versus no heparin among 12,490 patients with acute myocardial infarction. Gruppo Italiano per lo Studio della Sopravvivenza nell'Infarto Miocardico. *Lancet* 1990;336:65.

10. In-hospital mortality and clinical course of 20,891 patients with suspected acute myocardial infarction randomised between alteplase and streptokinase with or without heparin. The International Study Group. *Lancet* 1990;336:71.

11. ISIS-3: a randomised comparison of streptokinase vs tissue plasminogen activator vs anistreplase and of aspirin plus heparin vs aspirin alone among 41,299 cases of suspected acute myocardial infarction. ISIS-3 (Third International Study of Infarct Survival) Collaborative Group. *Lancet* 1992;339:753.

12. A comparison of reteplase with alteplase for acute myocardial infarction. The Global

Use of Strategies to Open Occluded Coronary Arteries (GUSTO III) Investigators. *N Engl J Med* 1997;337:1118.

13. Single-bolus tenecteplase compared with front-loaded alteplase in acute myocardial infarction: the ASSENT-2 double-blind randomised trial. Assessment of the Safety and Efficacy of a New Thrombolytic Investigators. *Lancet* 1999;354:716.

14. Randomised trial of late fibrinolysis in patients with suspected acute myocardial infarction. EMERAS (Estudio Multicentrico Estreptoquinas Republicas de America del Sur) Collaborative Group. *Lancet* 1993;342:767.

15. Late Assessment of Fibrinolytic Efficacy (LATE) study with alteplase 6-24 hours after onset of acute myocardial infarction. *Lancet* 1993;342:759.

16. Effectiveness of intravenous fibrinolytic treatment in acute myocardial infarction. Gruppo Italiano per lo Studio della Streptochinasi nell'Infarto Miocardico (GISSI). *Lancet* 1986;8478:397.

17. Grines CL, Browne KF, Marco J, et al. A comparison of immediate angioplasty with fibrinolytic therapy for acute myocardial infarction. The Primary Angioplasty in Myocardial Infarction Study Group. *N Engl J Med* 1993;328:673.

18. Ryan TJ, Antman EM, Brooks NH, et al. 1999 update: ACC/AHA guidelines for the management of patients with acute myocardial infarction. A report of the American College of Cardiology/ American Heart Association Task Force on Practice Guidelines (Committee on Management of Acute Myocardial Infarction). *J Am Coll Cardiol* 1999;34:890.

19. Braunwald E, Antman EM, Beasley JW, et al. ACC/AHA guidelines for the management of patients with unstable angina and non-ST-segment elevation myocardial infarction. A report of the American College of Cardiology/American Heart Association Task Force on Practice Guidelines (Committee on the Management of Patients with Unstable Angina). *J Am Coll Cardiol* 2000;36:970.

20. Wilcox RG, von der Lippe G, Olsson CG, et al. Trial of tissue plasminogen activator for mortality reduction in acute myocardial infarction. Anglo-Scandinavian Study of Early Fibrinolysis (ASSET). *Lancet* 1988;2:525.

21. Sgarbossa EB, Pinski SL, Barbagelata A, et al. Electrocardiographic diagnosis of evolving acute myocardial infarction in the presence of left bundle-branch block. GUSTO-1 (Global Utilization of Streptokinase and Tissue Plasminogen Activator for Occluded Coronary Arteries) Investigators. *N Engl J Med* 1996;334:481.

22. Effects of tissue plasminogen activator and a comparison of early invasive and conservative strategies in unstable angina and non-Q-wave myocardial infarction. Results of the TIMI-IIIB Trial. Thrombosis in Myocardial Ischemia. *Circulation* 1994;89:1545.

23. Tenaglia AN, Califf EM, Candela RJ, et al. Thrombolytic therapy in patients requiring cardiopulmonary resuscitation. *Am J Cardiol* 1991;68:1015.

24. van Campen LC, Leeuwen GR, Verheugt FW. Safety and efficacy of thrombolysis for acute myocardial infarction in patients with prolonged out-of-hospital cardiopulmonary resuscitation. *Am J Cardiol* 1994;73:953.

25. Bottiger BW, Bode C, Kern S, et al. Efficacy and safety of thrombolytic therapy after initially unsuccessful cardiopulmonary resuscitation: A prospective clinical trial. *Lancet* 2001;357:1583.

26. Wallentin L, Delborg DM, Lindahl B, et al. The low-molecular-weight heparin dalteparin as adjuvant therapy in acute myocardial infarction: the ASSENT PLUS study. *Clin Cardiol* 2001;24(3 Suppl):I12.

27. Kakkar VV, Iyengar SS, DeLorenzo F, et al. Low molecular weight heparin for the treatment of acute myocardial infarction (FAMI): Fragmin (dalteparin sodium) in acute myocardial infarction. *Indian Heart J* 2000;52:533.

28. Chamuleau SA, de Winter RJ, Levi M, et al. Low molecular weight heparin as an adjunct to thrombolysis for acute myocardial infarction: the FATIMA study. Fraxiparin Anticoagulant Therapy in Myocardial Infarction Study Amsterdam (FATIMA) Study Group. *Heart* 1998;80:35.

29. Baird SH, Menown IB, Mcbride SJ, et al. Randomized comparison of enoxaparin with unfractionated heparin following fibrinolytic therapy for acute myocardial infarction. *Eur Heart J* 2002;23:627.

30. Suryapranata H, van't Hof AW, Hoorntje JC, et al. Randomized comparison of coronary stenting with balloon angioplasty in selected patients with acute myocardial infarction. *Circulation* 1998;97:2502.

31. Schomig A, Kastrati A, Dirschinger J, et al. Coronary stenting plus platelet glycoprotein IIb/IIIa blockade compared with tissue plasminogen activator in acute myocardial infarction. Stent versus Thrombolysis for Occluded Coronary Arteries in Patients with Acute Myocardial Infarction Study Investigators. *N Engl J Med* 2000;343:385.

32. Brener SJ, Barr LA, Burchenal JE, et al. Randomized, placebo-controlled trial of platelet glycoprotein IIb/IIIa blockade with primary angioplasty for acute myocardial

infarction. ReoPro and Primary PTCA Organization and Randomized Trial (RAP-PORT) Investigators. *Circulation* 1998;98:734.

33. Montalescot G, Barragan P, Beauregard P, et al. Abciximab associated with primary angioplasty and stenting in acute myocardial infarction: The ADMIRAL study, 30 day final results. *Circulation* 1999;100:I-87.

34. Stone GW, Grines CL, Cox DA, et al. Comparison of angioplasty with stenting, with or without abciximab, in acute myocardial infarction. *N Engl J Med* 2002;346:957.

35. Brady WJ, Esterowitz D, Syverud SA. Consideration of primary angioplasty: impact on the door-to-drug time in AMI patients ultimately treated with thrombolytic agent. *Am J Emerg Med* 2001; 19:15.

36. Cannon CP, Gibson CM, Lambrew CT, et al. Relationship of symptom-onset-to-balloon time and door-to-balloon time with mortality in patients undergoing angioplasty for acute myocardial infarction. *JAMA* 2000;283:2941.

37. Ryan TJ, Anderson JL, Antman EM, et al. ACC/AHA guidelines for the management of patients with acute myocardial infarction: executive summary. A report of the American College of Cardiology/American Heart Association Task Force on Practice Guidelines (Committee on Management of Acute Myocardial Infarction). *Circulation* 1996;94:2341.

38. Antman EM, Cohen M, Bernink PJ, et al. The TIMI Risk Score for unstable angina/non-ST elevation MI: a method for prognostication and therapeutic decision making. *JAMA* 2000;284:835.

39. Poster presentation. American College of Cardiology Scientific Presentation. March 2001, Atlanta, GA. Royal Infirmary Investigators (Edinburgh).

40. Michalis LK, Papamichail N, Katsouras C, et al. Enoxaparin versus tinzaparin in the management of unstable coronary artery disease (EVET Study). *J Am Coll Cardiol* 2001;37:365a.

41. Cannon CP, Weintraub WS, Demoupoulos LA, et. al. Comparison of early invasive and conservative strategies in patients with unstable coronary syndromes treated with the glycoprotein IIb/IIIa inhibitor tirofiban. *N Engl J Med* 2001;344:1879.

42. Ferguson JJ. NICE-3 prospective, open label, non-randomized observational safety study on the combination of LMW heparin with the clinically available GP IIb/IIIa antagonists in 600 patients with acute coronary syndromes. *Eur Heart J* 2000;21:599.

43. Kereiakes DJ. Enoxaparin and abciximab adjunctive pharmacotherapy during percuta-

neous coronary intervention. *J Invasive Cardiol* 2001;13:272.

44. Lincoff AM, Tcheng JE, Califf RM, et al. Sustained suppression of ischemic complications of coronary intervention by platelet GP IIb/IIIa blockade with abciximab: One year outcome in the EPILOG trial. Evaluation in PTCA to Improve Long-term Outcome with abciximab GP IIb/IIIa blockade. *Circulation* 1999;99:1951.

45. Collet JP, Montalescot G, Lison L, et al. Percutaneous coronary intervention in unstable angina patients pretreated with subcutaneous enoxaparin. *Eur Heart J* 2000;21:599.

46. Dudek D, Zymek P, Bartus S, et al. Prospective randomized comparison of enoxaparin versus unfractionated heparin for elective percutaneous coronary interventions among ticlopidine-pretreated patients. *Eur Heart J* 2000;21:381.

47. Collet J, Montalescot G, Lison L, et al. Percutaneous coronary intervention after subcutaneous enoxaparin pretreatment in patients with unstable angina pectoris. *Circulation* 2001;103:658.

48. Invasive compared with non-invasive treatment in unstable coronary-artery disease: FRISC-II prospective randomised multicentre study. FRagmin and Fast Revascularization during InStability in Coronary artery disease investigators. *Lancet* 1999;354:708.

49. Goodman S. INTERACT Study, oral presentation. American College of Cardiology Annual Congress, Atlanta, GA; April 2002.

50. Cohen M, Demers C, Gurfinkel EP, et al. A comparison of low-molecular-weight heparin with unfractionated heparin for unstable coronary artery disease. Efficacy and Safety of Subcutaneous Enoxaparin in Non-Q-wave Coronary Events Study Group. *N Engl J Med* 1997;337:447.

51. Antman EM, McCabe CH, Gurkinel EP, et al. Enoxaparin prevents death and cardiac ischemic events in unstable angina/non-Q-wave myocardial infarction. Results of the thrombolysis in myocardial infarction (TIMI) 11B trial. *Circulation* 1999;100:1593.

52. Please see updated guidelines for NSTE ACS released March 15, 2002, at either www.acc.org or www.americanheart.org.

53. Young JJ, Kereiakes DJ, Grines CL. Low-molecular-weight heparin therapy in percutaneous coronary intervention: the NICE 1 and NICE 4 trials. National Investigators Collaborating on Enoxaparin Investigators. *J Invasive Cardiol* 2000;12(Suppl E):E14-

E18; discussion E25-E28.

54. Klein W, Buchwald A, Hillis SE, et al. Comparison of low-molecular-weight heparin with unfractionated heparin acutely and with placebo for 6 weeks in the management of unstable coronary artery disease. Fragmin in unstable coronary artery disease study (FRIC) [erratum appears in *Circulation* 1998;97:413]. *Circulation* 1997;96:61.

55. Cohen M. Low molecular weight heparins in the management of unstable angina/non-Q-wave myocardial infarction. *Semin Thromb Hemost* 1999;25(Suppl 3):113.

56. Antman EM, McCabe CH, Gurfinkel EP, et al. Enoxaparin prevents death and cardiac ischemic events in unstable angina/non-Q-wave myocardial infarction. Results of the thrombolysis in myocardial infarction (TIMI) IIB trial. *Circulation* 1999;100: 1593.

57. Wallentin L. Efficacy of low-molecular-weight heparin in acute coronary syndromes. *Am Heart J* 2000;139(2 Part 2):S29.

58. Balen RM, Marra CA, Zed PJ, et al. Cost-effectiveness analysis of enoxaparin versus unfractionated heparin for acute coronary syndromes. A Canadian hospital perspective. *Pharmacoeconomics* 1999;16(5 pt 2):533.

59. Mark DB, Cowper PA, Berkowitz SD, et al. Economic assessment of low-molecular-weight heparin (enoxaparin) versus unfractionated heparin in acute coronary syndrome patients: results from the ESSENCE randomized trial. Efficacy and Safety of Subcutaneous Enoxaparin in Non-Q wave Coronary Events [unstable angina or non-Q-wave myocardial infarction]. *Circulation* 1998;97:1702.

60. Fox KAA, Bosanquet N. Assessing the UK cost implications of the use of low molecular weight heparin in unstable coronary artery disease. *Br J Cardiol* 1998;5:92.

61. Detournay B, Huet X, Fagnani F, et al. Economic evaluation of enoxaparin sodium versus heparin in unstable angina. A French substudy of the ESSENCE trial. *Pharmacoeconomics* 2000;18:83.

62. Yusuf S, Zhao F, Mehta SR, et al. Effects of clopidogrel in addition to aspirin in patients with acute coronary syndromes without ST-segment elevation. *N Engl J Med* 2001;345:494.

63. Mehta SR, Yusuf S, Peters RJ, et al. Effects of pretreatment with clopidogrel and aspirin followed by long-term therapy in patients undergoing percutaneous coronary intervention: the PCI-CURE study. *Lancet* 2001;358:527.

64. Helft G, Osende JI, Worthley SG, et al. Acute antithrombotic effect of a front-loaded

regimen of clopidogrel in patients with atherosclerosis on aspirin. *Arterioscler Thromb Vasc Biol* 2000;20:2316.

CME QUESTIONS

23. PCI, which may include percutaneous transluminal coronary angioplasty (PTCA) and coronary stenting, have many theoretical and practical advantages, including which of the following?
    A. A larger patient eligibility pool for PCI
    B. A lower risk of intracranial bleeding
    C. A significantly higher initial reperfusion rate
    D. Earlier definition of coronary artery anatomy
    E. All of the above

24. Determining an optimal approach to coronary reperfusion requires a multifactorial assessment of clinical factors. Which of the following should be included in this assessment?
    A. Patient eligibility for specific interventions (medical vs invasive) based on risk stratification
    B. Adherence to risk-stratification protocols
    C. Availability of institutional resources and cardiologists with sufficient experience in percutaneous coronary reperfusion techniques
    D. The ability to provide prompt transfer to another hospital for patients who may require PCI and the presence of exclusion and inclusion factors that determine patient eligibility for fibrinolysis
    E. All of the above

25. The investigators of the ASSENT-3 trial concluded that the tenecteplase plus enoxaparin regimen reduced the frequency of ischemic complications in AMI, producing an overall relative reduction in primary adverse end points of what percentage in the enoxaparin-tenecteplase group as compared to the UFH group?

    A.   6% reduction

    B.   16% reduction

    C.   26% reduction

    D.   46% reduction

    E.   None of the above

26. Indications for transfer of a patient with AMI to a regional, tertiary care facility with PCI and cardiovascular surgery capabilities include which of the following subgroups?

    A.   Patients with contraindications to fibrinolytic therapy who may benefit from PCI or CABG

    B.   Patients with persistent hemodynamic instability or persistent ventricular dysrhythmias

    C.   Patients with postinfarction or post-reperfusion ischemia

    D.   Patients with contraindications to fibrinolytic therapy

    E.   All of the above

27. All of the following statements are true about the Integrilin and Enoxaparin Randomized assessment of Acute Coronary Syndromes Treatment (INTERACT) trial, except:

    A.   GP IIb/IIIa inhibitors are safer than enoxaparin in patients with NSTEMI.

    B.   The risk of bleeding at 48 and 96 hours for enoxaparin- and UFH-treated patients, respectively, was 1.1% vs. 3.8% (p = 0.014) and 1.8% vs. 4.6% (p = 0.03).

    C.   ECG-determined ischemic events were much less common in enoxaparin- (14.1% amd 12.7% at 0-48 and 48-96 hours, respectively) than UFH-treated patients.

    D.   This is the largest randomized study of the combination of a LMWH and a GP IIb/IIIa agent to date.

28. In the 2002 update (www.acc.org or www.americanheart.org), the ACC/AHA published new recommendations regarding the use of antico-

agulants. These include which of the following?

A.   Anticoagulation with subcutaneous LMWH or intravenous UFH should be added to antiplatelet therapy with ASA and/or clopidogrel (Class I, Level A).

B.   Enoxaparin is preferable to UFH as an anticoagulant in patients with UA/NSTEMI, unless CABG is planned within 24 hours (Class IIa, Level A).

C.   Both A and B

D.   None of the above

29. The issue of performing PCI in patients anticoagulated with LMWH, and therefore whose aPTT or activated clotting time (ACT) does not accurately reflect the extent of anticoagulation, was addressed in a study of 293 UA/NSTEMI patients. It showed that PCI can be performed safely with the usual dose of enoxaparin.

A.   True

B.   False

30. In the CURE study, the first primary outcome (a composite of death from cardiovascular causes, nonfatal myocardial infarction, or stroke) occurred in 31.3% of the patients in the clopidogrel group and 11.4% of the patients in the placebo group (RR with clopidogrel as compared with placebo, 0.80; 95% CI, 0.72-0.90; $p < 0.001$).

A.   True

B.   False

For instructions on how to participate in this CME activity, please see the back of this book (page 717).

QUICK CONSULT GUIDE:
PRIMARY CARE AND
EMERGENCY MEDICINE

PEDIATRIC EMERGENCIES

ACUTE OTITIS MEDIA

Organisms Isolated by Tympanocentesis in Acute Otitis Media

COMMON

Streptococcus pneumoniae

Haemophilus influenzae

Moraxella catarrhalis

LESS COMMON

Streptococcus pyogenes

*Staphylococcus aureus**

Gram-negative enteric bacteria*

Anaerobic bacteria

Viral pathogens:

- respiratory syncytial virus
- rhinovirus
- adenovirus
- influenza
- parainfluenza

* relatively common in neonates (< 1 month of age)

Risk Factors for Otitis Media

- Day care attendance
- Siblings at home
- Second-hand cigarette smoke
- Lack of exclusive breast feeding for the first four months
- Male sex
- White race
- Native American race
- Craniofacial abnormalities, including cleft palate
- Family history of otitis media
- Family history of atopy
- History of otitis media

Factors Considered in Determining Total Outcome Costs for Otitis Media in Children

- Cost of *initial* physician (or extended provider) visit

- Cost of the first antibiotic prescription

- Cost of subsequent human resource time (telephone consultations, reevaluations, etc.) expended by nurses, physicians, and other providers to service queries about the drug, its side effects, dosing schedule, and other questions

- Cost of practitioner reevaluation time to assess cause of treatment failures

- Cost of subsequent antibiotic prescriptions (i.e., additional courses of therapy) in response to treatment failures

- Economic opportunity costs sustained by parents or guardians because of time lost from work to care for child or administer medication

- Cost of medications or other measures (diapers) to service gastrointestinal side effects (diarrhea) of antibiotics

- Cost of managing sequelae related to treatment failure: recurrent infections, tympanostomy, mastoiditis, hearing loss, learning disability, otitis media with effusion, etc.

Common Signs and Symptoms of Inflammation and Fluid in the Middle Ear*

- Otalgia
- Ear pulling
- Diminished hearing
- Fever
- Loss of appetite

- Irritability
- Vomiting
- Vertigo
- Tinnitus
- Otorrhea

* O'Handley JG. Acute otitis media. In: Rakel RE (ed.) *Manual of Medical Practice.* 2nd ed. Philadelphia: WB Saunders; 1996:78-79.

Prescription, Parent, Patient and Drug Resistance (PPPD) Factors Influencing Antibiotic Selection for Acute Otitis Media in Children

PRESCRIPTION AND PHARMACY RESISTANCE BARRIERS

— Cost of course of therapy

— Prescription coverage by health plan

— Formulary status/availability

— Previous experience with medication

— Physician and pharmacist-based patient education

— Written instructions for parent/guardian regarding medication intake

— Emphasizing importance of medication compliance

PARENT RESISTANCE BARRIERS

— Number of days required to complete a course of therapy

— Daily dose frequency of medication (once-daily dosing optimal)

— Day care considerations: Can all doses of the antibiotic be given by the parent without reliance on day care personnel or other caretakers to ensure administration?

— Can medication be taken with or without food, or are special timing considerations required?

— Do side effects (diarrhea, GI discomfort, etc.) deter parents from completing a full course of therapy?

— Does the drug require refrigeration?

PATIENT RESISTANCE BARRIERS

— Taste of medication: Does the suspension have a pleasant and appealing flavor, and a palatable consistency? Or, is the taste excessively bitter and the consistency granular and unappealing for the child?

— Gastrointestinal tolerance profile: GI distress? Diarrhea? Nausea? Rash?

— Discontinuation rate of antibiotic

— Does child feel "forced" to take antibiotic?

DRUG RESISTANCE BARRIERS

— What are clinical cure rates in well-designed clinical trials?

— Does antibiotic show increasing in vitro resistance to *S. pneumoniae*?

— Does antibiotic show increasing in vitro resistance to beta-lactamase-+ middle ear pathogens, *H. influenzae*, and *M. catarrhalis*?

— What are regional or local antibiotic resistance patterns?

Prescription, Parent, Patient and Drug Resistance (PPPD) Approach to Selection of Antibiotic Suspensions for Treatment of Acute Otitis Media in Children[*]

ORAL ANTIBIOTIC SUSPENSION	PRESCRIPTION RESISTANCE	PARENTAL RESISTANCE
(Generic name)	(Cost for course of therapy < $40)	(Once-daily dosing)
Amoxicillin	++ ($7.49)	± (BID)
Amoxicillin-clavulanate	+ ($39.40)	± (BID)
Azithromycin	+ ($30.35)	+ (QD)
Cefaclor	+ ($39.40)	– (BID/TID)
Cefixime	– ($47.20)	+ (QD)
Cefpodoxime	– ($56.00)	+ (QD)
Cefprozil	– ($47.35)	± (BID)
Cefuroxime	– ($64.84)	± (BID)
Clarithromycin	– ($44.60)	± (BID)
Erythromycin-sulfisoxazole	+ ($23.60)	– (TID or QID)
Loracarbef	– ($57.20)	± (BID)
Trimethoprim-sulfamethoxazole	++ ($6.63)	± (BID)
Ceftriaxone	± ($24-72)	± QD (1-3 days)

Key:
[*] Finney JW, et al. *Am J Dis Child* 1985;139:89-95; Greenbery RN. *Clin Ther* 1984;6:592-599; Bosker G. St. Louis: Facts and Comparisons; 1996; Blondeau JM, et al. *Antimicrob Agents Chemother* 1999;43(Suppl A):25-30; Haddad JJR, et al. *Otolaryngol Clin North Am* 1994;27:431-441; McLinn S. *Pediatr Infect Dis J* 1995;14:S62-66; Demers DM, et al. *Pediatr Infect Dis J* 1994:13:87-89; Chinburapa V, Larson LN. *J Clin Pharm Ther* 1992;17:333-342; Beardon PH, et al. *BMJ* 1993;307:846-848; Berg JS, et al. *Ann Pharmacother* 1993;27:S1-24; Litchman HM. *R I Med* 1993;76:608-610; McNally DL, Wertheimer D. *Md Med J* 1992;41:223-225; Anonymous. *Can Med Assoc J* 1991;44:647-648; Coleman TJ. *BMJ* 1994;308:135; Roth HP, Caron HS. *Clin Pharm Ther* 1978;23:361-370.

PATIENT RESISTANCE	DRUG RESISTANCE
(Palatability and GI effect profile considered extremely favorable)	(Less than 30% of *S. pneumoniae* isolates from middle ear show in vitro resistance and drug show adequate coverage of beta-lactamase-producing *H. influenzae* and *M. catarrhalis*)
+	–
– (diarrhea)	+
+	+
+	±
+	±
– (poor taste)	+
– (poor taste)	+
+	+
– (poor taste)	+
– (poor taste, GI intolerance)	±
+	+
– (allergic reactions)	±
– (intramuscular injection)	+

(+) Satisfies specific PPPD category criterion

(-) Does not usually satisfy specific PPPD category criterion

(±) Possibly satisfies PPPD category criterion

Antibiotics of Choice for Pediatric Otitis Media

FIRST-LINE ANTIBIOTIC SUSPENSIONS FOR ACUTE OTITIS MEDIA IN CHILDREN (COST FOR COURSE OF THERAPY USUALLY LESS THAN $10)

GENERIC NAME	TRADE NAME	DOSAGE
Amoxicillin	Amoxil	45-90 mg/kg/d in two or three divided doses

SECOND-LINE ANTIBIOTIC SUSPENSION FOR AOM (COST < $10)

GENERIC NAME	TRADE NAME	DOSAGE
Trimethoprim-Sulfamethoxazole	Septra or Bactrim	8/40 mg/kg/d

FIRST-LINE ANTIBIOTIC SUSPENSIONS FOR ACUTE OTITIS MEDIA IN CHILDREN (COST FOR COURSE OF THERAPY USUALLY LESS THAN $45)

GENERIC NAME	TRADE NAME	DOSAGE
Amoxicillin-clavulanate	Augmentin	90/20 mg/kg/d
Azithromycin	Zithromax	30 mg/kg one dose, OR 10 mg/kg qd x 3 days

FIRST-LINE ANTIBIOTIC SUSPENSIONS FOR ACUTE OTITIS MEDIA IN CHILDREN (COST FOR COURSE OF THERAPY USUALLY MORE THAN $40)

GENERIC NAME	TRADE NAME	DOSAGE
Cefuroxime	Ceftin	30 mg/kg/d
Ceftriaxone	Rocephin	50 mg/kg/d IM

SECOND-LINE ANTIBIOTIC SUSPENSIONS FOR ACUTE OTITIS MEDIA IN CHILDREN (COST FOR COURSE OF THERAPY USUALLY MORE THAN $40)

GENERIC NAME	TRADE NAME	DOSAGE
Clarithromycin	Biaxin	15 mg/kg/d
Cefpodoxime	Vantin	10 mg/kg/d

DURATION	COST	COMMENTS
10 days	$6.02-$8.13	Significant resistance to beta-lactamase-producing *H. influenzae* and *M. catarrhalis*. Up to 25% of *S. pneumoniae* resistant at lower doses. Widely used as first-line agent.

DURATION	COST	COMMENTS
10 days	$5.36-$7.70	Increasing resistance (up to 30%) to *S. pneumoniae* species
		Allergic reactions: Stevens-Johnson (rare)

DURATION	COST	COMMENTS
10 days	$38.10-$44.30	Diarrhea common (16% of patients)
one dose OR 3 days	$28.40-$32.20	Compliance-enhancing. Good in vitro coverage of beta-lactamase-producing *H. influenzae* and *M. catarrhalis*. Clinical cure rates in pediatric otitis media comparable to those seen with amoxicillin/clavulanate.

DURATION	COST	COMMENTS
10 days	$62.84	
1-3 days	$24-$72	Intramuscular dosing may be inconvenient. IV dose also available.

DURATION	COST	COMMENTS
10 days	$42.40-$44.10	Palatability may be a consideration
10 days	$54.00-$57.20	Palatability may be a consideration

SHOULDER, ELBOW, AND FOREARM INJURIES

Summary of Fractures of Shoulder, Elbow, and Forearm

BONE	MECHANISM OF INJURY
CLAVICLE	
Middle	Fall onto shoulder or outstretched hand
Distal	Fall onto shoulder or outstretched hand
HUMERUS	
Proximal	Extension of arm in adduction
Shaft	Fall on elbow or hand/direct impact
ELBOW	
Supracondylar	Hyperextension fall
Lateral condyle	Fall on outstretched hand
Medial condyle	Fall on hand with valgus impact
Olecranon	Direct trauma
Radial head/neck	Fall on outstretched hand
RADIUS/ULNA	
Shaft	Fall on outstretched hand
Distal	Fall on outstretched hand
Monteggia	Fall on outstretched hand
Galeazzi	Fall on outstretched hand

TREATMENT

Figure-of-eight or sling/swathe

Sling/swathe

Sling/swathe

Sling/swathe
Sugar tong (adolescents)

Nondisplaced: Posterior splint with elbow at 90°
Displaced: Orthopedic reduction, pinning

Nondisplaced: Posterior splint
Displaced: > 2mm, reduction/pinning

Nondisplaced: Posterior splint
Displaced: Open reduction

Nondisplaced: Splint in partial extension
Displaced: Open reduction/fixation

Nondisplaced: Posterior splint
Displaced or > 15° angle: Reduction

Nondisplaced: Long arm cast or splint
> 10° angle: Reduction (open/closed)
Nondisplaced: Cast or splint
Displaced or > 10-15° angle: Reduction

Reduction

Reduction

Ossification Centers of the Elbow

Ossification Centers	Age of Appearance
Capitellum	1 yr.
Medial epicondyle	4-5 yrs.
Radial head	4-6 yrs.
Olecranon	6-9 yrs.
Trochlea	8-10 yrs.
Lateral epicondyle	10-12 yrs.

PEDIATRIC SEXUAL ABUSE

Behavioral Indicators of Pediatric Sexual Abuse*

BEHAVIORS SUGGESTIVE OF SEXUAL ABUSE

- Abrupt change in personality
- Age-inappropriate knowledge of sexual acts
- Aggression
- Appetite disturbances
- Clinging
- Depression
- Eating disturbances
- Low self-esteem
- Neurotic or conduct disorders
- Nightmares
- Phobias
- Excessive fear
- Problems at school
- Sexual behavior
- Sexual perpetration on others
- Self-injury
- Sleep disturbances
- Social problems with peers
- Substance abuse
- Suicidal ideation
- Suicide attempt
- Temper tantrums
- Withdrawal

* Bays J, Chadwick D. *Child Abuse Negl* 1993;17:91-110; De Jong AR, Finkel MA. *Curr Probl Pediatr* 1990;20:495-567; Hunter RS, Kilstrom N, Loda F. *Child Abuse Negl* 1985;9:17-25; Sidel JS, Elvik SL, Berkowitz CD, et al.*Pediatr Emerg Care* 1986;2: 157-164.

Complaint/Exam Indicators of Sexual Abuse*

COMPLAINTS/FINDINGS SUGGESTIVE OF SEXUAL ABUSE

- Abdominal pain

- Anogenital bleeding

- Anogenital discharge

- Anogenital itching

- Anogenital pain

- Anogenital trauma

- Bruises to hard palate

- Bruises to soft palate

- Chronic constipation

- Chronic pain

- Dysuria

- Encopresis

- Enuresis

- Foreign bodies in vagina or rectum

- Pregnancy

- Recurrent urinary tract infection

- Sexually transmitted disease

- Vulvovaginitis

* Bays J, Chadwick D. *Child Abuse Negl* 1993;17:91-110; De Jong AR, Finkel MA. *Curr Probl Pediatr* 1990;20:495-567; Hunter RS, Kilstrom N, Loda F. *Child Abuse Negl* 1985;9:17-25; Sidel JS, Elvik SL, Berkowitz CD, et al. *Pediatr Emerg Care* 1986;2: 157-164.

Interview Questions when Pediatric Sexual Abuse is Suspected*

SEXUAL ABUSE DISCLOSED

- I understand that something has happened to you.

- Do you hurt anywhere?

- Where do you hurt?

- What happened?

- Who did this?

SEXUAL ABUSE SUSPECTED

- Do you have private places on your body?

- What do you call them?

- Have you been touched in those private places? (Assign child's terminology.)

- Have you been hurt in those private places? (Assign child's terminology.)

* Jones DPH, McQuiaton M. *Interviewing the Sexually Abused Child.* 2nd ed. Denver, CO: C. Henry Kempe National Center for the Prevention and Treatment of Child Abuse and Neglect: 1986; Muram D. Child Sexual Abuse. In: Sanfilippo JS, Muram D, Dewhurst J, Lee PA (eds). *Pediatric and Adolescent Gynecology.* 2nd ed. Philadelphia, PA; W.B. Saunders Co.:2001:399-214.

Implications for Physicians when STDs are Encountered in Children

STD Confirmed	Sexual Abuse	Suggested Action
Gonorrhea*	Diagnostic‡	Report**
Syphilis*	Diagnostic	Report
HIV***	Diagnostic	Report
Chlamydia*	Diagnostic‡	Report
Trichomonas vaginalis	Highly suspicious	Report
Condylomata acuminata* (anogenital warts)	Suspicious	Report
Herpes (genital location)	Suspicious	Report#
Bacterial vaginosis	Inconclusive	Medical follow-up

* If not perinatally acquired

‡ Use definitive diagnostic methods such as culture or DNA probes

** To agency mandated in community to receive reports of suspected sexual abuse

*** If not perinatally or transfusion acquired

Unless there is a clear history of autoinoculation. Herpes 1 and 2 are difficult to differentiate by current techniques.

Findings in Suspected Child Abuse Commonly Classified as Normal*

NORMAL FINDINGS

- Periurethral bands
- Intravaginal ridges
- Hymenal tags
- Hymenal bumps
- Linea vestibularis
- Hymenal cleft/notch in anterior half of rim
- Urethral dilation (mild)

VARIANTS

- Septate hymen
- Failure of midline fusion
- Groove in fossa
- Diastasis ani
- Perianal skin tags in the midline
- Increased perianal pigmentation

* Monteleone JA, Glaze S, Bly KM. *Sexual Abuse: An overview.* In: Monteleone JA, Brodeur AE (eds). Child Maltreatment: A Clinical Guide and Reference. St. Louis, MO; G.W. Medical Publishing: 1998; Adams JA. *Pediatr Ann* 1997;26:299-304; Adams JA, Harper K, Knudson S. *Adolesc Pediatr Gynecol* 1992;5:73-75.

Findings in Suspected Child Abuse Commonly Classified as Nonspecific*

- Erythema of perineum
- Increased vascularity
- Labial adhesions
- Vaginal discharge
- Posterior fourchette friability
- Thickened hymen
- Anal fissures
- Flattened anal folds
- Anal dilation
- Venous congestion
- Venous pooling
- Vaginal bleeding
- Vaginitis
- Large hymenal opening
- Urethral dilation (moderate)
- Thickened perianal tissue
- Narrowed hymen

* Monteleone JA, Glaze S, Bly KM. *Sexual Abuse: An overview.* In: Monteleone JA, Brodeur AE (eds). Child Maltreatment: A Clinical Guide and Reference. St. Louis, MO; G.W. Medical Publishing: 1998; Adams JA. *Pediatr Ann* 1997;26:299-304; Adams JA, Harper K, Knudson S. *Adolesc Pediatr Gynecol* 1992;5:73-75.

Tanner Pubertal Staging*

PUBIC HAIR

Stage 1: Preadolescent. No pubic hair, or hair in pubic region is fine, like that over other areas of the body.

Stage 2: Appearance of few, long, lightly pigmented hairs. Straight or curled hair develops at the base of the penis or along the labia.

Stage 3: Hair increases in density, becomes coarse and curled, and darkens.

Stage 4: Hair is of adult color and texture but covering a smaller area, with no spread to the medial thighs.

Stage 5: Adult-like pattern

BREAST DEVELOPMENT

Stage 1: Preadolescent

Stage 2: Breast bud stage

Stage 3: Further enlargement and elevation of breast areola

Stage 4: Projection of areola and papilla to form secondary mound above the level of the breast

Stage 5: Adult stage, projection of papilla only, areola even with breast

MALE GENITALIA

Stage 1: Preadolescent

Stage 2: Enlargement of scrotum and testes, without enlargement of penis; scrotum reddens and changes texture

Stage 3: Continued enlargement of scrotum and testes, now with lengthening of penis

Stage 4: Increase in size of penis and glans

Stage 5: Adult stage

* Ludwig S. Child Abuse. In: Fleisher GR, Ludwig S (eds). *Textbook of Pediatric Emergency Medicine.* 4th ed. Philadelphia, PA; Lippincott Williams & Wilkins;2000:1669-1704.

Prophylaxis and Treatment for STDs

NEISSERIA GONORRHOEAE

Prophylaxis: Ceftriaxone 125 mg IM

Treatment:
- Child < 45 kg: Ceftriaxone 125 mg IM *or* spectinomycin 40 mg/kg (max 2 g) IM
- Child > 45 kg: Ceftriaxone 125 mg IM *or* cefixime 400 mg po x 1 or cipro floxacin 500 mg po *or* ofloxacin 400 mg po x 1 *or* spectinomycin 2 g IM

CHLAMYDIA

Prophylaxis: Child < 9 years: Erythromycin 50 mg/kg/d divided qid x 7 days (max dose 500 mg qid)

Treatment:
Infants < 6 months: Erythromycin 50 mg/kg/d divided qid 10-14 days
Child < 45 kg: Erythromycin 50 mg/kg/d divided qid x 10-14 days mg

SYPHILLIS

Treatment: Benzathine penicillin 50,000 U/kg IM (max. 2.4 million U)

HERPES SIMPLEX VIRUS

Treatment: Children: Acyclovir 80 mg/kg/d po divided qid po x 7-10 days

TRICHOMONAS

Treatment: Children: Metronidazole 15 mg/kg/d (max 250 mg) divided tid po x 7 days *or* metronidazole 40 mg/kg (max 2 g) po x 1

■ Adolescents: Ceftriaxone 125 mg IM x 1 *or* cefixime 400 mg po x 1 or ciprofloxacin 500 mg po x 1 *or* ofloxacin 400 mg po x 1 plus azithromycin 1 g po x 1 *or* doxycycline 100 mg po bid x 7 days

■ Child > 9 years or > 100 lbs: Tetracycline 50 mg/kg/d divided qid x 7 days (max dose = 500 mg qid) *or* doxycycline 4 mg/kg/d divided bid x 7 days (max dose 100 mg bid) *or* azithromycin 1 g po

Child > 45 kg but < 8 years of age: Azithromycin 1 g po x 1
Child ∅ to 8 years of age: Azithromycin 1 g po x 1 *or* doxycycline 100

po bid x 7 days

■ Adolescents: Acyclovir 400 mg po tid x 7-10 days *or* acyclovir 200 mg po 5 times per day for 7-10 days *or* famciclovir 250 mg po tid x 7-10 days *or* valacyclovir 1 g po bid x 7-10 days

■ Adolescents: Metronidazole 2 g po x 1 *or* metronidazole 500 mg po bid x 7 days

Table continued on next page

Prophylaxis and Treatment for STDs *(continued)*

HUMAN PAPILLOMA VIRUS

Referral to dermatology should be considered. Treatment dependent on age of

Treatment: Podophyllin 10-25% topically followed in 1-4 hours by bathing every week x 4 weeks.

- Trichloroacetic acid (TCA) or bichloroacetic acid (BCA) 80-90% applied topically and repeated weekly if necessary.
- Imiquimod 5% cream applied at bedtime 3 times per week for up to 16 weeks.

BACTERIAL VAGINOSIS

Treatment: Children: Metronidazole 15 mg/kg/d divided tid po x 7 days

HEPATITIS B

Prophylaxis: Fully vaccinated patient should not be revaccinated. If not vaccinated: Hepatitis B immune globulin (0.06 mL/kg IM) within 14 days of exposure and Hep. B vaccine.

HIV

Consider consultation of infectious disease specialist. Indications for prophylaxis are unclear and/or controversial.

Reprinted from: Leder MR, Leder MS. Emergency department evaluation and management of the sexually abused child or adolescent. *Pediatric Emergency Medicine Reports* 2000;5: 67.

child and location/number of lesions.

■ Podofilox 5% solution *or* gel atopically bid x 3 days followed by 4 days of no therapy.

■ Laser or cryotherapy

■ Adolescents: Metronidazole 500 mg po bid x 7 days

If vaccination status unclear, send hepatitis serology.

Prophylaxis: Option: Zidovudine (AZT) 200 mg po tid *or* 160 mg/m^2/dose po tid to a maximum of 200 mg po tid x 4 weeks plus lamivudine 4 mg/kg bid po to a maximum of 150 mg twice a day x 4 weeks.

INFECTIOUS DISEASE EMERGENCIES

INFLUENZA

Antiviral Agents for Influenza: Indications and Dosages

Generic Name	Trade Name	Indications
M2 INHIBITORS — INFLUENZA A		
Amantadine	Symmetrel	Treatment > age 9
		Prophylaxis > age 9
		Ages 1-9
Rimantadine	Flumadine	Treatment > age 10
		Prophylaxis < age 10
NEURAMINIDASE INHIBITORS — INFLUENZA A AND B		
Zanamivir	Relenza	Treatment ∅ age 7
Oseltamivir phosphate	Tamiflu™	Treatment ≥ age 1
		Prophylaxis ≥ age 13
		Treatment: ≤ 15 kg
		Treatment: > 15 kg-23 kg
		Treatment: > 23 kg-40 kg
		Treatment: > 40 kg

Dosage	Wholesale Cost - Treatment	Comments
100 mg bid ´ 7 days	$6.45 (generic)	CNS side effects
100 mg qd	$14.38 (branded)	> age 65: dose decreased
4.4-8.8 mg/kg/d to a		to 100 mg qd
max. dose of 150 mg		If CrCl < 80 mL/min:
		decrease dose
100 mg bid ↔ 7 days	$32.60	If CrCl < 20 mL/min:
5 mg/kg (max. 150 mg)		decrease dose
2 blisters bid ↔ 5 days	$46.18	Disk inhalation device
		Caution with history of
		bronchospasm
75 mg bid ↔ 5 days	$59.54	Mild GI side effects
75 mg qd x at least 7 days		
30 mg bid x 5 days		
45 mg bid x 5 days		
60 mg bid x 5 days		
75 mg bid x 5 days		

Candidates for Influenza Vaccine

INDICATED FOR:

- Health care workers

- Homeless persons

- Persons at high risk of severe consequences of contracting influenza

- Patients $\geq$ 50 years of age

- Presence of a chronic health condition including: asplenia, asthma, chronic pulmonary disease, diabetes, heart disease, hemoglobinopathy, HIV infection, immunosuppression, metabolic disease, renal disease

- Patients maintained on long-term aspirin therapy

- Pregnant women in the second or third trimester

- Public safety workers

- Staff and residents of nursing homes and residential facilities such as dormitories and prisons

- Travelers to foreign countries where influenza activity is reported

CONTRAINDICATED FOR:

- Persons with a history of anaphylactic reactions to eggs

- Persons with hypersensitivity to vaccine components

- Persons with acute febrile illness

Source: Recommendations of the Advisory Committee on Immunization Practices. *MMWR Morb Mortal Wkly Rep* 1999;48(RR-4); Update: Influenza activity-United States and worldwide, 1998-99 season and composition of the 1999-2000 influenza vaccine. *MMWR Morb Mortal Wkly Rep* 1999;48:374-378.

SKIN AND SOFT TISSUE INFECTIONS

Signs, Symptoms, and Microbiology of Folliculitis

- Reddened papules or pustules, 2 mm-5 mm in diameter

- Near hair follicles

- Common locations (beard, upper back, buttocks, chest, forearms)

- Pruritic or painful, especially when pustular

- Most common organisms: *S. aureus* or *S. pyogenes*

- "Hot tub" folliculitis: *P. aeruginosa*

Local and Antimicrobial Management of Folliculitis

INITIAL THERAPY

- Warm compresses and topical treatment.

- Area should be cleaned with a topical benzoyl peroxide soap, cleansing lotion, or an antibacterial soap.

- After thorough cleansing, a topical antibiotic (1% clindamycin) may be applied.

IF TOPICAL THERAPY FAILS:

- Systemic, oral anti-staphylococcal therapy (to methicillin-susceptiple *S. aureus*) may be necessary if local, skin-directed measures fail.

- Cephalexin 500 mg PO BID x 10 days continues to remain a standard and effective therapeutic option. Another initial, first-line option would be azithromycin (500 mg PO on day one, 250 mg PO days 2-5), which permits a relatively shorter course of therapy (5 days) and decreased daily dose frequency (once-daily) as compared to cephalexin or other cephalosporins (cefuroxime, cefadroxil).

Signs, Symptoms, and Microbiology of Furunculosis and Carbunculosis

- Furuncles (or boils) are deep-seated, painful nodules adjacent to hair follicles

- Confluence of several furuncles may create a carbuncle with confluent tracks

- Fluctuance and erythema are common

- Carbuncles may be associated with systemic signs (fever, malaise)

- When fluctuance develops, surgical drainage is advised

- Most common organisms: S. aureus or S. pyogenes

Management of Furunculosis: Initial Therapy

INITIAL THERAPY

- Initial topical measures are usually ineffective once furunculosis or carbunculosis has developed

- Systemic, oral anti-staphylococcal therapy (for methicillin-susceptiple S. aureus) may be necessary if local, skin-directed measures fail.

- Cephalexin 500 mg PO BID x 10 days continues to remain a standard and effective therapeutic option. Another initial, first-line option would be azithromycin (500 mg PO on day one, 250 mg PO days 2-5), which permits a relatively shorter course of therapy (5 days) and decreased daily dose frequency (once-daily) as compared to cephalexin or other cephalosporins (cefuroxime, cefadroxil).

- Large carbuncles with extensive sinus tracts and fluctuance will require surgical drainage.

Antibiotic Options for Uncomplicated Skin and Soft Tissue Infections in Adults

PREFERRED INITIAL AGENTS (WHEN COMPLIANCE AND/OR COST FACTORS PREDOMINATE)

- Cephalexin
- Azithromycin

ALTERNATIVE AGENTS

- Cefadroxil
- Cefuroxime
- Ciprofloxacin
- Clindamycin
- Dicloxacillin
- Levofloxacin
- Loracarbef

Clinical Signs Associated with Necrotizing Soft Tissue Infections

- Skin erythema, edema, warmth
- Blue, purple, or brown skin discoloration
- Skin necrosis and gangrene
- Bullae
- Subcutaneous crepitus
- Cutaneous numbness in the area of involvement
- Shock

Case Definition of Streptococcal Toxic Shock-Like Syndrome (STSS)*

ISOLATION OF GROUP A STREPTOCOCCUS:

- From a normally sterile site

- From a nonsterile site (throat, sputum, vagina, superficial skin lesion, etc.)

CLINICAL SIGNS OF SEVERITY:

Hypotension
BP < 90 mmHg in adults

< 5th percentile for children

Two or more of the following clinical signs:
1. Renal impairment
   - Creatinine greater than 177 micromoles/L (> 2 mg/dL)
   - Creatinine greater than twice upper limit of normal for age
   - Twofold elevation over the baseline level

2. Coagulopathy
   - Platelets less than 100,000/mm^3
   - Disseminated intravascular coagulopathy

3. Liver involvement
   - SGPT > 2 x normal
   - Total bilirubin > 2 x normal
   - Liver enzymes twice normal for age
   - Twofold elevation of liver enzymes

4. Adult respiratory distress syndrome

5. Generalized erythematous macular-papular rash

6. Soft tissue necrosis, including necrotizing fasciitis, myositis, or both

---

* Schurr M, Engelhardt S, Helgerson R. Limb salvage for streptococcal gangrene of the extremity. *Am J Surg* 1998;175:213-217.

Risk Factors Associated with Necrotizing Skin Lesions*

- Compromised immune status [+]

- Age older than 50 years

- Diabetes mellitus

- Arteriosclerosis

- Malnutrition

- Alcoholism[¶]

- Obesity

- Intravenous drug abuse

- Renal failure

- Trauma

- Malignancy

- Varicella infection [¶]

* Reference: Bosshardt TL, Henderson VJ, Organ CH. Necrotizing soft-tissue infections. *Arch Surg* 1996;131:846-854.

[+] Wolfson JS, Sober AJ, Rubin RH. Dermatologic manifestation of infections in immunocompromised patients. *Medicine* 1985;64:115-133.

[¶] Waldhausen JHT, Holterman MJ, Sawin RS. Surgical implications of necrotizing fasciitis in children with chickenpox. *J Ped Surg* 1996;31:1138-1141.

VIRAL AND BACTERIAL MENINGITIS

Differential Diagnosis of Bacterial Meningitis

INFECTIOUS	NON-INFECTIOUS
■ Parameningeal Focus	■ Systemic Disease
Brain Abscess	Sarcoidosis
Subdural Empyema	Kawasaki disease
Epidural Abscess	Systemic lupus erythematosus (SLE)
Pansinusitis	Multiple Sclerosis
■ Bacterial Infection	Migraine Headache
Partially treated ABM	Guillain-Barre
Lyme disease	Behcet's disease
Syphilis	Malignancy
Leptospirosis	Leukemia
Neurobrucellosis	Lymphoma
■ Fungal Infection	■ Vaccine Reaction
■ Mycobacterial Infection	Mumps
■ Parasitic Infection	MMR
■ Viral Infection	Polio
Adenovirus	Poison
Arbovirus	Lead
Cytomegalovirus (CMV)	Mercury
Coronavirus	■ Trauma
Enterovirus	Subarachnoid hemorrhage
Epstein Barr virus (EBV)	s/p Neurosurgery
Herpes simplex virus (HSV)	Traumatic LP
HIV	■ Drugs
Influenza Virus	Azathioprine
Parainfluenza virus	Ibuprofen
Rabies virus	Intravenous immune globulin (IVIG)
LCV	Isoniazid
Rhinovirus	OKT3
Rotavirus	Sulfamethizole
Varicella-zoster virus	Trimethoprim-sulfamethoxazole

Typical Cerebrospinal Fluid (CSF) Findings in Patients with Bacterial Meningitis

CSF PARAMETER	TYPICAL FINDINGS
Opening pressure	> 180 mm H_2O[a]
White blood cell count	1000-5000/mcL (range, < 100 to > 10,000)[b]
Percentage of neutrophils	> 80% [c]
Protein	100-500 mg/dL
Glucose	< 40 mg/dL[d]
Lactate	> 35 mg/dL
Gram's stain	Positive in 60-90%[e]
Culture	Positive in 70-85%[f]
Bacterial antigen detection	Positive in 50-100%

[a] Values over 600 mm H_2O suggest the presence of cerebral edema, intracranial suppurative foci, or communicating hydrocephalus.

[b] Patients with very low CSF white blood cell counts (0 to 20/uL) tend to have a poor prognosis.

[c] About 30% of patients with *Listeria monocytogenes* meningitis have an initial lymphocyte predominance in CSF.

[d] The CSF-serum glucose ratio is < 0.31 in ~70% of patients.

[e] The likelihood of detecting the organism by Gram's stain correlates with the concentration of bacteria in the CSF; concentrations of < 103 cfu/mL is associated with positive Gram's stain ~25% of the time and concentrations > 105 cfu/mL leads to positive microscopy in up to 97% of cases.

[f] Yield of CSF cultures may decrease in patients who have received prior antimicrobial therapy.

Adapted from: Tunkel AR, Scheld WM. Acute bacterial meningitis in adults. In: Remington JS, Swartz MN, eds. *Current Clinical Topics in Infectious Diseases.* Boston: Blackwell Science, 1995:220.

Cerebrospinal Fluid Parameters in Meningitis

	NORMAL	BACTERIAL	VIRAL
WBC count (WBC/uL)	0-5	> 1000	100-1000
% PMN	0-15	90	< 50
% lymph		> 50	> 50
Glucose (mg/dL)	45-65	<40	45-65
CSF:blood glucose ratio	0.6	< 0.4	0.6
Protein (mg/dL)	20-45	>150	50-100
Opening pressure (cm H$_2$0)	6-20	++	NL or +

Recommended Dosages of Antibiotics for Meningitis

ANTIBIOTIC*	DOSAGE
Ampicillin	2g IV q 4 h
Cefotaxime	2g IV q 4-6 h
Ceftazidime	2g IV q 8 h
Ceftriaxone	2g IV q 12 h
Gentamycin	Load 1.5mg/kg IV then 1-2mg/kg q 8 h
Nafcillin/ Oxacillin	1.5-2g IV q 4 h
Penicillin G	4 million units IV q 4 h
Rifampin	600 mg po q 12-24 h
Trimethoprim-sulfa-methoxazole	10 mg/kg IV q 12 h
Vancomycin	1.5-2 g IV q 12 h

* May need to adjust for renal or hepatic disease

FUNGAL	TB	PARAMENINGEAL FOCUS OR ABSCESS
100-500	100-500	10-1000
< 50	< 50	< 50
> 80		
30-45	30-45	45-65
< 0.4	< 0.4	0.6
100-500	100-500	> 50
++	++	N/A

Antibiotic Chioce for Meningitis Based on Gram's Stain

STAIN RESULTS	ORGANISM	ANTIBIOTIC
Gram (+) cocci	S. pneumoniae, S. aureus, S. agalactiae (Group B)	Vancomycin and third-generation cephalosporin
Gram (-) cocci	N. meningitidis	Penicillin G
Gram (-) cocco-bacilli	H. influenzae	Third-generation cephalosporin
Gram (+) bacilli	Listeria monocytogenes	Ampicillin, Pen G + Gentamycin
Gram (-) bacilli	E.coli, Klebsiella Serratia, Pseudomonas	Ceftazidime +/- amino-glycoside

Antibiotic Choice in Bacterial Meningitis Based on Age and Comorbid Illness

AGE	ORGANISM
NEONATE	E. coli, Group B strep, *Listeria monocytogenes*
1-3 MONTHS	S. pneumoniae, N. meningitidis, H. influenzae, S. agalactiae Listeria, E. coli
3 MONTHS TO 18 YEARS	N. meningitidis, S. pneumoniae, H. influenzae
18-50 YEARS	S. pneumoniae, N. meningitidis
OLDER THAN 50 YEARS	N. meningitidis, S. pneumoniae Gram negative bacilli, *Listeria*, Group B strep

MEDICAL ILLNESS	ORGANISM
NEUROSURGERY/HEAD INJURY	S. aureus, S. epidermidis Diphtheroids, Gram negative bacilli
IMMUNOSUPPRESSION	Listeria, Gram negative bacilli S. pneumoniae, N. meningitidis (consider adding Vancomycin)
CSF SHUNT	S. aureus, Gram negative bacilli

Third generation cephalopsorin = ceftriaxone or cefotaxime

ANTIBIOTIC

Ampicillin and third-generation cephalosporin

Ampicillin and third-generation cephalosporin

Third-generation cephalosporin

Third-generation cephalosporin

Vancomycin and third-generation
cephalosporin

ANTIBIOTIC

Vancomycin and
Ceftazidime

Ampicillin and Ceftazidime

Vancomycin and Ceftazidime

Algorithm for Evaluation of Patients with Probable Viral Meningitis

Patient complains of fever, headache, nausea, and vomiting with accompanying or preceding viral illness. Patient is nontoxic, has no alteration of mental status nor neurologic abnormalities. The patient is not in the extremeties of age, has no immunocompromising illness or drugs and has not recently taken antibiotics.

Lumbar

WBC count greater than 1000/mcL, greater than 50% PMN, glucose less than 40 mg/dL, protein greater than 100 mg/dL, + or - Gram's stain

WBC count less than 500/mcL, greater than 50% PMN, glucose 45-65 mcg/dL, protein 20-100 mg/dL, — Gram's stain

Admit, two sets of blood cultures, and IV antibiotics

Observe, no antibiotics.

Patient improves subjectively and objectively in 8-12 hours?

No   Yes

Repeat LP (second LP should not be done before 24 hours have passed since the initial onset of symptoms, if possible).

No

Shift from polymorphic to monomorphic?

Puncture

WBC count less than
1000/mcL, greater than
50% lymphocyte, glucose
45-65 bd/dL, protein 50-100
mg/dL, — Gram's stain

WBC count less than
5/mcL, greater than 50%
lymphocyte, glucose 45-65
mg/dL, protein 20-45
mg/dL, — Gram's stain

If IV antibiotics were given to patient upon presentation
(i.e., a high pretest probability for ABM, consider admitting the patient for observation to rule out other
life-threatening illnesses

Discharge, no antibiotics,
follow
cultures, repeat LP if clinical
deterioration

Yes

COMMUNITY-ACQUIRED PNEUMONIA

IDSA—Year 2000 Guidelines. Empirical Selection of Antimicrobial Agents for Treating Patients with Community Acquired Pneumonia (CAP)

OUTPATIENTS

- Generally preferred are (not in any particular order): doxycycline, a macrolide, or a fluoroquinolone.

- These agents have activity against the most likely pathogens in this setting, which include *Streptococcus pneumoniae, Mycoplasma pneumoniae,* and *Chlamydia pneumoniae.*

- Selection should be influenced by regional antibiotic susceptibility patterns for *S. pneumoniae* and the presence of other risk factors for drug-resistant *S. pneumoniae.*

- Penicillin-resistant pneumococci may be resistant to macrolides and/or doxycycline.

- For older patients or those with underlying disease, a fluoroquinolone may be a preferred choice; some authorities prefer to reserve fluoroquinolones for such patients.

HOSPITALIZED PATIENTS

- General medical ward

- Generally preferred are: an extended spectrum cephalosporin combined with a macrolide or a β-lactam/β-lactamase inhibitor combined with a macrolide or a fluoroquinolone (alone).

Note:

IDSA = Infectious Disease Society of America

β-lactam/β-lactamase inhibitor: ampicillin-sulbactam or piperacillin-tazobactam.

Extended-spectrum cephalosporin: cefotaxime or ceftriaxone.

Macrolide: azithromycin, clarithromycin, or erythromycin.

± with or without.

INTENSIVE CARE UNIT

- Generally preferred are: an extended spectrum cephalosporin or β-lactam/β-lactamase inhibitor plus either a fluoroquinolone or macrolide.

ALTERNATIVES OR MODIFYING FACTORS

- Structural lung disease: antipseudomonal agents (piperacillin, piperacillin-tazobactam, imipenem, or cefepime) plus a fluoroquinolone (including high-dose ciprofloxacin)

- β-lactam allergy: fluoroquinolone ± clindamycin

- Suspected aspiration: fluoroquinolone with or without clindamycin, metronidazole, or a β-lactam/β-lactamase inhibitor

---

Fluoroquinolone: gatifloxacin, levofloxacin, moxifloxacin, or other fluoroquinolone with enhanced activity against *S. pneumoniae* (for aspiration pneumonia, some fluoroquinolones show in vitro activity against anaerobic pulmonary pathogens, although there are no clinical studies to verify in vivo).

Recommended Dosages of Antibiotics in Community-Acquired Pneumonia (CAP)

	Penicillin	
Empiric treatment**	**≤ 0.06**	**0.12–1**
	Outpatients	
Macrolide (erythromycin, clarithromycin, or azithromycin)	+++	+
Doxycycline (or tetracycline)	+++	++
Oral β-lactam (cefuroxime axetil, amoxicillin, or amoxicillin-clavulanate potassium)	+++	++
Fluoroquinolones (levofloxacin, moxifloxacin, or gatifloxacin)†	+++	+++
	Hospitalized (Nonintensive	
Parenteral β-lactam (cefuroxime, cefotaxime sodium, ceftriaxone sodium, or ampicillin sodium-sulbactam sodium) plus macrolide (erythromycin, clarithromycin, or azithromycin)	+++	+++
Fluoroquinolones (e.g., moxifloxacin, levo-floxacin, gatifloxacin, or trovafloxacin)†	+++	+++
	Intubated or	
Intravenous β-lactam (ceftriaxone or cefotaxime sodium) plus intravenous macrolide (erythromycin or azithromycin)	+++	+++
Intravenous β-lactam (ceftriaxone or cefotaxime) plus fluoroquinolone (e.g., gatifloxacin, levo-floxacin, moxifloxacin, or trovafloxacin)†	+++	+++
Fluoroquinolones (e.g., moxifloxacin, levofloxacin, gatifloxacin, or trovafloxacin)†	++	++

MIC mcg/mL			
2	4	∅ 8	Comments
±	-	-	Covers atypical pathogens (*Mycoplasma* spp, *Chlamydia* spp, and *Legionella* spp)
+	-	-	Covers atypical pathogens; not FDA-approved for children younger than 8 years
+	-	-	Does not cover atypical pathogens, alternatively cefpodoxime or cefprozil may be used
+++	++	++	Not first-line treatment because of concerns about emerging resistance; not FDA-approved for use in children; covers atypical pathogens

Care Unit) Patients

++	±	-	Ceftriaxone and cefotaxime have superior activity against resistant pneumococci in comparison with ampicillin-sulbactam and with cefuroxime.
+++	++	++	See previous comments about fluoroquinolones.

Intensive Care Unit Patients‡

++	±	-	Ceftriaxone or cefotaxime are preferred over other β-lactams because of their superior activity against resistant pneumococci; clarithromycin has no intravenous formulation.
++	++	++	Ceftriaxone or cefotaxime are preferred over other β-lactams; see previous comments about fluoroquinolones.
++	++	++	See previous comments about fluoroquinolones; efficacy of monotherapy for critically ill persons with pneumococcal pneumonia has not been established.

Table continued on next page

Recommended Dosages of Antibiotics in Community-Acquired Pneumonia (CAP) *(continued)*

Key:

 * FDA indicates Food and Drug Administration. Ratings estimate clinical
   efficacy and in vitro susceptibility among persons with pneumococcal
   pneumonia. In-depth information on empiric treatment of pneumonia
   is given by the Infectious Disease Society of America and the
   American Thoracic Society guidelines.

 † The relative antipneumococcal activity of these agents differs slightly,
   with that of trovafloxacin equal or superior to that of grepafloxacin,
   which equals that of sparfloxacin, which is superior to that of levofloxacin. Because of new data showing an association with serious
   liver damage, the FDA issued a public health advisory recommending
   that trovafloxacin be used only for patients with serious and life- or
   limb-threatening infections who receive initial treatment in an inpatient health care facility and for whom physicians believe that the
   benefit of the agent outweighs its potential risk.

 ‡ Vancomycin hydrochloride may be indicated for the treatment of
   selected critically ill children with community-acquired pneumonia for
   whom coverage of drug-resistant *Streptococcus pneumoniae* must be
   ensured.

 ** Adaptations made to reflect introduction of new agents since report
    was published.

ASCAP 2003 Guidelines — Empiric Antimicrobial Therapy of Choice for Outpatient and In-Hospital Management of Patients with CAP

PATIENT PROFILE/ETIOLOGIC AGENTS

Otherwise Healthy

< 60 years of age (Patients deemed to be suitable for outpatient/oral therapy, i.e., no systemic toxicity, high likelihood of compliance, and supportive home environment)*

Otherwise Healthy

> 60 years of age (Patients deemed to be suitable for outpatient/oral therapy, i.e., no systemic toxicity, high likelihood of compliance, and supportive home environment)*

In-Hospital (not in intensive care unit)
underlying risk factors or comorbid conditions:
In-Hospital management (COPD, history of pneumonia, diabetes, etc.)

CAP acquired in the nursing home environment
(increased likelihood of gram-negative, *E. coli*, *Klebsiella pneumoniae*)

CAP in the elderly individual with chronic alcoholism
(Increased likelihood of *Klebsiella pneumoniae* infection)

Severe bacteremic CAP with documented
***S. pneumoniae* species showing high-level**
resistance to macrolides and/or penicillin, but maintaining high sensitivity to extended spectrum quinolones and cephalosporins

Severe CAP complicated by structural disease
of the lung (bronchiectasis): Increased likelihood of *Pseudomonas* and polymicrobial infection

FIRST-LINE ANTIBIOTIC THERAPY[†]	ALTERNATIVE FIRST-LINE ANTIBIOTIC THERAPY
Azithromycin PO	Moxifloxacin PO (preferred) OR Levofloxacin PO OR Clarithromycin OR Gatifloxacin PO
Azithromycin PO	Moxifloxacin PO (preferred) OR Levofloxacin PO OR Clarithromycin OR Gatifloxacin PO
Ceftriaxone IV plus azithromycin IV[†††]	Moxifloxacin OR Levofloxacin IV OR Gatifloxacin IV
Ceftriaxone IV plus azithromycin IV	Moxifloxacin OR Levofloxacin IV OR Gatifloxacin IV
Ceftriaxone IV plus azithromycin IV	Cefotaxime[††] plus erythromycin IV OR Levofloxacin IV OR Cefepime IV plus azithromycin IV
Ceftriaxone IV plus moxifloxacin OR Ceftriaxone IV plus levofloxacin IV	Vancomycin[¶] plus azithromycin IV
Cefepime IV plus levofloxacin IV plus/minus aminoglycoside OR Ciprofloxacin IV plus amino-glycoside IV plus azithromycin IV	Ciprofloxacin IV plus cefepime IV plus azithromycin IV OR Carbapenem IV plus azithromycin IV plus aminoglycoside

Table continued on next page

ASCAP 2003 Guidelines — Empiric Antimicrobial Therapy of Choice for Outpatient and In-Hospital Management of Patients with CAP *(continued)*

PATIENT PROFILE/ETIOLOGIC AGENTS

CAP in a patient with suspected aspiration
(increases the likelihood of gram-negative
and anaerobic infection**)

Severe CAP in a compromised host with a
previous hospitalization for, or who resides in
a community or facility with a high reported
incidence of methicillin-resistant *S. aureus*
(MRSA)***

**CAP patient with severe pneumonia
requiring ICU hospitalization*****

---

* Oral therapy/outpatient treatment recommendations are appropriate
  only for those otherwise healthy patients with CAP of mild enough
  severity that they are judged to be suitable candidates for outpatient
  management with oral antibiotics.

§ Quinolones are restricted for use in patients > 18 years of age.

¶ If *S. pneumoniae* demonstrates complete resistance to extended spec
  trum quinolones (very rare), third-generation cephalosporins, and
  macrolides, then vancomycin may be required as part of initial therapy,
  although this would be necessary only in rare circumstances.

† First-line therapy recommendations take into consideration cost of the
  drug (which may vary from one institution to another), convenience of
  dosing, daily dose frequency, spectrum of coverage, side effects, and risk
  of drug-drug interactions.

†† Cefotaxime IV should be dosed on a q 8Υ basis when used for treatment of CAP.

FIRST-LINE ANTIBIOTIC THERAPY[†]	ALTERNATIVE FIRST-LINE ANTIBIOTIC THERAPY
Ceftriaxone IV plus azithromycin IV plus clindamycin IV	Levofloxacin IV plus clindamycin IV OR Levofloxacin IV plus metronidazole IV OR Gatifloxacin IV plus clindamycin IV
Moxifloxicin IV plus vancomycin IV OR Levofloxacin IV vancomycin IV	Gatifloxacin IV plus vancomycin IV
Ceftriaxone IV plus levofloxacin IV +/- aminoglycoside (*Pseudomonas* strongly suspected) OR Ceftriaxone IV plus azithromycin IV plus/minus anti-pseudomonal agent	Cefepime IV plus aminoglycoside IV plus azithromycin IV OR Carbepenem IV plus aminoglycoside IV plus azithromycin IV

[†††] Some institutions may use oral macrolide therapy for patients with mild-to-moderate CAP.

[**] When anaerobic organisms are suspected as one of the possible etiologic pathogens in a patient with CAP, clindamycin or a β-lactam/β-lactamase inhibitor (ampicillin/sulbactam, tricarcillin/clavulanate, or ticarcillin/tazobacatam) is recommended.

[***] High community prevalence of, previous history of hospitalization, or increasing local incidence of methicillin-resistant *S. aureus* (MRSA) in a patient with a clinical presentation consistent with *S. aureus* pneumonia; vancomycin should be considered as component for initial therapy.

[§§] Cefotaxime may be substituted for ceftriaxone, although ceftriaxone is preferred because of its once-daily dosing.

URINARY TRACT INFECTION

Pathogens Responsible for Uncomplicated and Complicated Urinary Tract Infections§

1. *Escherichia coli*
2. *Staphylococcus aureus**
3. *Klebsiella pneumoniae*
4. *Proteus mirabilis*
5. *Enterococcus* faecalis*
6. *Pseudomonas aeruginosa*
7. *Enterobacter cloacae*
8. *Citrobacter*

§ = Listed in order of decreasing frequency

* = Gram-positive organisms

Urinary Tract Infections in the Elderly—Definitions and Classification

Bacteriuria: Bacteria in the urine without symptoms

Uncomplicated UTI: Symptomatic bacteriuria without anatomical, functional, or drug-related factors, cystitis, lower urinary tract infection

Complicated UTI: UTI associated with anatomical, functional, or pharmacological factors predisposing patients to persistent infections, recurrent infections, or treatment failures

Recurrent infection: New infections with different organisms

Relapse: Infection with the same organism

Pyuria: Presence of white blood cells in the uring

Pyelonephritis: Infection of the kidneys

Urosepsis: Hypotension, confusion, bacteremia, multi-organ involvement, and systemic toxicity secondary to urinary tract source

Treatment of Pediatric Patients with UTI

ACUTE, UNCOMPLICATED UTI (3-5 DAYS)

Amoxicillin	30-50 mg/kg/day PO divided tid [a]
Amoxicillin/ clavulinic acid	45 mg/kg/day PO divided bid [b]
Trimethoprim/ sulfamethoxazole	8-10 mg/kg/day of TMP PO divided bid
Nitrofurantoin	5-7 mg/kg/day PO divided qid [c,d]
Cefixime	8 mg/kg/day PO divided bid
Cephalexin	25-50 mg/kg/day PO divided qid
Cefuroxime	20 mg/kg/day PO bid (max, 1 g/day) [e]
Cefaclor	20-40 mg/kg/day PO divided tid [e,f]
Cefprozil	15-30 mg/kg/day PO divided bid (max, 1 g/kg/day) [e,f]
Loracarbef	15-30 mg/kg/day PO divided bid (max, 0.8 g/day) [e,f]

COMPLICATED UTI OR UTI REQUIRING ADMISSION (14 DAYS)

Ampicillin ± Tobramycin	100 mg/kg/day IV divided qid 6-7.5 mg/kg/day IV divided tid [g,h]
Ceftriaxone	50-100 mg/kg/day IV or IM [i]
Ceftazidime	30-50 mg/kg IV tid [i]
Cefotaxime	150 mg/kg/day IV divided tid [i]

[a] Increasing resistance rates limiting efficacy; trimethoprim/sulfamethoxazole is superior in recent studies.

[b] Reserved for patients with amoxicillin-resistant organism.

[c] Not used in patients younger than 6 weeks of age.

[d] Avoid in patients with G6PD deficiency.

[e] Not as effective in patients with enterococcus infection.

[f] Only in patients older than 28 days.

[g] Associated with ototoxicity and nephrotoxicity; adjust according to renal function and follow serum levels.

[h] Intramuscular form may be used in outpatient setting for patients with a history of allergy to cephalosporins.

[i] Significant concern about resistant enterococci; not recommended as first-line drug for recurrent infections.

Recommended Oral Antibiotics for Uncomplicated UTI and Intravenous Agents for Hospital-Based Management of Pyelonephritis

ACUTE UNCOMPLICATED UTI IN ADULTS, CYSTITIS (3-DAY REGIMEN)

First-line agents

Fluoroquinolone (initial agent of choice)

Ciprofloxacin extended release (cipro XR) (preferred)
500 mg PO qd x 3 days

Fluoroquinolone (alternative)

Enoxacin	200 mg PO bid x 3 days
Gatifloxacin	200-400 mg PO qd x 3 days
Levofloxacin	250 mg PO qd x 3 days
Ofloxacin	200 mg PO bid x 3 days
Lomefloxacin	400 mg PO qd x 3 days
Norfloxacin	400 mg PO bid x 3 days

Secondary alternatives

Trimethoprim/ sulfamethoxazole*	160/800 mg PO bid x 3 days

* Only if *E. coli* resistance is < 5-8% in patient population.

** Alternatives: Oral cephalosporin, nitrofurantoin, doxycycline, trimethoprim, or amoxicillin/clavulinic acid.

ACUTE UNCOMPLICATED PYELONEPHRITIS, OUTPATIENT TREATMENT

A fluoroquinolone for 7 days*:

Preferred:

Ciprofloxacin	500 mg PO bid x 7 days

Alternative:

Enoxacin	400 mg PO bid x 7 days
Gatifloxacin	400 mg PO qd x 7 days
Levofloxacin	500 mg PO qd x 7 days
Ofloxacin	400 mg PO bid x 7 days
Lomefloxacin	500 mg PO bid x 7 days

* Recommendations for other (alternative) fluoroquinolones based on limited studies and generalization of efficacy of ciprofloxacin, which has greatest body of evidence-based trials in UTI.

** Secondary Alternatives: Amoxicillin/clavulinic acid, cephalosporin, TMP/SMX-DS for 14 days.

ACUTE UNCOMPLICATED PYELONEPHRITIS, INPATIENT TREATMENT

Fluoroquinolone IV (initial empiric agent of choice)
Preferred:

Ciprofloxacin	400 mg IV bid

Alternative:

Gatifloxacin	400 mg IV qd
Levofloxacin	500 mg IV qd
Ofloxacin	400 mg IV bid
Ampicillin	150-200 mg/kg/day divided q 3-4 h
(+ gentamicin)	(+ 5-7 mg/kg qd)
Cefotaxime	1-2 g q 4-12 h
Ceftriaxone	1-2 g IV qd
Pipercillin	3 g IV q 6 h

Complicated Pyelonephritis, Urosepsis, or Indwelling Catheter

Ciprofloxacin	400 mg IV q 8 h
(+ tobramycin)	(+ 5-7 mg/kg/day)
Ampicillin (+ tobramycin)	150-200 mg/kg/day IV divided q 4 h
	(+ 5-7 mg/kg/day)
Pipercillin/tazobactam	3.4 g IV q 6 h or 4.5 g q 8 h
Ticarcillin/clavulinic acid	3.1 g IV q 6 h
Imipenim	0.5S g IV q 6 h

Note: Any patients receiving advanced generation penicillins and aminoglycosides or fluoroquinolones may need adjustments of their dosing and
or intervals if they have renal impairment.

Adverse Effects of Fluoroquinolones

	Ciprofloxacin	Levofloxacin
SKIN//MUCOCUTANEOUS		
Photosensitivity[a,b]	✓	✓
Rash	✓	✓
Pruritus	✓	✓
GASTROINTESTINAL		
Dyspepsia	✓	✓
Gastrointestinal upset	✓	✓
Diarrhea	✓	✓
Vomiting		
LFT abnormalities[c,d]	✓	
Taste perversion		
Abdominal pain		✓
Nausea		✓
NEUROLOGIC		
Headache	✓	✓
Insomnia		
Somnolence	✓	
Dizziness	✓	✓
Seizure[e]	✓	✓

Lomefloxacin	Ofloxacin	Gatifloxacin
✓	✓	
✓		
✓	✓	
		✓
		✓
		✓
	✓	✓
		✓
		✓
		✓
✓	✓	✓

Table continued on next page

Adverse Effects of Fluoroquinolones (continued)

	Ciprofloxacin	Levofloxacin
CARDIOVASCULAR		
Prolongation of QT interval[f,g]		
Theophylline toxicity	✓	
Digoxin toxicity[g]	✓	✓
Warfarin potentiation[hP]	✓	✓
MUSCULOSKELETAL		
Arthritis	✓	✓
Tendonitis	✓	✓
Tendon rupture[i]	✓	✓
GENITOURINARY		
Vaginitis	✓	✓

Key:

* Other, very infrequent side effects include drug fever, serum-sickness-like reaction, angioedema, anaphylaxis, vasculitis.

[a] Photosensitivity is rare in association with ciprofloxacin and levofloxacin (< 1.0%) and high with sparfloxacin (8%).

[b] Caveat to Note a: Up to 50% photosensitivity in patients with cystic fibrosis.

[c] LFT abnormalities are mild and of unclear significance. No clear evidence of hepatitis or hepatotoxicity except in association with trovafloxacin.

Lomefloxacin	Ofloxacin	Gatifloxacin
		✓
	✓	
✓	✓	✓
✓	✓	✓
	✓	
	✓	
	✓	
		✓

^d LFT, liver function test

^e Seizures are rare. Concomitant use of NSAIDS may lower seizure
  threshold.

^f Sparfloxacin, moxifloxacin, and gatifloxacin are contraindicated in
  patients taking medications that prolong the QT interval.

^g Fluoroquinolones may elevate digoxin levels. Watch for signs of toxicity
  (nausea, vomiting, CNS disturbances, arrythmias).

^h Closely monitor PTT and INR to prevent bleeding complications.

ⁱ Rare.

Antibiotic Treatment Guidelines for Outpatient and Inpatient UTI Syndromes in the Elderly

ASYMPTOMATIC BACTERIURIA

Evaluation and monitoring for symptoms, renal function, continuing bacteriuria

URINARY INCONTINENCE PLUS OTHERWISE ASYMPTOMATIC BACTERIURIA

Evaluate and treat underlying cause of incontinence

ACUTE, SYMPTOMATIC CYSTITIS

Ciprofloxacin extended release (Cipro XR) 500 mg PO qd x 3 d (preferred)

TMP/SMX DS, one tab DS PO bid x 3 days (alternative, avoid in areas where *E. coli* resistance to TMP/SMX is > 10-20%)

CATHETERIZED PATIENT

Lower abdominal pain or new symptoms suggestive of UTI/ without fever or systemic signs
Ciprofloxacin 250 mg PO bid x 7 days (preferred)

Lower abdominal pain with fever or systemic signs:
Ciprofloxacin 500 mg PO bid x 7-10 days (preferred)
Norfloxacin/ofloxacin/levofloxacin (alternatives)

ACUTE PYELONEPHRITIS—MILD:

Ciprofloxacin 500 mg PO bid x 7-10 days (preferred)
Norfloxacin/ofloxacin/levofloxacin (alternatives)
Amoxicillin/clavulanate 500 mg PO bid x 10-14 days

ACUTE PYELONEPHRITIS—SYSTEMIC TOXICITY AND SIGNS OF BACTEREMIA:

Ciprofloxacin 400 mg IV q 12 hrs (preferred)
Ceftriaxone 1 g IV/IM q 24 hrs
Cefotaxime 1-2 g IV q 8 hrs
Levofloxacin 250 mg IV q 24 hrs
Gatifloxacin 400 mg IV q 24 hrs

Diagnostic Approaches for Identifying Elderly Patients with UTI: Assessment Strategies in the Long Term Care Facility

RISK FACTORS—INCREASED SUSPICION FOR UTI

- Frail elderly
- Previous history of UTI
- Indwelling catheter
- Recent GU manipulation
- Anticholinergic medications
- Bacteriuria

CLASSICAL FINDINGS

- Dysuria
- Urgency
- Frequency
- Flank pain
- Back pain
- Shaking chills/rigors
- Fever
- Tachycardia
- Hypotension (urosepsis)

ATYPICAL FINDINGS

- Fatigue
- Lethargy
- Confusion
- Cough
- Weakness
- Dyspnea
- Afebrile
- Abdominal pain

LABORATORY AND MICROBIOLOGICAL EVALUATION

- Urine collection
- Midstream clean-catch or catheterization
- Leukocyte esterase
- Microscopic bacteriuria
- Pyuria
- Urine culture
- Blood culture

FINDINGS SUGGESTIVE OF BACTEREMIC UTI

- Elevated serum creatinine
- Increased leukocyte count
- Fever
- Presence of diabetes mellitus
- Low serum albumin

Risk Factors for Developing UTI in the Elderly Patient Residing in a Long Term Care Facility

- Previous urinary tract infection

- Prolonged stay in long-term care facility

- Immobilization

- Less frequent urination

- Incomplete bladder emptying

- Prostate disease (men)

- Neuropathic diseases

- Immune response deterioration

- Increased incidence of renal/bladder/prostatic calculi

- Iatrogenic genitourinary instrumentation

HUMAN IMMUNODEFICIENCY VIRUS (HIV)

Factors that Increase HIV Transmission Risk After Occupational Percutaneous Exposure

- Deep injury
- Percutaneous exposure to a visibly bloody device
- Percutaneous exposure to a needle previously inserted into an artery or vein
- Terminal illness or AIDS in the source patient

Factors that Increase Risk of HIV Acquisition Through Sexual Activity

- Presence of ulcerative genital lesions
- Presence of inflammatory genital lesions
- Cervical ectopy
- Absence of circumcision

Determining Appropriate Post Exposure Prophylaxis (PEP) Regimen

Small inoculum ≪ Low titer	≪	PEP may not be necessary
Small inoculum ≪ High titer	≪	Consider basic PEP regimen
Moderate inoculum ≪ Low titer	≪	Basic PEP regimen recommended
Moderate inoculum ≪ High titer	≪	Expanded PEP regimen recommended
Large inoculum ≪ Low or high titer	≪	Expanded PEP regimen recommended

Risk of HIV Transmission Per Episode of Contact

BLOOD TRANSFUSION	
(recipient of 1 unit)	95%

NON-SEXUAL, NON-OCCUPATIONAL	
IV drug abuse/needle sharing/other percutaneous	0.67%

OCCUPATIONAL	
(Percutaneous)	< 0.5%

SEXUAL	
Penile—anal contact (receptive partner)	0.1-3%
Penile—anal contact (insertive partner)	0.03%
Penile—vaginal contact (receptive partner)	0.1-0.2%
Penile—vaginal contact (insertive partner)	0.03-0.09%

Source Factors that Increase the Risk of HIV Transmission

- High viral titer
    Primary HIV infection
    Advanced or pre-terminal AIDS

- Menstruation

- Other vaginal bleeding

- Presence of inflammatory or ulcerative genital lesions

Most Commonly Reported Symptoms in Patients with Acute Retroviral Syndrome (ARS)

REFERENCE NUMBER§	1	2	3	4	5	6
Fever	95%	100%	77%	87%	92%	96%
Fatigue	90%	51%	66%	26%	*	61%
Sore throat	70%	43%	16%	48%	75%	*
Weight loss	68%	20%	*	13%	*	*
Myalgias	60%	*	18%	42%	92%	*
Headache	58%	*	51%	39%	58%	61%
Nausea	58%	*	*	26%	67%	*
Cervical adenopathy	55%	80%	16%	*	75%	*
Night sweats	50%	33%	*	*	92%	*
Diarrhea	50%	7%	*	32%	33%	*
Vomit	40%	*	*	23%	67%	*
Rash	35%	20%	56%	67%	50%	67%
Abdominal pain	*	*	*	32%	*	*
Arthralgia	*	*	*	29%	*	*
Cough	*	*	*	26%	*	*
Oral ulcers	*	*	*	13%	*	*

* = Symptom/sign not reported

§ = References

1. Schacker T, Collier A, Hughes J, et al. Clinical and epidemiologic features of primary HIV infection. *Ann Int Med* 1996;125:257-264.

2. Dorrucci M, Rezza G, Vlahov D, et al. Clinical characteristics and prognostic value of acute retroviral syndrome among injecting drug users. *AIDS* 1995;9:597-604.

3. Vanhems P, Allard R, Cooper DA, et al. Acute human immunodeficiency virus type 1 disease as a mononucleosis-like illness: Is the diagnosis too restrictive? *Clin Infect Dis* 1997;24:965-970.

4. Kinloch-de Loes S. Symptomatic primary infection due to human immunodeficiency virus type 1: Review of 31 cases. *Clin Infect Dis* 1993;17:59-65.

5. Cooper DA. Acute AIDS retrovirus infection. Definition of a clinical illness associated with seroconversion. *Lancet* 1985;1:537-540.

6. Perrin LU, Balavoine JF, Schockmell GA, et al. Post-exposure prophylaxis and sexual HIV transmission between husband and wife. Int Conf AIDS 1998;12:630(abstract no. 33189).

Differential Diagnosis of Acute Retroviral Syndrome (ARS)

- Epstein-Barr viral mononucleosis
- Cytomegalovirus infection
- Toxoplasmosis
- Secondary syphilis
- Viral hepatitis
- Enteroviral infection
- Primary herpes simplex virus infection
- Drug reaction

Medications Used for Treatment of HIV Infection

GENERIC	BRAND
NUCLEOSIDE REVERSE TRANSCRIPTASE INHIBITORS (NRTI)	
Zidovudine (AZT)	(Retrovir)
Stavudine (d4T)	(Zerit)
Didanosine (ddl)	(Videx)
Lamivudine (3TC)	(Epivir)
Zalcitabine (ddC)	(Hivid)
Zidovudine plus lamivudine	(Combivir)
Abacavir (ABC)	(Ziagen)
NON-NUCLEOSIDE REVERSE TRANSCRIPTASE INHIBITORS (NNRTI)	
Nevirapine	(Viramune)
Delavirdine	(Rescriptor)
Efavirenz	(Sustiva)
PROTEASE INHIBITORS (PI)	
Saquinavir	(Invirase, Fortovase)
Ritonavir	(Norvir)
Indinavir	(Crixivan)
Nelfinavir	(Viracept)
Amprenavir	(Agenerase)

Web Sites of Interest for HIV

- **Centers for Disease Control and Prevention:**
    www.cdc.gov

- **HIV/AIDS Treatment Information Service:**
    www.hivatis.org

- **HIV InSite (University of California at San Francisco):**
    hivinsite.ucsf.edu

- **Pediatric AIDS Clinical Trials Group:**
    pactg.s-3.com

- **AIDS Education and Research Trust:**
    www.avert.org

- **Joint United Nations Programme on HIV/AIDS:**
    www.unaids.org

Symptoms Associated with Abacavir Hypersensitivity Reaction

- Fever

- Skin rash

- Fatigue

- Gastrointestinal symptoms
    Nausea
    Vomiting
    Diarrhea
    Abdominal pain

- Respiratory symptoms
    Pharyngitis
    Dyspnea
    Cough

Side Effects of Nucleoside Reverse Transcriptase Inhibitors (NRTIs)

MEDICATION	SIDE EFFECTS
ZIDOVUDINE (AZT, ZDV, RETROVIR)	
	Headache
	Insomnia
	Asthenia
	Bone Marrow Suppression (anemia +/- neutropenia)
	Lactic acidosis with hepatic steatosis
	Myopathy
DIDANOSINE (DDI, VIDEX)	
	Peripheral neuropathy
	Pancreatitis
	Nausea
	Diarrhea
	Lactic acidosis with hepatic steatosis
	Retinal depigmentation
ZALCITABINE (DDC, HIVID)	
	Peripheral neuropathy
	Pancreatitis
	Stomatitis
	Rash
	Lactic acidosis with hepatic steatosis
	Esophageal ulceration
	Fever
STAVUDINE (D4T, ZERIT)	
	Peripheral neuropathy
	Pancreatitis
	Transaminitis
	Agitation
LAMIVUDINE (3TC, EPIVIR)	
	Peripheral neuropathy
	Pancreatitis
	Nausea
ABACAVIR (ZIAGEN)	
	Nausea
	Headache
	Hypersensitivity syndrome

Side Effects and Contraindicated Drug Interactions of Protease Inhibitors

	SIDE EFFECTS	DRUG INTERACTIONS
NEVIRAPINE (VIRAMUNE)		
	Rash	Protease inhibitors
	Nausea	Rifampin, rifabutin
	Transaminitis	Oral contraceptives
	Hepatitis	Triazolam, midazolam
DELAVIRDINE (RESCRIPTOR)		
	Rash	Terfenadine, astemizole
	Nausea	Alprazolam, midazolam, triazolam
	Transaminitis	Rifampin, rifabutin
		Ergot derivatives
		Amphetamines
		Nifedipine
		Anticonvulsants
		Cisapride
EFAVIRENZ (SUSTIVA)		
	Altered dreams	Astemizole, cisapride
	Dizziness	Midazolam, triazolam
	Somnolence	Ergot derivatives
	Insomnia	
	Transaminitis	
	Impaired concentration	
	Confusion	
	Hallucinations	
	Amnesia	

Evaluation of HIV Exposure

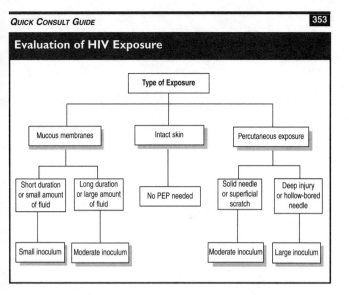

Evaluation of HIV Status

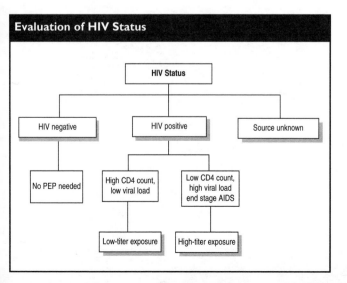

BITE WOUNDS

Complications of Animal Bites

- Localized cellulitis
- Abscess formation
- Septic arthritis
- Tenosynovitis
- Osteomyelitis
- Sepsis
- Endocarditis
- Meningitis

Microbiology of Bite Wounds: Most Common Pathogens

DOG AND CAT BITES	HUMAN BITES
P. multocida	*Streptococcus* species
S. aureus	*S. aureus*
Streptococcus	*E. corrodens*
Corynebacterium	*Bacteroides*
Fusobacterium	*Fusobacterium*
Bacteroides	*Peptostreptococcus*
Porphyromonas	
Prevotella	

Assessment of Low- Vs. High-Risk Bite Wounds

LOWER RISK
- Larger lacerations
- Wounds on face or scalp

HIGHER RISK
- Punctures
- Cat bites
- Most human bites
- Bites or wounds on hand, wrist, or foot
- Immunocompromised patients
- Diabetic patients
- Patients with vascular disease

General Bite Wound Management Techniques

1. Cleanse the wound. Povidone-iodine solution is recommended for periphery cleansing. The standard solution is diluted 10:1 with saline and can serve as both the cleansing agent and irrigant.

2. After thoroughly scrubbing the wound periphery, irrigate copiously with high pressure using a 19-gauge needle, catheter, or splash shield attached to a 20 mL or 35 mL syringe. Deliver diluted povidone-iodine solution directly into the wound.

3. Debride all devitalized tissue and wound edges. This is essential to reduce the possibility of wound infection.

4. Irrigate after debridement to provide greater exposure of the wound.

5. To facilitate effective irrigation of fang wounds, particularly slender cat teeth wounds, the entry site can be widened with a simple 1 to 1.5 cm incision across the puncture with a #15 knife blade. Retract the new wound with a hemostat or forceps to permit irrigation. Leave these incisions to close without sutures. If the edges are devitalized, trim back to viable skin.

6. Culture purulence or suspected infection. If antibiotics appear advisable, a beta-lactam with lactamase inhibitor or second-generation cephalosporin is recommended.

7. Ensure proper tetanus immunization.

8. Assess and treat for rabies exposure if necessary.

Source: Trott A. *Wounds and Lacerations: Emergency Care and Closure.* 2nd ed. St. Louis: Mosby; 1997.

NEUROLOGICAL EMERGENCIES

STATUS EPILEPTICUS

Clinical Classification of Status Epilepticus (SE)*

OVERT GENERALIZED CONVULSIVE STATUS EPILEPTICUS

Continuous convulsive activity and intermittent convulsive activity without regaining full consciousness

- Convulsive (tonic-clonic)
- Tonic
- Clonic
- Myoclonic

SUBTLE GENERALIZED CONVULSIVE STATUS EPILEPTICUS

Coma following generalized convulsive status epilepticus with or without motor activity

SIMPLE STATUS EPILEPTICUS (CONSCIOUSNESS PRESERVED)

- Simple motor status epilepticus
- Sensory status epilepticus
- Aphasic status epilepticus

NONCONVULSIVE STATUS EPILEPTICUS

Consciousness impaired; twilight or fugue state
- Petit mal status
- Complex partial status epilepticus

Note: There is no uniform or consensus of classification at this time.
*Includes both primary and secondarily generalized seizures

Rationale for Aggressive Treatment in Status Epilepticus

1. The longer generalized convulsive status epilepticus (GCSE) persists, the harder it is to control.

2. Neuronal damage is primarily caused by continuous excitatory activity, not systemic complications of GCSE.

3. Systemic complications of seizure activity, particularly hyperpyrexia, may exacerbate neuronal damage.

4. Every seizure counts in terms of making GCSE more difficult to control and for causing neuronal damage.

Etiology of Status Epilepticus (Partial List)

Status Epilepticus (SE) in a patient with a history of seizure disorder

- noncompliance with prescribed medical regimen
- withdrawal seizures from anticonvulsants
- breakthrough seizures

New onset seizure disorder presenting with SE

SE secondary to medical, toxicologic, or structural symptoms

- Hypoxic injury
  post-resuscitation
  others

- Stroke syndromes
  ischemic
  acute
  delayed

- Subarachnoid hemorrhage

- Intracranial tumor

- Trauma

- Toxicologic
  theophylline
  cocaine
  amphetamines
  isoniazid
  alcohol withdrawal

- Metabolic
  hyponatremia
  hypernatremia
  hypercalcemia
  hepatic encephalopathy

- Infectious
  meningitis
  brain abscess
  encephalitis
  CNS
  cysticercosis

Generalized Convulsive Status Epilepticus Treatment in Adults

REGIMENS*	GENERIC	PROPRIETARY	ROUTE
Initial drug of choice—a benzodiazepine administered IV	Lorazepam	Ativan	IV
	Diazepam	Valium	IV
	Midazolam	Versed	IM
If IV route unavailable, alternative regimens for benzodiazepine administration	Midazolam	Versed	Intranasal
	Diazepam	Valium	P.R.
	Lorazepam	Ativan	P.R.
Second Agent: A phenytoin. Administer If seizures fail to stop within five minutes of drug administration	Phenytoin	Dilantin	IV
	Fosphenytoin	Cerebyx	IV or IM
	Phenytoin Fosphenytoin	Dilantin Lerebyx	IV
Third Agent: If seizures fail to stop after optimal dosing of a benzodiazepine and phenytoin, no clear pathway exists. A variety of agents are summarized here.	Midazolam	Versed	IV
	Phenobarbital		IV
	Pentobarbital		
	Propofol	Diprivan	IV
	Lidocaine		
	Etomidate		

* = All drugs ideally administered intravenously.
† = Also true for pentobarbital, propofol, lidocaine, and etomidate.

DOSE	RATE	COMMENTS
0.1 mg/kg	2 mg/min	Doses higher than 8 mg likely ineffective. Begin w/ 4 mg then repeat x 1 after 10 min if seizure continues
0.2-0.5 mg/kg	4 mg/min	30 mg max. dose considered by some. 5-10 mg initially. Repeat in 10 min if necessary
10 mg		Case report in adult, limited clinical information
10 mg		Case reports dose for adult
0.5 mg/kg		Return administration reported in children. Repeat dose of 0.25 mg/kg P.R. if seizure fails to stop
0.1 mg/kg		Limited case reports in children
20 mg/kg	50 mg/min	Must be administered in normal saline. Hypotension, arrhythmias may necessitate slowing administration rate further. Soft-tissue necrosis reported with extravasation. Cardiac and BP monitoring necessary.
20 PE**/kg	150 PE/min	Increased cost ($70-$100). Soft-tissue reactions thought to be eliminated with near-physiologic pH. Cardiac and BP monitoring necessary
Increase to total 30 mg/kg or 30 PE/kg	*(Same as above)*	Consensus recommendation
0.2 mg/kg loading dose	0.1-0.4 mg/kg (max rate infusion is 4 mg/min)	Continuous intubation, pressure support ICU admission, and EEG monitoring†
20 mg/kg	Max rate is 100 mg/min	One recommendation: Additional 10 mg/kg every 30 minutes until seizures stop.
Loading dose 5-12 mg/kg	0.5 mg/kg/h (max rate of infusion is 50 mg/min)	*(Same as above)*
Loading dose 0.2 mg/kg	Infusion 0.1-2.0 mg/kg/h	Doses as high as 7.5 mg/kg/h reported
1-1.5 mg/kg bolus		Anecdotal reports; Repeat dose once reported
0.3 mg/kg bolus	Infusion 20 mcg/kg/min	

** PE = phenytoin equivalent

Classification of Status Epilepticus (SE) According to the Need for Aggressive Treatment

SE REQUIRING IMMEDIATE, AGGRESSIVE TREATMENT

- Continuous generalized convulsive activity with impaired consciousness lasting greater than five minutes*

- Serial seizures without return to full consciousness between seizures

- Subtle GCSE—Coma with minimal or no associated motor activity. †
  (Consider if post-ictal state is not improving in 20 minutes.* May evolve from generalized convulsive status epilepticus.)

SE THAT POSSIBLY BENEFITS FROM AGGRESSIVE TREATMENT

Evidence of CNS injury from seizures is not as clear.

- Complex partial status epilepticus (twilight or fugue state)†

SE REQUIRING TREATMENT

No data to suggest time of stopping is critical to prevent CNS damage.

- Absence status epilepticus (spike-wave status epilepticus)†

- simple motor status epilepticus (epilepsia partialis continua)†

* time is arbitrary

† EEG may be required for diagnosis

Differential Diagnosis of Generalized Convulsive Status Epilepticus (GCSE)

— Nonepileptic (psychogenic) seizures

— Repetitive abnormal posturing (extensor, flexor)

— Tetanus

— Neuroleptic malignant syndrome

— Rigors due to sepsis

— Myoclonic jerks

— Tremors

— Hemiballism

— Involuntary movements

STROKE

Inclusion and Exclusion Criteria for Administration of t-PA

INCLUSION CRITERIA

- Ischemic stroke
- t-PA can be administered within 3 hours of symptom onset
- Neurological deficit measured by NIH Stroke Scale
- Clearly defined time of symptom onset

EXCLUSION CRITERIA

- Evidence of acute intracerebral or intracranial hemorrhage on non-contrast CT of the head
- Early CT evidence of acute infarction
- Other stroke, serious head trauma, or intracranial surgery in past three months
- Intracranial neoplasm, arteriovenous malformation, or aneurysm
- Uncontrolled hypertension, i.e. not reduced to 185/110 or lower within 30 minutes by oral agents, nitroglycerine paste, labetalol, or esmolol
- Rapidly improving or minor neurological symptoms
- Symptoms suggesting subarachnoid hemorrhage
- History of intracranial hemorrhage
- Major surgery in past 14 days
- Known bleeding diathesis
- Gastrointestinal or genitourinary tract bleeding in the past 3 weeks
- Arterial puncture at a noncompressible site in the past 7 days
- Seizure at the onset of stroke
- Patients with a prothrombin (PT) time greater than 15 seconds
- Patients on warfarin (coumadin) with a PT time greater than 15 seconds
- Heparin within the past 48 hours and elevated activated partial thromboplastin time (aPTT)
- Platelet count less than 100,000
- Serum glucose less than 50mg/dL or greater than 400 mg/dL

Algorithm for Emergency Department Evaluation of Acute Stroke

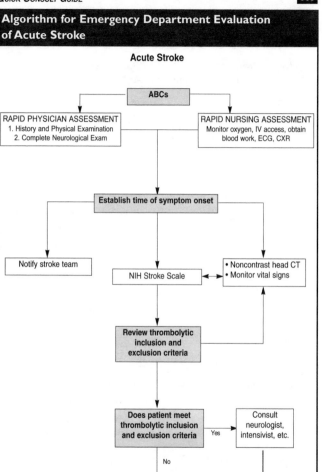

Acute Stroke

ABCs

RAPID PHYSICIAN ASSESSMENT
1. History and Physical Examination
2. Complete Neurological Exam

RAPID NURSING ASSESSMENT
Monitor oxygen, IV access, obtain blood work, ECG, CXR

Establish time of symptom onset

Notify stroke team

NIH Stroke Scale

• Noncontrast head CT
• Monitor vital signs

Review thrombolytic inclusion and exclusion criteria

Does patient meet thrombolytic inclusion and exclusion criteria

Yes → Consult neurologist, intensivist, etc.

No

Follow accepted stroke critical pathway/coordinated care track

Administer t-PA

Modified Version of the National Institutes of Health Stroke Summary Scale

ITEM	NAME	RESPONSE
1A	**Level of Consciousness**	0=Alert
		2=Not alert
		3=Unresponsive
1B	**Level of Questions**	0=Answers both correctly
		1=Answers one correctly
		2=Answers neither correctly
1C	**Level of Commands**	0=Performs both tasks correctly
		1=Performs one task correctly
		2=Performs neither task
2	**Best Gaze**	0=Normal
		1=Partial gaze palsy
		2=Total gaze palsy
3	**Visual Fields**	0=No visual loss
		1=Partial hemianopsia
		2=Complete hemianopsia
		3=Bilateral hemianopsia
4	**Facial Palsy**	0=Normal
		1=Minor paralysis
		2=Partial paralysis
		3=Complete paralysis
5	**Motor Arm** a. Left b. Right	0=No drift 1=Drift before 10 seconds 2=Falls before 10 seconds 3=No effort against gravity 4=No movement

ITEM	NAME	RESPONSE
6	**Motor leg**	0=No drift
	a. Left	1=Drift before 5 seconds
	b. Right	2=Falls before 5 seconds
		3=No effort against gravity
		4=No movement
7	**Ataxia**	0=Absent
		1=One limb
		2=Two limbs
8	**Sensory**	0=Normal
		1=Mild loss
		2=Severe loss
9	**Language**	0=Normal
		1=Mild aphasia
		2=Severe aphasia
		3=Mute or global aphasia
10	**Dysarthria**	0=Normal
		1=Mild
		2=Severe
11	**Extinction/inattention**	0=Normal
		1=Mild
		2=Severe
12	**Distal Motor**	0=Normal
	a. Left arm	1=Some extension after 5 seconds
	b. Right arm	2=No extension after 5 seconds

Typical Stroke Syndromes

VASCULAR TERRITORY	CLINICAL PICTURE
Internal carotid artery	Variable but may involve hemiparesis and aphasia in dominant hemisphere
Anterior watershed	Hemiparesis greatest in leg with sensory loss
Posterior watershed	Hemianopia
MCA watershed	Hemiparesis, hemisensory loss, aphasia in dominant hemisphere
Superficial ACA	Contralateral leg weakness, sensory loss Hemianopia
Deep ACA	Movement disorders Dysesthesia
Lacunar	Pure motor or sensory loss
Vertebral Artery	Impaired contralateral pain and thermal sense, ipsilateral Horner syndrome, nystagmus, vertigo, ipsilateral limb ataxia
MCA, Superior division	Contralateral face, arm, leg sensory and motor deficit, ipsilateral head and eye deviation, Broca aphasia
MCA, Inferior division	Homonymous hemianopia, Wernicke aphasia
Basilar artery	Coma, quadriplegia, "locked-in" syndrome.

Key: ACA = anterior cerebral artery
ICA = internal carotid artery
MCA = middle cerebral artery

Risk Factors for Stroke

RISK FACTORS	COMMENTS
Hypertension	Primary risk factor
Increased age	Over age 65
Male gender	In patients under 60
Atrial fibrillation	Particularly with CHF or valvular disease
Cigarette use	
Diabetes	Particularly with women
Family history	Both paternal and maternal alcohol use
Prior TIA	Highest risk in first year
Hyperlipidemia	Possible role

MOVEMENT DISORDERS

Important Hisotrical Questions for Evaluation of a Patient with Suspected Movement Disorder

1. Manner and temporal nature of symptom onset

2. Location of symptoms; body parts most affected

3. Factors that alleviate or exacerbate the symptoms

4. Whether symptoms are present at rest, with sustained posture, with movement, or only during the execution of specific tasks

5. Exposure to toxins or environmental factors and medication use

6. History of premature birth, perinatal injury, or behavioral problems

Cardinal Features of Parkinsonism

BRADYKINESIA

Slowness of movement with a paucity of normal spontaneous movements such as arm swing when walking

RIGIDITY

Form of increased resistance to passive manipulation in which the increased tone has a "plastic" (constant resistance to passive manipulation) quality or "cogwheel" rigidity (in which resistance has a ratchet-like characteristic)

TREMOR

Typically a "resting tremor" of the hands/arms, legs, or chin that improves with use of the affected body part

IMPAIRMENT OF POSTURAL REFLEXES

Manifested by falls or near falls, and in difficulty in maintaining a stable stance when displaced gently backward on examination

Classification of Movement Disorders

HYPOKINETIC MD/PARKINSONISM

Parkinson's disease

Drug-induced parkinsonism

Parkinsonian syndromes

TREMORS

Resting tremors

Postural tremors

Kinetic tremors

Task-related tremors

HYPERKINETIC/CHOREIC MOVEMENT DISORDERS

Chorea

Athetosis

Ballism (Hemiballism is more common)

Dystonia

Tics

MYOCLONUS

Generalized

Segmental

Focal

Used with permission from: Shah S, Albin R. Movement Disorders. In: Shah S, Kelly K, eds. *Emergency Neurology: Principles and Practice.* New York: Cambridge University Press; 1999. Reprinted with the permission of Cambridge University Press.

Phenomenology of Movement Disorders

MOVEMENT DISORDER	FEATURES
Parkinsonism	Bradykinesia, rigidity, often resting tremor, often postural instability, stooped posture masked facies, hypophonia
Dystonia	Sustained, spasmodic, repetitive contractions causing involuntary abnormal postures
Tremor	Involuntary, rhythmic and roughly sinusoidal movements: some are action induced
Chorea	Involuntary, irregular, rapid, jerky movements without a rhythmic pattern; dance-like
Athetosis	Akin to chorea but with distinct "writhing" movements
Myoclonus	Brief, rapid, shock-like jerks
Tics	Intermittent, brief, sudden, repetitive, stereo-typed movements or sounds
Hemiballism	Uncontrollable, rapid, large amplitude flinging movements of a limb

Used with permission from: Shah S, Albin R. Movement Disorders. In: Shah S, Kelly K, eds. *Emergency Neurology: Principles and Practice*. New York: Cambridge University Press; 1999. Reprinted with the permission of Cambridge University Press.

AREAS OF INVOLVEMENT	ANATOMIC LOCALIZATION
Often asymmetric at onset, but can be generalized	Basal ganglia—Interruption of or interference with nigrostriatal dopaminergic neurotransmission
Any voluntary muscle can be affected (usually head, neck, face, and limbs)	Presumed to be basal ganglia— Associated with putamen lesions in some cases.
Head, hands, limbs, and voice	In parkinsonian resting tremor— Basal ganglia Most other tremors may involve cerebellar dysfunction
Generally limbs, but any body part can be affected	Basal ganglia—Striatum or subthalamic nucleus
Limbs, but any body part can be involved	Identical to chorea
Generally involves very small muscles	Can result from dysfunction at any level of the central nervous system
Any body part can be affected; phonation/sounds	Presumed to be basal ganglia
Generally a limb	Basal ganglia—Subthalamic nucleus or striatum

Common Presentations of the Parkinsonian Patient

COMPLICATIONS OF PARKINSONISM

1. Falls due to impaired postural reflexes (consider subdural hematoma in a patient with mental status changes)

2. Orthostatic hypotension from autonomic instability resulting in syncope and falls

3. Painful muscle spasms

4. Paresthesias

5. Severe localized limb pain, chest pain, or abdominal pain

COMPLICATIONS OR SIDE EFFECTS OF DRUG THERAPY FOR PARKINSONISM

1. Nausea: Common with carbidopa/L-dopa or dopamine agonists

2. Flushing and orthostasis resulting from the therapy

3. Mental status changes, particularly hallucinations, delirium, and dementia

4. Neuroleptic malignant syndrome can result from discontinuation of dopamine replacement therapy

Forms of Parkinsonism

IDIOPATHIC PARKINSONISM

Involves basal ganglia but no discernible degenerative conditions

DRUG-INDUCED PARKINSONISM

Neuroleptics, phenothiazine, haloperidol, tricyclic antidepressants, methyldopa, lithium, metoclopramide

NEURODEGENERATIVE DISORDERS

(Clinically indistinguishable from other forms of parkinsonism.) Involve basal ganglia. Discernible degenerative conditions

Etiologies of Selected Dystonias

DYSTONIA DUE TO DEGENERATIVE DISORDERS OF CNS

Parkinson's disease

Huntington's disease

Progressive supranuclear palsy

Other degenerative disorders of the basal ganglia and midbrain

Wilson's disease

Storage diseases

GTP cyclohydrolase deficiency

Lesch-Nyhan disease

Mitochondrial disorders

Leigh's syndrome

DYSTONIA DUE TO NON-DEGENERATIVE DISORDERS OF CNS

Traumatic brain injury

History of perinatal anoxia

Kernicterus

Stroke (cerebral infarction)

Arteriovenous malformation

Encephalitis

Toxins (e.g., manganese)

Brain tumors

Multiple sclerosis

Drugs

Peripheral trauma

Used with permission from: Shah S, Albin R. Movement Disorders. In: Shah S, Kelly K, eds. *Emergency Neurology: Principles and Practice.* New York: Cambridge University Press; 1999. Reprinted with the permission of Cambridge University Press.

Disorders Simulating Dystonic Torticollis (Cervical Dystonia)

NEUROLOGICAL DISORDERS

Posterior fossa tumor

Focal seizures

Bobble-head syndrome (third ventricular cyst)

Syringomyelia

Congenital nystagmus

Extraocular muscle palsies

Arnold-Chiari malformation

MUSCULOSKELETAL/ STRUCTURAL

Herniated cervical disc

Rotational atlantoaxial subluxation

Congenital muscular or ligamentous absence, laxity, or injury

Bony spinal abnormalities: Degenerative; neoplastic; infectious

Cervical soft-tissue lesions: Adenitis, pharyngitis

Labyrinthine disease

Abnormal posture in utero

Adapted from: Wiener W, Lang A. *Movement Disorders: A comprehensive Survey.* Mount Kisco, NY: Futura Publishing Co.; 1989.

Neuroleptic Medication-Induced Movement Disorder

1. Acute dystonic reaction (ADR)

2. Akathisia

3. Drug-induced parkinsonism

4. Neuroleptic malignant disorder

5. Tardive disorders

Differential Diagnosis of Chorea

HEREDITARY CHOREAS

Huntington's disease (classic choreiform movement)

Neuroacanthocytosis

Wilson's disease

Benign familial chorea

Inborn errors of metabolism

Porphyria

Ataxia-telangiectasia

Tuberous sclerosis

METABOLIC CHOREAS

Hyper- and hypothyroidism

Hyper- and hypoparathyroidism

Hypocalcemia

Hyper- and hyponatremia

Hypomagnesemia

Hepatic encephalopathy

Renal encephalopathy

INFECTIOUS OR IMMUNOLOGICAL CHOREAS

Sydenham' chorea (post rheumatic fever)

Chorea gravidarum

Systemic lupus erythematosus

Polycythemia vera

Multiple sclerosis

Sarcoidosis

Viral encephalitis

Tuberous meningitis

CEREBROVASCULAR CHOREAS

Basal ganglia infarction

Arteriovenous malformation

Venous angiomata

Polycythemia

STRUCTURAL CHOREAS

Posttraumatic

Subdural and epidural hematoma

Tumor (primary CNS or metastatic)

DRUGS/MEDICATIONS

Phenytoin

Phenothiazines

Lithium

Amphetamines

Oral contraceptives

Levodopa

TOXINS

Mercury

Carbon monoxide

INFECTIONS

Neurosyphilis

Lyme's disease

Subacute sclerosing panencephalitis

Used with permission from: Shah S, Albin R. Movement Disorders. In: Shah S, Kelly K, eds. *Emergency Neurology: Principles and Practice.* New York: Cambridge University Press; 1999. Reprinted with the permission of Cambridge University Press.

Causes of Hemiballism

CAUSES	SUBTYPES
Cerebrovascular accidents	Ischemic, hemorrhagic Arteriovenous malformation Subarachnoid hemorrhage
Space occupying lesions	Metastatic cancer Subthalamic nucleus cyst
Infections	Tuberculous meningitis
Cerebral trauma	
Metabolic disorders	Non-ketotic hyperosmolar state
Multiple sclerosis	
Drugs	Phenytoin toxicity Oral contraceptives and estrogens Levodopa
Complications of stereotactic surgery	

Adapted from: Wiener WM J, Lang Anthony L, eds. Movement Disorders: A Comprehensive Survey. Mount Kisco, NY: Futura Publishing Co.; 1989.

Conditions that Can Enhance Physiologic Tremor

- **Mental state:** Anger, anxiety, stress, fatigue, excitement

- **Metabolic:** Fever, thyrotoxicosis, pheochromocytoma, hypoglycemia

- **Drugs and toxins**

- **Miscellaneous:** Caffeinated beverages, monosodium glutamate, nicotine

Adapted from: Weiner W, Lang A. In: Movement Disorders: A Comprehensive Survey. Mount Kisco, NY: Futura Publishing Company, Mount Kisco; 1989.

Features of Psychogenic Tremor

1. History of many undiagnosed conditions

2. History of multiple somatization

3. Absence of significant finding on physical examination or imaging study

4. Presence of secondary gain (pending compensation or litigation)

5. Spontaneous remissions and exacerbations

6. Employment in the health care delivery field

7. History of psychiatric illness

Used with permission from: Shah S, Albin R. Movement Disorders. In: Shah S, Kelly K, eds. *Emergency Neurology: Principles and Practice.* New York: Cambridge University Press; 1999. Reprinted with the permission of Cambridge University Press.

Etiological Classification of Tics

PRIMARY TIC DISORDERS

Tourette's syndrome

Various chronic tic disorders

SECONDARY TIC DISORDERS

Inherited: Huntington's disease

             Neuroacanthocytosis

             Torsion dystonia

             Chromosomal abnormalities

             Other

Acquired: *Drugs:* Neuroleptic, anticonvulsants, levodopa, stimulants

             Trauma

             Infections: Encephalitis, Creutzfeldt-Jakob disease, Sydenham's chorea

             Developmental: Mental retardation, static encephalopathy, autism, pervasive developmental disorder

             Stroke

             Degenerative: Parkinsonism, progressive supranuclear palsy

             Toxic: Carbon monoxide

Adapted from: Kurlan R, ed. *Treatment of Movement Disorders*. Philadelphia, PA: J.B.Lippincott Co.; 1995.

Well-Known Causes of Tremor

- **Physiologic**
- **Pathologic**

    Essential tremor

    Parkinson's disease

    Wilson's disease

    Midbrain tremor

    Peripheral neuropathy

    Multiple sclerosis

    Cerebellar infarction

    Cerebellar degenerative disorders

- **Psychogenic tremors**
- **Drugs and toxins**

    Neuroleptics

    Lithium

    Adrenocorticosteroids

    Beta-adrenergic agonists

    Theophylline

    Ethanol

    Calcium channel blockers

    Valproic acid

    Thyroid hormone

    Caffeine

    Nicotine

    Tricyclic antidepressants

Used with permission from: Shah S, Albin R. Movement Disorders. In: Shah S, Kelly K, eds. *Emergency Neurology: Principles and Practice.* New York: Cambridge University Press; 1999. Reprinted with the permission of Cambridge University

PAIN MANAGEMENT

Commonly Used NSAIDs and Over-the-Counter Medications: Doses and Comments

Drug Name	Usual Adult oral Dose (mg)	Usual Dose Interval (h)	Pediatric Dose (mg/kg)
Aspirin			
	325-1000	4-6	10-15 q 4-6
Acetaminophen			
	500-1000	4-6	10-15 q 4-6
Choline Magnesium Trisalicylate			
	1000-1500	12	25 bid
Ibuprofen			
	200-800	6	10 q 6-8
Naproxen			
	250-500	6-12	5 bid
Ketoprofen			
	12.5-50	6-8	Not recommended
Flurbiprofen			
	50-100	Bid-tid	Not recommended
Oxaprozin			
	1200	24	Not recommended

MAXIMAL DAILY DOSE (mg/d)	OTHER COMMENTS
4000	Not for use in children younger than age 12 with possible viral illness due to Reye's syndrome
4000	Significant liver toxicity in overdose. May increase INR in patients taking warfarin.
2000-3000	No effect on platelet function. Avoid in children younger than age 12 with possible viral illness.
2400-3200	Relatively infrequent GI side effects
750-1250	May be beneficial for headaches or migraines
300	Slightly increased GI side effects
300	Potent anti-inflammatory properties
1800	Onset delayed for 3-6 hours

Table continued on next page

Commonly Used NSAIDs and Over-the-Counter Medications: Doses and Comments *(continued)*

DRUG NAME	USUAL ADULT ORAL DOSE (mg)	USUAL DOSE INTERVAL (h)	PEDIATRIC DOSE (mg/kg)
SULINDAC			
	150-200	Bid	Not recommended
ETODOLAC			
	200-400	6-12	Not recommended
INDOMETHACIN			
	25-50	8-12	Not recommended
KETOROLAC			
	30 mg IV/IM	6	None
PIROXICAM			
	20	24	Not recommended
NABUMETONE			
	500-1000	12	Not recommended
CELECOXIB			
	100-200	12-24	Not recommended
ROFECOXIB			
	12.5-50	24	Not recommended

Key: INR = International Normalized Ratio; GI = Gastrointestinal

MAXIMAL DAILY DOSE (mg/d)	OTHER COMMENTS
400	Prodrug with decreased GI side effects
1000	Balanced COX-1/COX-2 with decreased GI side effects
150-200	Limit use to 2 weeks if possible
120, except 150 first day	Efficacy similar to 4 mg morphine. Not for use for more than 5 days
20	About half of patients intolerant of GI effects
2000	Low incidence of GI effects
400	Primarily COX-2 inhibitor
50	Primarily COX-2 inhibitor. Increased incidence of cardiac events in VIGOR trial

Equivalent Doses of Common Opioids: Typical Starting Doses

Drug Name	Adult Oral Dose	Adult Parenteral
Morphine	30-60 mg q 3-4 hours	10 mg
Codeine	130 mg q 3-4 hours	75 mg
Hydromorphone	2-4 mg q 3-4 hours	1-2 mg
Levorphanol	2 mg q 6-8 hours	1 mg
Meperidine	50-150 mg q 2-3 hours	100 mg
Methadone	2.5-10 mg q 6-8 hours	10 mg
Oxycodone	30 mg q 3-4 hours	N/A
Oxymorphone	N/A	1 mg q 3-4 hours
Buprenorphine	N/A	0.3 mg q 6-8 hours
Butorphanol	N/A	2 mg q 3-4 hours
Nalbuphine	N/A	10 mg q 3-4 hours

From Acute Pain Management in Adults — U.S. Department of Health and Human Services, AHCPR Publication 92-0019. These represent typical starting doses. Individual adjustments may be necessary. N/A = Not available.

ORAL PEDIATRIC	PARENTERAL PEDIATRIC
0.3 mg/kg	0.1 mg/kg
1 mg/kg	Not recommended
0.06 mg/kg	N/A
0.04 mg/kg	0.02 mg/kg
0.5-0.8 mg/lb	0.75 mg/kg
0.2 mg/kg	0.1 mg/kg
0.2 mg/kg	N/A
N/A	Not recommended
N/A	0.004 mg/kg
N/A	Not recommended
N/A	0.1 mg/kg

Skeletal Muscle Relaxants: Dose, Duration of Action, and Side Effects

Drug Name	Usual Dose (mg)	Duration of Action (Hours)
Baclofen	Start 3-5 tid, then increase by 5 mg every 3 days	Highly variable
Carisoprodol	350 qid	4-6
Chlorphenesin	400 tid-qid	—
Chlorzoxazone	250-750 tid-qid	3-4
Cyclobenzaprine	10 tid	12-24
Diazepam	2-10 tid-qid	Highly variable
Metaxalone	800 tid-qid	2-4
Methocarbamol	1000-1500 qid	4-6
Orphenadrine	100 bid	8-12

OTHER SIDE EFFECTS	COMMENTS
Dizziness, ataxia, confusion	Usual maintenance dose is 50-60 mg/d divided tid. Not first-line treatment in most cases. Possible severe withdrawl following abrupt cessation, including seizures.
Dizziness, ataxia, headache, tremor, syncope	Contraindicated for patients with history of acute intermittent porphyria. Possible severe withdrawl following abrupt cessation, including seizures.
Confusion, headache, dizziness	Avoid in patients with hepatic disease. Limit use to eight weeks.
Dizziness, paradoxical stimulation	Associated with significant hepatotoxicity in rare instances
Primarily aticholinergic; also hypotension and cardiac arrhythmias	Contraindicated with recent MAOI use. Avoid in patients with hyperthyroidism, CHF, history of arrhythmia, glaucoma, urinary retention, history of suicide attempts, or severe depression.
Dizziness, paradoxical CNS stimulation, cardio-pulmonary depression	Not indicated as first-line therapy in acute musculoskeletal injury unless significant anxiety is present. Possible severe withdrawal following abrupt cessation.
Liver function impairment, rash, dizziness, headache	Contraindicated in patients with history of drug-induced anemia.
Dizziness, headache, rash	Available in parenteral form
Anticholinergic; headache, dizziness	Antihistamine analog; Avoid in patients with glaucoma and urinary retention. Available in parenteral form. Rarely associated with aplastic anemia.

PULMONARY EMERGENCIES

CHRONIC OBSTRUCTIVE PULMONARY DISEASE (COPD)

Factors Influencing Patient Disposition in Acute Exacerbations of Chronic Obstructive Pulmonary Disease (AECOPD)

- Age of patient

- Overall respiratory status

- Respiratory rate

- O_2 saturation

- Degree of hypercarbia

- Patient's status compared to baseline

- Mental status

- Home environment

- Likelihood of acceptable medication compliance

- Nighttime emergency department visit

- Previous pattern of frequent relapse

- Pulmonary function tests

- FEV_1 less than 40% of predicted normal

- Multiple ED courses of aerosolized β-agonist

SERF (Severity of Exacerbation and Risk Factor) Risk-Stratification Pathway for Antibiotic Selection in Acute Bacterial Exacerbations of Chronic Obstructive Pulmonary Disease

SEVERITY OF EXACERBATION AND RISK FACTOR (SERF) SUPPORT TOOL

Rationale:

The need for intensification and amplification of antimicrobial coverage in patients with acute exacerbations of chronic obstructive lung disease (ABE/COPD) depends on:

- Likelihood of infection with gram-negative enterobacteria

- Colonization status

- Patient's history of exacerbations and antimicrobial treatment response record

- Ability of patient to tolerate a treatment failure given his or her respiratory status

- Other factors requiring sound clinical judgment.

THE SERF PATHWAY

- Based on evidence-based trials and consensus opinion

- Designed as a clinical decision support tool to help guide empiric antibiotic therapy for outpatients with ABE/COPD.

Final decisions regarding drug selection should be made by the clinician on a patient-by-patient basis using on a comprehensive database including history, physical examination, and other diagnostic information.

SERF (Severity of Exacerbation and Risk Factor) Pathway: Intensification of Treatment Trigger (IOTT) Criteria for Risk-Stratification in Acute Bacterial Exacerbations of Chronic Obstructive Pulmonary Disease

INTENSIFICATION-OF-TREATMENT TRIGGER (IOTT) CRITERIA SHOULD BE CONSIDERED WHEN SELECTING AN ANTIBIOTIC FOR EMPIRIC OUTPATIENT TREATMENT OF ABE/COPD.

WHEN IOTT CRITERIA ARE PRESENT, CLINICIANS SHOULD CONSIDER NEWER AGENTS WITH EVIDENCE-BASED SUPPORT AS INDICATED AND RECOGNIZE POSSIBLE LIMITATIONS OF OLDER AGENTS SUCH AS SULFONAMIDES, PENICILLINS, AND TETRACYCLINES

IOTT criteria include the following:

- History of multiple bacterial exacerbations of COPD within a short time period (more than 3 exacerbations in < 4 months)

- Multiple antimicrobial treatment exposures

- Documentation of gram-negative (enterobacteria, pseudomonas, Klebsiella, etc.) respiratory tract colonization

- History of requiring mechanical ventilation after treatment failure of ABE/COPD

- History of gram-negative nosocomial lower respiratory tract infection

- Chronic, systemic corticosteroid use

- Multiple emergency department visits with relapse within a 10-day period

- Supplemental home oxygen

- Smoking

- High prevalence (documented) S. pneumoniae resistance to penicillin

- Chronic alcoholism associated with history of gram-negative (Klebsiella) lower respiratory tract infection

- Serious co-morbidity (immunosuppression, HIV, underlying malignancy, etc.)

Technique for Using a Metered-Dose Inhaler

1. Invert inhaler so that opening is downward after shaking briskly.

2. Hold inhaler about four finger-widths in front of open mouth.

3. Exhale normally to functional residual capacity.

4. Activate inhaler at beginning of inspiration.

5. Inhale slowly and deeply to total lung capacity.

6. Hold breath for 10 seconds.

7. Exhale slowly.

Indications for Chronic Supplemental Oxygen for Chronic Obstructive Pulmonary Disease (COPD)*

RECOMMENDED INDICATIONS

$PAO_2 \leq 55$ mmHg or $SaO_2 \leq 89\%$ at rest, with exercise, or during sleep.

Evidence of pulmonary hypertension or cor pulmonale, mental or psychological impairment, or polycythemia, and a PaO_2 of 56-59 mmHg or $SaO_2 < 90\%$ at any time.

MEDICARE CRITERIA FOR REIMBURSABLE OXYGEN SUPPLEMENTATION

$PaO_2 \leq 55$ mmHg or $SaO_2 \leq 88\%$

PaO_2 of 56-59 mmHg or $SaO_2 \leq 89\%$ if evidence of cor pulmonale (P pulmonale, polycythemia, or congestive heart failure)

*PaO_2 denotes the partial pressure of arterial oxygen, and SaO_2 denotes arterial oxygen saturation.

Antibiotics for Acute Exacerbations of COPD: Dose, Frequency, and Duration

ANTIBIOTIC

FIRST-LINE

Generics

Trimethoprim-sulfamethoxazole (Bactrim, Septra)

Amoxicillin (Amoxil, Wymox)

Tetracycline

Doxycycline (Doryx, Vibramycin)

Macrolides/Azalides

Azithromycin (Zithromax)

Clarithromycin (Biaxin)

SECOND-LINE

Quinolones

Ofloxacin (Floxin)

Ciprofloxacin (Cipro)

Lomefloxacin (Maxaquin)

Cephalosporins

Cefixime (Suprax)

Cefprozil (Cefzil)

Cefaclor (Ceclor)

Penicillins

Amoxicillin/clavulanate (Augmentin)

RECOMMENDED DOSE	FREQUENCY	DURATION
I DS tab po	bid	7-14 d
500 mg	tid	7-14 d
500 mg	qid	7-14 d
100 mg	bid	7-14 d
500 mg po	qd	3 d
250 mg bid (for *S. pneumoniae*/ *M. catarrhalis*)		
500 mg bid (for *H. influenzae*)	bid	7-14 d
400 mg	bid	10 d
500 mg	bid	10 d
400 mg	qd	10 d
400 mg	qd	
200 mg	bid	10 d
500 mg	bid	10 d
250 mg	tid	10 d
500 mg	tid	10 d

Characteristics of Bronchodilators Delivered by Metered-Dose Inhalers

MEDICATION	DOSE (MG)/PUFF	Level of Activity* BETA-1-AGONIST	Level of Activity* BETA-2-AGONIST
Isoproterenol	0.08	+ + +	+ + +
ISOETHARINE	0.34	+ +	+ +
Metaproterenol	0.65	+	+ + +
TERBUTALINE	0.20	+	+ + + +
Albuterol	0.09	+	+ + + +
BITOLTEROL	0.37	+	+ + + +
Pirbuterol	0.20	+	+ + +
SALMETEROL	0.04	+	+ + + +
Ipratropium	0.18	-	-

*The number of plus signs denotes the relative level of activity

Level of Activity*	Time of Effect		
ANTICHOLINERGIC	ONSET (MIN))	PEAK (MIN)	DURATION (MIN)
-	3-5	5-10	60-90
-	3-5	5-20	60-150
-	5-15	10-60	60-180
-	5-30	60-120	180-360
-	5-15	60-90	240-360
-	5-10	60-90	300-480
-	5-10	30-60	180-240
-	10-20	180	720
+ + + +	5-15	60-120	240-480

THE DIFFICULT AIRWAY

Suggested Contents of Bedside Storage Unit for the Difficult Airway

1. Rigid laryngoscope blades of varied design and size, laryngoscope handles

2. Endotracheal tubes of assorted sizes with preinserted stylets and attached syringes for cuff inflation

3. Fiberoptic intubation equipment

4. Devices for nonsurgical airway

5. Equipment for emergency surgical airway (scalpel, tracheal dilator, tracheal hooks, and tracheostomy tubes)

6. An exhaled CO_2 detector

7. Magill forceps

8. Oropharyngeal and nasopharyngeal airways

9. Water soluble lubricant, anesthetic topicals, vasoconstrictive topicals

LMA-Fastrach Sizes and Patient Sizes

SIZE	PATIENT
3	Small adults
4	Normal adults
5	Large adults

LMA Sizes and Patient Sizes, and Endotracheal Tube Mnemonic

LMA Size	Patient
1	Neonates/infants up to 5 kg
1 1/2	Infants between 5 and 10 kg
2	Infants/children between 10 and 20 kg
2 1/2	Children between 20 and 30 kg
3	Children heavier than 30 kg and small adults
4	Normal and large adults
5	Large adults

ENDOTRACHEAL TUBE SIZE MNEMONIC FOR CHILDREN > 2 YEARS OLD

$$\text{ETT size (mm)} = \frac{16 + \text{Age in years}}{4}$$

Mallampati Airway Classification: Oropharyngeal View

Class I	Soft palate, fauces, uvula, anterior and posterior tonsillar pillars
Class II	Soft palate, fauces, uvula
Class III	Soft palate, base of uvula
Class IV	Soft palate not visible at all

Reproduced from: Deem S, Bishop MJ. Evaluation and management of the difficult airway. *Crit Care Clin* 1995;11:1-27, with permission from Elsevier Science.

Head Positioning for Tracheal Intubation in an Adult

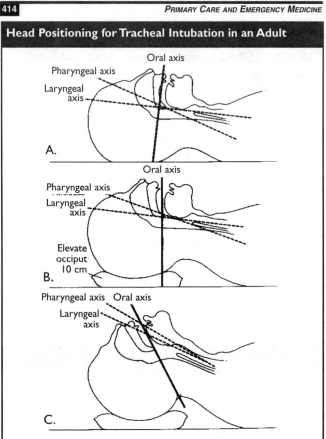

A = Neutral position. B = Head elevated. C = "Sniffing" position, flexed neck, extended head. Note how flexing the neck and extending the head to line up the various axes allows for intubation. Position C creates the shortest distance and straightest line between the teeth and vocal cords.

Rprinted from: Clinton JE, Ruiz E. Emergency airway management procedures. Roberts JR, Hedges JR, eds. *Clinical Procedures in Emergency Medicine*. 2nd edition. Philadelphia: WB Saunders; 1991:13, with permission from Elsevier Science.

Head Positioning for Tracheal Intubation in a Child

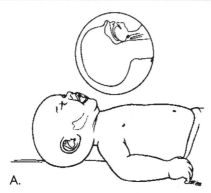

A.

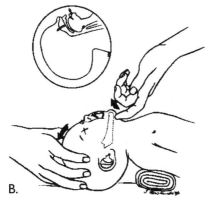

B.

A = Neutral position (laryngeal view obstructed).

B = Placement of folded towel beneath shoulders provides unobstructed view.

ACUTE ASTHMA

Evaluation of the Patient with Asthma: History

GENERAL

- Age
- Gender

MEDICATION USE AND COMPLIANCE

- Steroids
- Leukotriene antagonists
- Theophylline

MEDICAL HISTORY

- Cardiovascular disease

PAST EPISODES

- ICU admissions
- Number of emergency department visits in last year
- Any history of pneumothorax

CURRENT EPISODE

- Onset
- Time course (crescendo pattern)
- Characterization of symptoms
      Dyspnea
      Fever
      Chest tightness
      Wheezing
      Cough or sputum production
- Prior treatment
- Recent upper respiratory infection (URI) symptoms
- Occupational exposures

FAMILY HISTORY

- Other family members with asthma
- Other pulmonary disease
- History of atopy (eczema, dermatitis)

SOCIAL HISTORY

- Tobacco history or second-hand exposure
- Drug history, especially inhaled drugs/inhalants

Evaluation of the Patient with Asthma: Important Aspects of the Physical Examination

GENERAL APPEARANCE

- Anxiety
- Mental status
- Level of respiratory distress:
    Retractions
    Accessory muscle use

VITAL SIGNS

- Temperature
- Heart rate
- Respiratory rate
- Pulse oximetry
- Blood pressure (pulsus paradoxus)

PULMONARY

- Hyperresonance
- Prolonged expiratory phases (increased I:E)
- Air flow
- Wheeze distribution
- Any focal findings

ASSOCIATED FINDINGS

- Ear, nose, and throat (increased nasal secretions, sinusitis, mucosal swelling)
- Cardiac (S_3, S_4, diffuse apical impulse, murmurs)
- Skin (dermatitis, eczema, atopy, urticaria)
- Extremities (edema, cyanosis, clubbing)
- Upper airway (inspiratory stridor, localized wheeze, dysphonia)
- Lymphadenopathy

Drugs for Acute Management of Asthma

DRUG	ROUTE	DOSE
ADRENERGIC		
Epinephrine	SQ	0.3-0.5 mg repeated q20 min to 1 mg
BETA ADRENERGIC		
Terbutaline	SQ	0.25-0.5 mg repeated q30 min to total of 5 mg over 4 hr
	MDI	200 mcg/spray 2 inhalations q20 min
Albuterol	Nebulization	0.5 cc in 3-6 cc normal saline q20 min
	MDI	90 mcg/spray 1-2 puffs q20 min
Metaproterenol	Nebulization	0.3 cc in 3-6 cc normal saline
	MDI	1-2 puffs q20 min 0.65 mg per actuation
Pirbuterol	MDI	0.2 mg/actuation 1-2 puffs q20 min
Bitolterol	MDI	370 mcg/spray 1-2 puffs q20 min
STEROIDS		
Prednisone	Oral	Typically 40-60 mg po
Methyl-prednisolone	IV	Typically 80-120 mg
OTHER AGENTS		
Magnesium sulfate	IV	1-2 g over 20 minutes
Aminophylline		5.6 mg/kg loading dose then 0.9 mg/kg/hr maintenance
Ipratropium	MDI	18 mcg/spray 1-2 puffs with beta-agonists
	Nebulization	0.02% solution with beta-agonist (500 mcg [1 unit dose vial])

ADVANTAGES	DISADVANTAGES
Does not require patient cooperation	Pain at injection site, Needle exposure
Does not require patient cooperation	Pain at injection site, Needle exposure
Mimics home therapy	Staff time to demonstrate proper use
Duration of action 4-6 hr	Requires nebulizer setup
Mimics home therapy	Should be used with a spacer
Duration of action 4-6 hr	Less B_2 specific than albuterol
Duration of action 4-6 hr	Less B_2 specific than albuterol
Maximum onset of action 30-60 minutes	Only available as MDI
Rapid onset of action, duration 8 hours	Only available as MDI
Inexpensive	Hours for onset of action
Intravenous	No advantage over oral therapy
Some studies show benefit	Typically only beneficial in severe asthma
Modest bronchodilation	Must check levels before administration and adjust dose for medications and chronic illnesses
Modest bronchodilation	Not all studies have demonstrated effect
Modest bronchodilation	Not all studies have demonstrated effect

Additional Agents for Post ED Asthma Therapy

DRUG	ROUTE	DOSE
INHALED STEROIDS		
Triamcinolone	MDI	2 puffs bid-qid
Beclomethasone	MDI	2 puffs bid-qid
Budesonide	MDI	1-2 puffs bid
Fluticasone	MDI varying strengths	1-2 puffs bid
LEUKOTRIENE ANTAGONISTS		
Zafirlukast	Oral	20 mg bid
Montelukast	Oral	10 mg qd
OTHER AGENTS		
Cromylyn	MDI nebulizer	2 puffs qid 20 mg minutes before exercise
Nedocromil	MDI	2 puffs qid
Sustained release theophylline	Oral	Start 200-300 mg bid and adjust based on levels
Levalbuterol	Nebulizer	0.63-1.25 mg q6-8 h
Salmeterol	MDI	2 puffs bid

COMMENTS	TYPICAL COST
Rinse mouth after use	$52 per cannister
Rinse mouth after use	$52 per cannister
Rinse mouth after use	$108 per cannister
Rinse mouth after use	$44-91 per cannister
Caution with hepatic disease	$58 for 1-month supply
4 or 5 mg dose in children	$71 for 1-month supply
Use 10-60 minutes before exercise	$56/month
Tailor dose to clinical effect	$40/month
Monitor theophylline levels	$20/month
Not currently approved for acute therapy	$176/month
Not for rescue therapy	$65/month

Differential Diagnosis in Asthma

ADULTS

Chronic obstructive pulmonary disease (COPD)

Foreign body aspiration

Allergic reaction

Congestive heart failure (CHF)

Neoplasms

Toxic inhalation

Tracheal stenosis

PEDIATRICS

Tracheobronchitis

Foreign body aspiration

Tracheomalacia

Bronchopulmonary dysplasia

Cystic fibrosis

Allergic reaction

Beta-Agonist Dosages

Albuterol (Proventil, Ventolin)	2-4 puffs q4h	0.5 cc (2.5 mg) in 2.5 cc NS
Bitolterol Tornalate)	2 puffs q8h	0.5 cc (0.2% [1mg]) in 2 cc NS
Isoetharine (Bronkosol)	4 puffs q4h	0.5 cc (0.25%) in 3 cc NS
Isoproterenol (Isuprel)	5-15 puffs (1:200) q4h	0.5 cc (0.5%) in 3 cc NS
Metaproterenol (Alupent, Metaprel)	2-3 puffs q3-4h	0.3 cc (1.5 mg) in 2.5 cc NS
Pirbuterol (Maxair)	2 puffs q4-6h	
Terbutaline (Brethine)	2 puffs q4-6h	
Salmeterol (Serevent)	2 puffs q12h	

Laboratory Testing for Asthma

PULMONARY FUNCTION (PEFR OR FEV$_1$)

Initially and after treatment in all patients

CHEST RADIOGRAPH

Consider if focal findings or signs of pneumonia (fever, purulent sputum) are present, or if uncertain of diagnosis

ELECTROCARDIOGRAM

Not routinely indicated;

May consider for patients with known cardiac history

COMPLETE BLOOD COUNT

Not routinely indicated

ELECTROLYTES

Not routinely indicated

THEOPHYLLINE LEVEL

Prior to bolus administration of aminophylline or tachyarrhythmias in patient on therapy

ARTERIAL BLOOD GASES

Very severe obstruction that is not responsive to therapy or during mechanical ventilation

CARDIAC, THROMBOTIC, AND VASCULAR EMERGENCIES

ACUTE CORONARY SYNDROMES

Antithrombin and Antiplatelet Agent Choices

ANTITHROMBIN AGENTS

AT III dependent
Heparin
LMWH
Dalteparin (Fragmin)
Enoxaparin (Lovenox)
Nadroparin (Fraxiparine)

AT III independent
Hirudin
Hirulog

ANTIPLATELET AGENTS

Cyclooxygenase inhibitor
Aspirin

GP IIb/IIIa inhibitors
Abciximab (Reopro)
Eptifabitide (Integrilin)
Tirofiban (Aggrastat)

ADP inhibitors
Ticlopidine (Ticlid)
Clopidogrel (Plavix)

Thromboxane synthetase inhibitor
Ridogrel

THROMBOLYTIC AGENTS

Alteplase (t-PA)

Reteplase (r-PA)

Streptokinase

Tenecteplase (TNK-tPA)

The Blood Coagulation Cascade

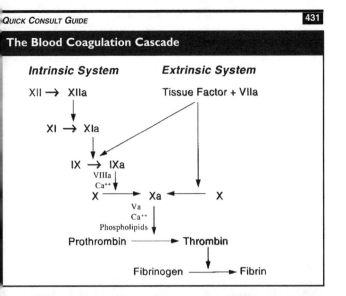

Intrinsic System

XII → XIIa

XI → XIa

IX → IXa

VIIIa
Ca++

X → Xa ← X

Va
Ca++
Phospholipids

Prothrombin ──────→ Thrombin

Extrinsic System

Tissue Factor + VIIa

Fibrinogen ──────→ Fibrin

Common Markers Used to Identify Acute Myocardial Infarction

Marker	Initial Elevation after AMI	Mean Time to Peak Elevations	Time to Return to Baseline
Myoglobin	1-4 h	6-7 h	18-24 h
CTnl	3-12 h	10-24 h	3-10 d
CTnT	3-12 h	12-48 h	5-14 d
CKMB	4-12 h	10-24 h	48-72 h
CKMBiso	2-6 h	12 h	38 h
LD	8-12 h	24-48 h	10-14 d

CTnl, CTnT = troponins of cardiac myofibrils; CPK-MB, MM = tissue isoforms of creatine kinase; LD = lactate dehydrogenase.

Adapted from: Adams JE III, Abendschein DR, Jaffee S. Biochemical markers of myocardial injury: Is MB creatine kinase the choice for the 1990s? Circulation 1993;88:750-763.

Comparison of Parenteral GP IIb/IIIa Inhibitors

AGENT		ABCIXIMAB (REOPRO)
Size		Large (~ 48 kDal)
Binding		High affinity
Clearance		Splenic and renal
Drug to receptor ratio		1.5-2.0
Mechanism		Monoclonal antibody
Antibody response		Yes
Binding to related integrins		Yes
Plasma T½ (mins)		10
Biologic[1] T½ (hours)		12-24
Indications (per the FDA)		PCI or refractory angina when PCI is planned within 24 hr
FDA approved dose	PCI	0.25 mg/kg bolus before PCI; 0.125 mcg/kg/min (max, 10mcg/min) infusion x 12 hr after PCI
	UA	0.25 mg/kg bolus and then 10 mcg/min infusion x 18-24 hrs. before PCI, continued 1 hr after PCI[2]

UA = unstable angina;

NQMI = non-Q wave myocardial infarction;

PCI = procedural coronary intervention;

T½ = half-life

[1] Is the platelet-bound half-life

[2] This approval is for patients who are not responding to conventional medical therapy when PCI is planned within 24 hours.

EPTIFIBATIDE (INTEGRILIN)	TIROFIBAN (AGGRASTAT)
Small (< 1 kDal)	Small (< 1 kDal)
Competitive	Competitive
Renal	Renal
250-2500	> 250
Peptide inhibitor	Nonpeptide inhibitor
No	No
No	No
150	120
~ 2.5	~ 2
ACS (UA and non-Q MI) with or without PCI	ACS (UA and non-Q MI) with or without PCI
135 mcg/kg bolus, 0.5 mcg/kg/min infusion for 20-24 hr (IMPACT II dose)[3] 180 mcg/kg bolus, 2.0 mcg/kg/min infusion x 72-96 hr (PURSUIT dose)	0.4 mcg/kg/min x 30 min, then then 0.1 mcg/kg/min x 48-108 hr

[3] FDA approved dose may not be optimal. The larger dose of eptifibatide used in the PURSUIT trial is recommended for use in the setting of PCI.

Comparison of Unfractionated Heparin (UFH) and Low Molecular Weight Heparin (LMWH)

Effect	UFH	LMWH
Mean molecular weight	12,000-15,000 Daltons	4000-6500 Daltons
Mean saccharide units	40-50	13-22
Anti-Xa:Antithrombin activity	1:1	2-4:1
Nonspecific protein binding	Much	Minimal
Neutralization by Platelet factor 4	Yes	Minimal
Inhibition of Fibrin-bound thrombin	No	Yes
Binding to endothelium	Yes	Minimal
Binding to macrophages	Yes	Minimal
Inactivation of platelet-bound Xa	Weak	Strong
Inhibition of platelet function	++++	++
Interaction with platelets	More	Less
Causes thrombocytopenia	Not rare	Very rare
Dose response	Poor	Fair
Bioavailability	~ 30%	> 90%

UFH = Unfractionated heparin;

LMWH = Low molecular weight heparin;

SC = Subcutaneous

[1] = Interaction with endothelial cells causes increased vascular permeability, resulting in potentially increased bleeding.

[2] = Hepatic macrophage uptake of an agent results in increased hepatic metabolism

Significance of Difference
On LMWH

- Bioavailability
- Antithrombin potency

- Antithrombin potency

- Antithrombin potency

- Bioavailability
- Bleeding[1]

- Bioavailability
- Half-life[2]

- Antithrombin potency

- Bleeding

- Bioavailability

- Bleeding

- Safety and consistency

- Safety and consistency

From: Garrison R, Kleinschmidt K. Use of Low molecular weight heparins. *Crit Decis Emerg Med* 1999;13:11-19. Reprinted with permission from the American College of Emergency Physicians.

Low Molecular Weight Heparins: Effect on Triple End Points in Comparison to Heparin

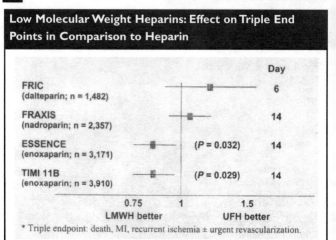

* Triple endpoint: death, MI, recurrent ischemia ± urgent revascularization.

The use of LMWH in unstable angina/NSTEMI on the triple end point of death, AMI, and recurrent Ischemia with or without revascularization. Early (6 day) and intermediate outcomes of the four trials that compared LMWH and heparin: ESSENCE, TIMI IIB, FRIC, and FRAXIS. Nadroparin in FRAXIS was given for 14 days.

UNSTABLE ANGINA

Predictors of High Risk of Complications in Unstable Angina

HISTORY

- Prior CAD
- Pain worse than usual or like prior MI
- Pressure, burning, or indigestion-like pain
- Pain > 1 hour, but < 48 hours
- Radiation to left or both shoulders
- Nausea, diaphoresis, or dyspnea
- High clinical suspicion
- History of CHF, DM, or loss of consciousness
- Age: M > 60, F > 70

PHYSICAL EXAM

- S3 or S4
- Rales
- Cyanosis
- Diaphoresis

ECG

- Transient ST depression, T-wave inversion, or ST elevation during pain
- ST segment depression > 1 mm
- Marked symmetrical T-wave inversion in multiple precordial leads

LABORATORY

- Elevated CK-MB
- Elevated cardiac index (CK-MB/total CPK)
- Elevated troponin I or T

Algorithm for Management of Unstable Angina

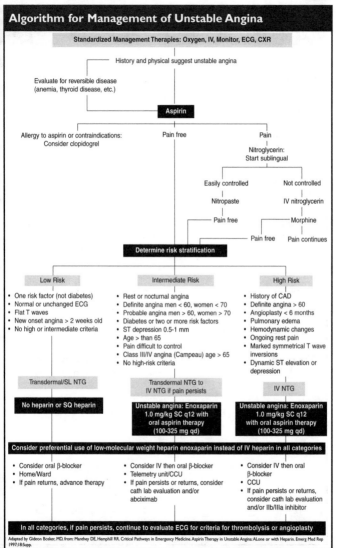

Standardized Management Therapies: Oxygen, IV, Monitor, ECG, CXR

History and physical suggest unstable angina

Evaluate for reversible disease
(anemia, thyroid disease, etc.)

Aspirin

Allergy to aspirin or contraindications:
Consider clopidogrel

Pain free

Pain

Nitroglycerin:
Start sublingual

Easily controlled

Not controlled

Nitropaste

IV nitroglycerin

Pain free

Morphine

Pain free

Pain continues

Determine risk stratification

Low Risk	Intermediate Risk	High Risk
• One risk factor (not diabetes) • Normal or unchanged ECG • Flat T waves • New onset angina > 2 weeks old • No high or intermediate criteria	• Rest or nocturnal angina • Definite angina men < 60, women < 70 • Probable angina men > 60, women > 70 • Diabetes or two or more risk factors • ST depression 0.5-1 mm • Age > than 65 • Pain difficult to control • Class III/IV angina (Campeau) age > 65 • No high-risk criteria	• History of CAD • Definite angina > 60 • Angioplasty < 6 months • Pulmonary edema • Hemodynamic changes • Ongoing rest pain • Marked symmetrical T wave inversions • Dynamic ST elevation or depression
Transdermal/SL NTG	Transdermal NTG to IV NTG if pain persists	IV NTG
No heparin or SQ heparin	**Unstable angina: Enoxaparin 1.0 mg/kg SC q12 with oral aspirin therapy (100-325 mg qd)**	**Unstable angina: Enoxaparin 1.0 mg/kg SC q12 with oral aspirin therapy (100-325 mg qd)**

Consider preferential use of low-molecular weight heparin enoxaparin instead of IV heparin in all categories

• Consider oral β-blocker • Home/Ward • If pain returns, advance therapy	• Consider IV then oral β-blocker • Telemetry unit/CCU • If pain persists or returns, consider cath lab evaluation and/or abciximab	• Consider IV then oral β-blocker • CCU • If pain persists or returns, consider cath lab evaluation and/or IIb/IIIa inhibitor

In all categories, if pain persists, continue to evaluate ECG for criteria for thrombolysis or angioplasty

Adapted by Gideon Bosker, MD; from: Manthey DE, Hemphill RR. Critical Pathways in Emergency Medicine. Aspirin Therapy in Unstable Angina: ALone or with Heparin. Emerg Med Rep 1997;18:Supp.

Medications for Unstable Angina: Route, Dose, Frequency, and Contraindications

MEDICATION	ROUTE	DOSE
Aspirin	PO	81-325 mg
Heparin	IV	80 U/kg IV bolus
LMWH Enoxaparin	SC	1 mg/kg SC
GRI (GIIb/IIa receptor inhibitor) abciximab	IV	0.25 mg/kg IV bolus
Nitroglycerin	SL to chest wall IV	0.4 mg one-half - 2 in. 50 mg in 250 D5W
Metoprolol	IV	5 mg
Morphine	IV	2-5 mg
Diltiazem	IV	bolus: 20 mg over 2 min

FREQUENCY	CONTRAINDICATIONS
daily	Major hemorrhage, distinct allergy
18 U/kg/h infusion	Active hemorrhage
q 12 hours	Active hemorrhage, pre-disposition to hemorrhage
10 mcg/min infusion x 12 hours	Active hemorrhage, pregnancy, predisposition to hemorrhage
q 5 min x 3 q 8 hours 10-20 mcg/min (3-6 mL/h), titrate to relieve pain, keep SBP > 90	SBP < 90
q 5 min x 3	COPD, CHF, AV block, asthma, hypotension, bradycardia
q 5-30 min prn	Allergy, hypotension
infusion: 5-15 mg/h	AV block, CHF, bradycardia, hypotension

Management and Triage of Emergency Department Chest Pain Syndromes

Category	Criteria
I. Acute myocardial infarction	1mm ST elevation in 2 or more contiguous leads or new LBBB in symptomatic patient
II. Unstable angina	Accelerating or rest pain with known CAD, post MI pain, chest pain with new 1 mm ST depression in 2 or more contiguous leads or reversible T wave inversions, chest pain with CHF or hypotension
III. Probable unstable angina	Typical symptoms with non-specific ECG changes or history of diabetes mellitus or multiple risk factors
IV. Possible unstable angina	Low risk patient with typical symptoms with normal ECG or atypical symptoms with nonspecific ECG changes
V. Non-cardiac chest pain	Atypical symptoms in very low risk patient or symptoms explained by another diagnosis

MEDICATIONS	MEDICATIONS TO CONSIDER	DISPOSITION
ASA, nitroglycerin, TNK-TPA (or PTCA), LMWH	Morphine	CCU
ASA, nitroglycerin, LMWH (enoxaparin); or as second-line alternative: heparin (UFH) IIb/IIIa inhibitor	Morphine, GRI, (especially prior to PCI), beta-blocker, diltiazem, clopidogrel	CCU
ASA, nitrates, beta-blocker	Enoxaparin or UFH, morphine	Telemetry unit or ED observation unit
ASA, nitrates		ED observation unit or discharge with rapid outpatient work-up
		Treat other cause of pain, discharge or admit as indicated by diagnosis

Provocative Testing Algorithm for Unstable Angina

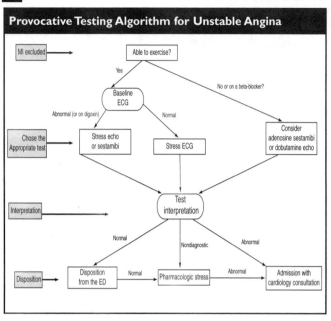

Predictors of Low Risk of Complications in Unstable Angina

- Reproducible chest pain

- Pleuritic chest pain

- Stabbing pain

- Radiation to back, legs, or abdomen

- Normal ECG

HEART FAILURE

Diastolic Heart Failure: Etiologies

- Restrictive Cardiomyopathy
    Cardiac amyloidosis

- Constrictive Pericarditis

- Ischemic Heart Disease
    Post-infarction scarring/remodeling

- Hypertropic Heart Disease
    Hypertrophic cardiomyopathy
    Chronic hypertenison
    Aortic stenosis

- Mitral or Tricuspid Stenosis

Major Etiologies of Heart Failure

- Coronary artery disease

- Complications of myocardial infarction
    Acute mitral regurgitation (papillary muscle rupture)

- Sustained cardiac arrhythmia

- Poorly controlled hypertension

- Valvular rupture or disease

- Myocarditis

- Postpartum cardiomyopathy

- Acute pulmonary embolus

- Pericardial disease/tamponade
    Effusion
    Constrictive pericarditis

- Hyperkinetic states
    Anemia
    Thyrotoxicosis
    A-V fistula (e.g., dialysis)

- Infiltrative disorders

Forrester Classification for Cardiac Patients

CLASS	DESCRIPTION	CARDIAC INDEX	PCWP*	MORTALITY (%)
I	No congestion/peripheral hypo-perfusion	2.7	12	2
II	Isolated congestion	2.3	23	10
III	Isolated peripheral hypoperfusion	1.9	12	22
IV	Both congestion and peripheral hypoperfusion	1.7	27	55

* PCWP = Pulmonary capillary wedge pressure

Cardiogenic Shock Criteria

- Systolic blood pressure < 90 mmHg (higher if chronically hypertensive)

- Urine output < 0.5 cc/kg/hr

- Evidence of end organ dysfunction:
  - Renal failure
  - Cerebral (confusion)
  - Peripheral hypoperfusion (cool extremities)

- If hemodynamic monitoring is available:
  - PCWP > 18 mmHg and CI < 1.8 L/min/m^2

Key: PCWP = Pulmonary capillary wedge pressure; CI = Cardiac index

Pathophysiological Cycle of Acute Decompensated Heart Failure

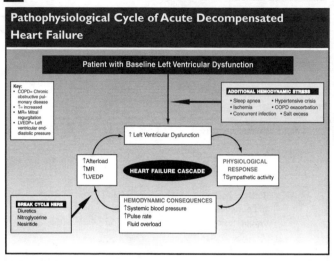

Common Causes of Heart Failure Decompensation

- Acute myocardial ischemia or infarction

- Uncontrolled hypertension

- Obesity

- Superimposed infection

- Atrial fibrillation or other arrythmia

- Excessive alcohol

- Worsening valvular lesion

- Endocrine abnormalities (e.g., diabetes, hyperthyroidism, etc.)

- Negative inotropic medications (e.g., verapamil, nifedipine, etc.)

- Non-steroidal anti-inflammatory drugs

- Treatment and dietary non-compliance

Heart Failure Differential Diagnosis

DYSPNEIC STATES

- Chronic obstructive pulmonary disease exacerbation
- Asthma exacerbation
- Pulmonary embolus
- Acute myocardial infarction
- Physical deconditioning
- Obesity
- Pleural effusions
- Pneumonia/pulmonary infection
- Pneumothorax

FLUID RETENTIVE STATES

- Renal failure/nephrotic syndrome
- Liver failure/cirrhosis
- Portal vein thrombosis
- Hypoproteinemia
- DVT
- Dependent edema

LOW CARDIAC OUTPUT STATES

- Acute myocardial infarction
- Tension pneumothorax
- Pericardial tamponade
- Sepsis

ACC/AHA Heart Failure Classification

ACC/AHA CLASS	STAGE
A	High risk for developing left ventricular dysfunction (LVD)
	Diabetes mellitus
	Family history of cardiomyopathy
B	Asymptomatic LVD
	LV systolic dysfunction
	Asymptomatic valvular disease
C	Symptomatic LVD
	Shortness of breath and fatigue
	Reduced exercise tolerance
D	Refractory end-stage HF

New York Heart Association Heart Failure Classes

CLASS	LIMITATIONS	DAILY LIVING SYMPTOMS	BNPL (PG/ML)
I	No limitation	Asymptomatic during usual daily activities	100
II	Slight limitation	Mild symptoms during ordinary daily activities	200
III	Moderate limitation	Symptoms noted with minimal activities	450
IV	Severe limitation	Symptoms present even at rest	> 1000

PATIENT DESCRIPTION	NYHA CLASS
Hypertension Coronary artery disease	—
Previous MI	I
Known structural heart disease	II-III
Marked symptoms at rest despite maximal medical therapy	IV

Accuracy of Various Heart Failure Parameters*

VARIABLE	SENSITIVITY	SPECIFICITY	ACCURACY
History of HF	62	94	90
Dyspnea	56	53	54
Orthopnea	47	88	72
Rales	56	80	70
S3	20	99	66
JVD+	39	94	72
Edema	67	68	68

+ JVD = Jugular venous distention

* Dao Q, Krishnaswamy P, Kazanegra R, et al. Utility of B-type natriuretic peptide in the diagnosis of congestive heart failure in an urgent-care setting. *J Am Coll Cardiol* 2001; 37:379-385.

Most Common Portable CXR Findings* in Heart Failure (Descending Order of Frequency)

1. Dilated upper lobe vessels
2. Cardiomegaly
3. Interstitial edema
4. Enlarged pulmonary artery
5. Pleural effusion
6. Alveolar edema
7. Prominent superior vena cava
8. Kerley's lines

* Chait A, Cohen HE, Meltzer LE, et al. The bedside chest radiograph in the evaluation of incipient heart failure. *Radiology* 1972;105:563-566.

Etiologies of Cardiogenic Shock

EXTENSIVE MYOCARDIAL INFARCTION (MI)

MI WITH MECHANICAL COMPLICATIONS
— Ventricular septal defect
— Acute mitral regurgitation
— Myocardial free wall rupture

SEPTIC SHOCK WITH MYOCARDIAL DEPRESSION

PERICARDIAL TAMPONADE

LV OUTFLOW OBSTRUCTION
— Hypertrophic obstructive cardiomyopathy (HOCM)
— Aortic stenosis

MYOCARDITIS

END-STAGE CARDIOMYOPATHY

CARDIAC CONTUSION

Initial Therapy for Acute Pulmonary Edema (APE)

1. Sit the patient upright with legs dependent (to reduce venous filling), if possible.

2. Administer 100% oxygen.

3. Administer nitrates if systolic BP > 100.
   — Sublingual nitroglycerin 0.4 mg q 1-5 minutes (monitor BP closely)
   — IV nitroglycerine or nitroprusside if needed.

4. Administer IV furosemide (or ethacrynic acid if sulfa allergy)

5. Administer IV morphine 2-6 mg (if no respiratory acidosis/depression)

6. Cardioversion to restore sinus rhythm

Contraindications to Angiotensin-Converting Enzyme Inhibitors (ACEIs)

■ Angioedema

■ Progressive azotemia (> 3 mg/dL, especially if progressively increasing)

■ Bilateral renal artery stenosis

■ Systemic hypotension (systolic blood pressure < 80, especially in ambulatory patients)

■ Hyperkalemia

■ Pregnancy

■ Hemodynamic instability

■ Intolerance secondary to **severe** cough

Angiotensin-Converting Enzyme Inhibitors (ACEIs)/Adrenergic Receptor Blockers (ARBs) for Chronic Systolic Heart Failure Agents*

DRUG	START	TARGET DOSE	TRIAL DATA
CAPTOPRIL			
	6.25 mg tid	50 mg tid	SAVE
LISINOPRIL			
	2.5 mg qd	40 mg qd	ATLAS
ENALAPRIL			
	5 mg qd	20 mg qd	SOLVD
RAMIPRIL			
	2.5 mg qd	10 mg bid	AIRE
LOSARTAN			
	50 mg qd	50 mg bid	ELITE
VALSARTAN			
	40 mg bid	160 mg bid	Val-HeFT

* Dosing data from major clinical trials

Indications for Admission to Cardiac ICU in Patients with Heart Failure (HF)

- Worsening hypoxemia or increasing oxygen requirements

- Hypercarbia

- Myocardial ischemia (by ECG or cardiac enzymes)

- Concomitant severe infection (i.e., pneumonia, sepsis)

- Evidence of end organ dysfunction (oliguria, obtundation)

- Severe structural/valvular lesions (aortic stenosis, hypertrophic obstructive cardiomyopathy [HOCM])

Nesiritide Effect Summary

HEMODYNAMICS

— Decreases afterload
— Decreases preload
— Vasodilator (including corornary arteries)

DIURETIC

— Promotes free water loss
— Promotes sodium loss
— Minimal kaliuretic effect

SYMPTOMATIC IMPROVEMENT

— Dyspnea
— Global clinical status

IMPORTANT LACK OF EFFECT

— Not inotropic
— Not arrhythmogenic

NEUROHORMONAL ANTAGONIST

— Endothelin
— Sympathetic nervous system
— Renin angiotensin system

Possible Causes of Hypotension after Initiating Therapy with Nitrates

■ Right ventricular infarction

■ Aortic stenosis

■ Hypertrophic obstructive cardiomyopathy

■ Anaphylaxis

■ Cardiogenic shock

■ Intravascular volume depletion

Diuretics for Acute Heart Failure: Dosing, Effects, and Side Effects

AGENT	DOSING (IV)
FUROSEMIDE	
	<u>**No prior use:**</u> 40 mg IVP
	<u>**If prior use:**</u> Double last 24-hour usage (max 180 mg)
	If no effect by 20-30 min: Re-double dose
BUMETANIDE	
	1-3 mg
	1 mg ~ 40 mg furosemide
TORSEMIDE	
	10-20 mg
ETHACRYNIC ACID	
	50 mg
METOLAZONE	
	5-10 mg po 20-30 min before IV furosemide

EFFECT	SIDE EFFECTS
■ Diuresis starts within 15-20 min ■ Duration of action is 4-6 hrs	■ Reduced K+ and Mg++; ■ Hyperuricemia; ototoxicity ■ Sulfa allergy; hypovolemia; ■ Pre-renal azotemia; ■ Myalgia
■ Diuresis starts within 10 min ■ Peak action at 60 min	■ Same as above
■ Diuresis starts within 10 min ■ Duration of action is 6-8 hrs ■ Better oral bioavailability than furosemide	■ Same as above
■ Similar to furosemide	■ Same as above ■ Non-sulfa agent ■ Increased ototoxicity
■ Additive to loop diuretic	■ Similar to furosemide except no ototoxicity ■ Has liver disease caution

Vasodilators for Acute Heart Failure: Dosing, Titration, and Side Effects

AGENT	DOSING
Nitroglycerin Sublingual	0.4 mg SL q 1-5 min
Nitroglycerin Intravenous	0.2-0.4 mcg/kg/min (starting dose)
Nitroprusside	0.1-0.2 mcg/kg/min (starting dose)
	10 mcg/kg/min (maximum)
Nesiritide	2 mcg/kg bolus then infusion of 0.01 mcg/kg/min

Beta-Blockers for Chronic Systolic Heart Failure: Starting and Target Doses*

DRUG	STARTING DOSE	TARGET DOSE	TRIAL DATA
Metoprolol xl/cr	12.5 mg qd	100 mg qd	MERIT-HF
Carvedilol	3.125 mg bid	25-50 mg bid	US-TRIALS COPERNICUS
Bisoprolol	1.25 mg qd	10 mg qd	CIBIS II

* Dosing data from major clinical trials

TITRATION	SIDE EFFECTS
Blood pressure symptoms	■ Hypotension ■ Headache
Blood pressure symptoms	■ Hypotension ■ Headache
Blood pressure symptoms	■ Hypotension ■ Possibility of coronary steal ■ Cyanide toxicity ■ Thiocyanate toxicity
Titration usually unnecessary	■ Hypotension

Contraindications to Beta-Blockers

- Unstable hemodynamics, or congested and requiring IV diuresis (most ED patients)

- Severe bronchospastic airway disease

- Symptomatic bradycardia

- Advanced heart block

- Acute vascular insufficiency or worsening claudication/rest pain

- Class IV stable HF (therapy should be provided by HF specialist)

- Inotropic therapy/cardiogenic shock

- Severe conduction system disease (unless protected by a pacemaker)

Inotrope Characteristics: Mechanism, Dosing, and Comments

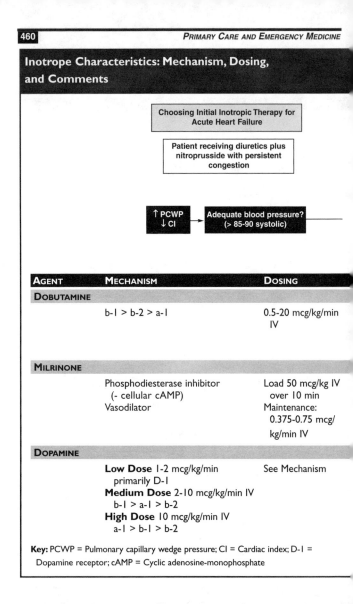

Choosing Initial Inotropic Therapy for Acute Heart Failure

Patient receiving diuretics plus nitroprusside with persistent congestion

↑ PCWP
↓ CI
→ **Adequate blood pressure? (> 85-90 systolic)** →

AGENT	MECHANISM	DOSING
DOBUTAMINE		
	b-1 > b-2 > a-1	0.5-20 mcg/kg/min IV
MILRINONE		
	Phosphodiesterase inhibitor (- cellular cAMP) Vasodilator	Load 50 mcg/kg IV over 10 min Maintenance: 0.375-0.75 mcg/kg/min IV
DOPAMINE		
	Low Dose 1-2 mcg/kg/min primarily D-1 **Medium Dose** 2-10 mcg/kg/min IV b-1 > a-1 > b-2 **High Dose** 10 mcg/kg/min IV a-1 > b-1 > b-2	See Mechanism

Key: PCWP = Pulmonary capillary wedge pressure; CI = Cardiac index; D-1 = Dopamine receptor; cAMP = Cyclic adenosine-monophosphate

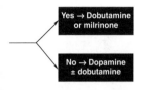

Yes → Dobutamine
or milrinone

No → Dopamine
± dobutamine

COMMENTS

- Primarily β-1 stimulation
- Less vasodilation than milrinone
- Less effective if β-receptor downregulation
- Quicker onset than milrinone

- Risk of hypotension especially when use loading dose
- Needs adjustment for renal insufficiency
- Effective in states of β-receptor downregulation
- Possibly less ischemic potential than dobutamine

- Agent of choice when shock or unacceptable hypotension
- Prefer a central line to prevent skin extravasation
- Lower doses promote renal blood flow
- Can ℘ PCWP
- Goal is to bring systolic blood pressure to acceptable range

DEEP VENOUS THROMBOSIS (DVT) AND PULMONARY EMBOLISM (PE)

Risks for Venous Thromboembolism (VTE)

INHERITED

- Antithrombin deficiency
- Proteins C & S deficiencies
- Factor V Leiden
- Prothrombin mutation

ACQUIRED (PERSISTENT)

- Age
- Malignancy
- Antiphospholipid antibodies
- History of VTE
- Lupus anticoagulant factor

ACQUIRED (TRANSIENT)

- Surgery and major trauma
- Pregnancy
- Oral contraceptives/hormone replacement therapy
- Prolonged immobilization:
  - Bed rest
  - Paralysis
  - Travel

Adapted from: Martinelli I. Risk factors in venous thromboembolism. *Thromb Haemost* 2001;86:395-403.

Differential Diagnosis of Deep Vein Thrombosis (DVT)

- Abscess
- Baker's cyst
- Cellulitis
- Claudication
- Musculoskeletal injury
- Venous stasis

Differential Diagnosis of Pulmonary Embolism (PE)

- Acute myocardial infarction (AMI)

- Aortic dissection

- Musculoskeletal disorders
    Chest contusion
    Costochondritis
    Rib fracture

- Obstructive pulmonary disease (including asthma)

- Pericardial disease

- Pneumonia

- Pneumothorax

Pitfalls in Diagnosis of Venous Thromboembolism (VTE)

FAILURE TO CONSIDER PRE-TEST PROBABILITY

RELYING ON PHYSICAL EXAM ALONE:

- Homan's sign in DVT

- Heart rate or respiratory rate in PE

- Pulse oximetry in PE

RELYING ON ONE TEST TO EXCLUDE VTE:

- Normal ABG, especially in COPD

- Normal ultrasound in DVT (calf veins)

- Relying on ultrasound in those with previous DVT

- Normal V/Q (saddle embolus)

- Relying on V/Q in those with COPD/asthma

Predicting Pre-Test Probability for Deep Vein Thrombosis (DVT)

CLINICAL FEATURES*	SCORE**
Cancer (treatment ongoing or within 6 months, or palliative)	1
Paralysis, paresis, plaster immobilization of lower extremities	1
Bedridden for more than 3 days or major surgery within 4 weeks	1
Tenderness localized along the deep venous system	1
Entire leg swollen	1
Calf swelling > 3 cm compared to asymptomatic leg (measure at 10 cm below tibial tuberosity)	1
Pitting edema (greater in the symptomatic leg)	1
Collateral superficial veins (non-varicose)	1
Alternative diagnosis as likely or greater than DVT	-2

* In patients with symptoms in both legs, the more symptomatic leg is used.

** Analysis: High probability > 3, moderate 1-2, low probability ≤ 0

Reprinted with permission from Elsevier Science (Wells PS, Anderson DR, Bormanis J, et al. Value of assessment of pretest probability of deep-vein thrombosis in clinical management. *Lancet* 1997;350:1795-1798.)

Predicting Pre-Test Probability for Pulmonary Embolism (PE)

CLINICAL FEATURES	SCORE**
Clinical signs and symptoms of DVT	3.0
Heart rate > 100 beats/min	1.5
Immobilization (for $\varnothing$ 3 consecutive days)	1.5
Surgery in the previous 4 weeks	1.5
Previous diagnosis of DVT or PE	1.5
Hemoptysis	1.0
Cancer (treatment ongoing or within 6 months, or palliative)	1.0
PE as likely or more likely than another diagnosis	3.0

** Analysis: High probability, score > 6.0; moderate, 2.0-6.0; low, < 2.0

Used with permission from: Wells PS, Anderson DR, Rodger M, et al. Excluding pulmonary embolism at the bedside without diagnostic imaging: Management of patients with suspected pulmonary embolism presenting to the emergency department by using a simple clinical model and D-dimer. *Ann Int Med* 2001;135:98-107.

Diagnostic Algorithm for Pulmonary Embolism (PE) Evaluation

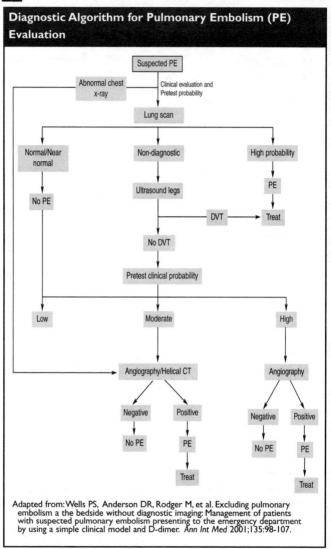

Adapted from: Wells PS, Anderson DR, Rodger M, et al. Excluding pulmonary embolism a the bedside without diagnostic imaging: Management of patients with suspected pulmonary embolism presenting to the emergency department by using a simple clinical model and D-dimer. *Ann Int Med* 2001;135:98-107.

Proposed Algorithm Using D-dimer for Evaluation of Suspected Pulmonary Embolism (PE)

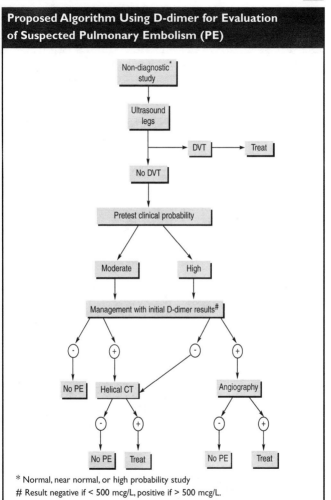

* Normal, near normal, or high probability study

\# Result negative if < 500 mcg/L, positive if > 500 mcg/L.

Adapted from: Wells PS, Anderson DR, Rodger M, et al. Excluding pulmonary embolism a the bedside without diagnostic imaging: Management of patients with suspected pulmonary embolism presenting to the emergency department by using a simple clinical model and D-dimer. *Ann Int Med* 2001;135:98-107.

Diagnostic Algorithm for Deep Venous Thrombosis (DVT) Evaluation

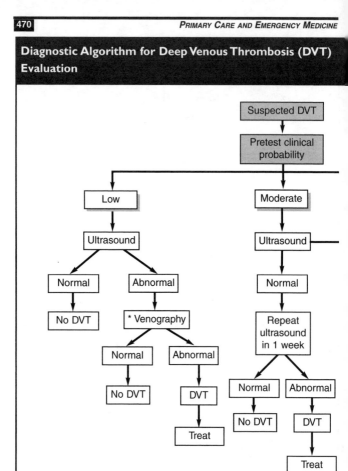

* Individualize for each patient. Consider repeat ultrasound.

+ Discordant probability and test result: Serial ultrasound also may be a possibility.

Reprinted with permission from Elsevier Science (Wells PS, Anderson DR, Bormanis J, et al. Value of assessment of pretest probability of deep-vein thrombosis in clinical management. *Lancet* 1997;1795-1798).

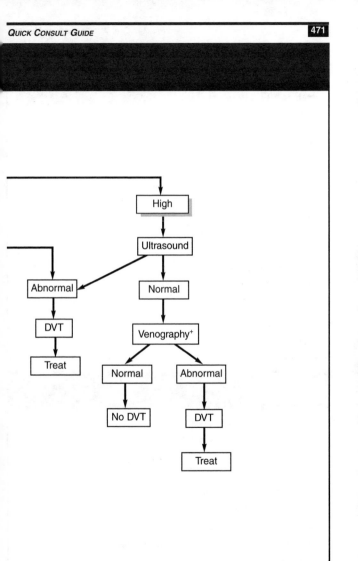

Deep Venous Thrombosis (DVT) Risk Factors for Hospitalized Patients

MEDICALLY ILL PATIENTS

- Respiratory failure
- Congestive heart failure
- Serious infection
- Malignancy
- Elderly
- History of DVT
- Immobilization
- ICU setting
- Hypercoagulability syndromes
- Inflammatory rheumatic disorders

SURGICAL PATIENTS

- Abdominal surgery
- Orthopedic surgery
- Lower extremity trauma
- Immobilization
- Elderly

Exclusionary Criteria for DVT Prophylaxis in Seriously Ill Medical Patients

- Pregnancy or possible pregnancy
- Major surgery in past 3 months
- Breast feeding
- Bleeding disorder
- Uncontrolled hypertension
- Conditions conferring risk for hemorrhage
- Abnormal clotting tests
- Hypersensitivity to heparin, LMWHs, or heparin products
- Severe renal failure

Patients with Serious Medical Illnesses who Should be Considered for DVT Prophylaxis*

SEVERE RESPIRATORY FAILURE

- Acute exacerbations of Chronic Obstructive Pulmonary Disease (ABE/COPD)
- Adult respiratory distress syndrome
- Community-acquired pneumonia
- Noncardiogenic pulmonary edema
- Pulmonary malignancy
- Interstitial lung disease

CLASS III-IV CONGESTIVE HEART FAILURE

- Ischemic cardiomyopathy
- Non-ischemic cardiomyopathy
- CHF secondary to valvular disease
- Chronic idiopathic cardiomyopathy
- CHF secondary to arrythmias

SERIOUS INFECTIONS

- Pneumonia
- Urinary tract infection
- Abdominal infection

ELDERLY PATIENTS

- All hospitalized elderly patients who are immobilized for 3 days or more and who have serious underlying medical conditions known to be risk factors for DVT should be strongly considered for prophylaxis with enoxaparin.

* Enoxaparin (Lovenox®) 40 mg subcutaneoulsly, QD is indicated providing there are no contraindications and immobilization period of 3 or more days is anticipated.

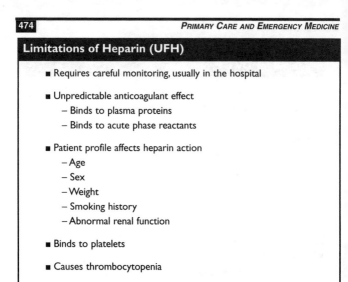

Limitations of Heparin (UFH)

- Requires careful monitoring, usually in the hospital

- Unpredictable anticoagulant effect
  - Binds to plasma proteins
  - Binds to acute phase reactants

- Patient profile affects heparin action
  - Age
  - Sex
  - Weight
  - Smoking history
  - Abnormal renal function

- Binds to platelets

- Causes thrombocytopenia

Heparin Dose for Prevention of Venous Thromboembolism (VTE) in Medical Patients

PRODUCT	DOSAGE	FREQUENCY
HEPARIN (UFH)		
	5000 Units	Every 8-12 hours
ENOXAPARIN		
	40 mg	Once daily

BRADYCARDIA

Vascular Supply of the Cardiac Conduction System*

STRUCTURE	IMMEDIATE BLOOD SUPPLY	CORONARY VASCULAR SUPPLY
SA node	sinus nodal artery	RCA 60%
		LCX 40%
AV node	AV nodal artery	PDA (of RCA) 90%
		LCX 10%
Bundle of His	AV nodal artery	PDA (of RCA) 90%
		LCX 10%
	Septal perforating arteries	LAD
Right bundle branch	AV nodal artery	PDA (of RCA) 90%
		LCX 10%
	Septal perforating arteries	LAD
Left bundle branch		
Anterior fascicle	Septal perforating arteries	LAD
Posterior fascicle		LAD
		PDA (of RCA)

Key: RCA = right coronary artery; LCX = left circumflex artery; PDA = posterior descending artery; LAD = left anterior descending artery

Percentages refer to inter-, rather than intra-individual variations in blood supply.

* References: Josephson ME, Zimetbaum P, Marchinski FE, et al. The bradyarrhythmias: Disorders of sinus node function and AV conduction disturbances. In: Fauci AS, Braunwald E, Isselbacher KJ, et al, eds. *Harrison's Principles of Internal Medicine.* 14th ed. New York: McGraw Hill; 1998:1253-1261; Woodburne RT. *Essentials of Human Anatomy.* 7th ed. New York: Oxford University Press; 1983.

Infectious Causes of Myocarditis with Potential for Bradydysrhythmia

VIRAL

Coxsackie B virus	Influenza	Mononucleosis
Hepatitis	Mumps	Rubella
Rubeola	Varicella	Respiratory syncytial virus

BACTERIAL

Streptococcus	Meningococcus	Mycoplasma
Staphylococcus	Diphtheria	

OTHER

Trypanosomiasis (Chagus disease)	Syphilis	Lyme disease

Rheumatologic Diseases Affecting the Heart with Potential for Bradydysrhythmia*

- Rheumatoid arthritis
- Scleroderma
- Systemic lupus erythematosus
- Polymyositis
- Reiter's syndrome
- Ankylosing spondylitis
- Sjögren's syndrome
- Behcet's disease
- Wegener's granulomatosis

* References: Coblyn JS, Weinblatt ME. Rheumatic diseases and the heart. In: Braunwald E, ed. *Heart Disease: A Textbook of Cardiovascular Medicine*. 5th ed. Philadelphia: WB Saunders; 1997:1776-1785; Lee LA, Pickrell MB, Reichlin M. Development of complete heart block in an adult patient with Sjögren's syndrome and anti-Rho/SS autoantibodies. *Arthritis Rheum* 1996;39:1427-1429; Handa R, Wali JP, Aggarwal P, et al. Wegener's granulomatosis with complete heart block. *Clin Exp Rheumatol* 1997;15:97-99.

Electrocardiographic Waveforms Seen During Transvenous Pacemaker Placement*

LOCATION	WAVEFORM	
	P wave	*QRS complex*
Superior vena cava	negative	negative
High right atrium	larger/negative	smaller/negative
Mid-right atrium	larger/biphasic	smaller/negative
Low right atrium	smaller/positive	larger/negative
Right ventricle, free	smaller/positive	larger/negative
Right ventricle, against wall		ST segment elevation
Inferior vena cava	smaller/positive	smaller again/negative

* References: Benjamin GC. Emergency transvenous cardiac pacing. In: Roberts JR, Hedges JR, eds. *Clinical Procedures in Emergency Medicine*. 3rd ed. Philadelphia:WB Saunders;1998:210-225;Vukmir RB. Emergency cardiac pacing. *Am J Emerg Med* 1993;11:166-176; Jafri SM, Kruse JA. Temporary transvenous cardiac pacing. *Crit Care Clin* 1992;8:713-725.

Algorithm for Treatment of Atrial Fibrillation

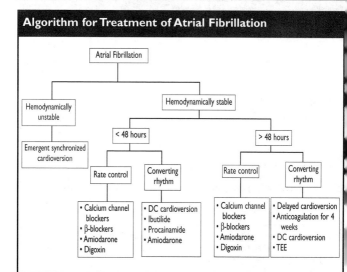

THORACIC AORTIC DISSECTION

Risk Factors for Aortic Dissection*

- Increased age—peak incidence > 50 and < 70 years

- Male sex (3:1)

- History of hypertension (60-90% of patients)

- Connective tissue disorders (Marfan's, Ehlers-Danlos)

- Turner's syndrome

- Aortic coarctation

- Third trimester pregnancy

- Congenital bicuspid or unicuspid aortic valve

- Ebstein's anomaly

- Aortic valve stenosis

- Familial incidence

- Illicit drugs (cocaine and methamphetamine)

- Iatrogenic (surgery or cardiac catheterization)

- Trauma (though blunt trauma usually produces aortic rupture)

* References: Chen K, Varon J, Wenker OC, et al. Acute thoracic aortic dissection: The basics. *J Emerg Med* 1997;15:859-867; Pansini S, Gagliardotto PV, Pompei F, et al. Early and late risk factors in surgical treatment of acute type A aortic dissection. *Ann Thorac Surg* 1998;66:779-784.

Difference Between Aortic Aneurysm and Aortic Dissection

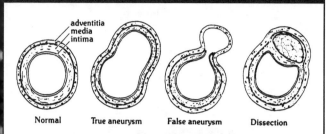

Normal   True aneurysm   False aneurysm   Dissection

Reproduced with permission from: Galloway AC, Miller JS, Spencer FC, et al. Thoracic aneurysms and aortic dissection. In: Schwartz GR, et al, eds. *Principles and Practice of Emergency Medicine*. Philadelphia: The McGraw-Hill Companies; 1992:924.

Chest X-ray Findings Suggestive of Aortic Dissection

MEDIASTINAL FINDINGS

- Widened mediastinum (most common)
- Extension of aortic shadow beyond calcified wall (most specific)
- Blurred aortic knob or localized bulge
- Aortic enlargement
- Double density of the aorta (false lumen less radiopaque)
- Loss of space between aorta and pulmonary artery

RIGHT SIDE OF FILM

- Deviation of trachea/NG tube to the right
- Shift and elevation of right mainstem bronchus
- Deviation of right paraspinal line

LEFT SIDE OF FILM

- Depressed left mainstem bronchus
- New pleural effusion
- Apical cap (localized apical hemothorax)

Frequency of Peripheral Vascular Complications in Acute Aortic Dissection

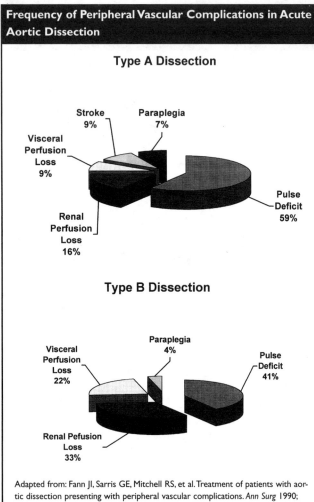

Adapted from: Fann JI, Sarris GE, Mitchell RS, et al. Treatment of patients with aortic dissection presenting with peripheral vascular complications. *Ann Surg* 1990; 212:705-713.

Summary of ED Management of Acute Aortic Dissection

A. MEDICAL THERAPY FOR AORTIC DISSECTION

Combination Therapy:

- Beta-blocker—Goal of heart rate between 60 bpm and 80 bpm
- Propranolol 1 mg IV slow push every 5 minutes, or
- Metoprolol 5 mg IV push every 5 minutes up to 15 mg, or
- Esmolol 500 mcg/kg bolus over 12 minutes followed by 50 mcg/kg/min to 200 mcg/kg/min infusion, with
- Nitroprusside—Goal of systolic blood pressure between 100 mmHg and 120 mmHg or BP sufficient to maintain mentation and urine output
- Begin 0.5 mcg/kg/min and titrate up to reach target blood pressure

Monotherapy:

- Labetalol 20 mg IV bolus initially followed by 20-80 mg every 5-10 minutes until target heart rate reached, and then start infusion at 1-2 mg per hour

B. INDICATIONS FOR SURGICAL REPAIR OF AORTIC DISSECTION

- All Type A dissections
- Type B dissections with complications of (rupture, severe distal ischemia, intractable pain, progression, uncontrolled hypertension)
- Aortic rupture
- Severe distal ischemia
- Intractable pain
- Uncontrolled hypertension
- Progression of dissection

C. KEY POINTS TO REMEMBER

- All patients receive medical therapy initially, regardless of dissection type
- Start beta-blocker therapy before or simultaneously with nitroprusside to avoid reflex tachycardia
- Lifelong medical therapy is required

Final Diagnosis in Patients Initially Misdiagnosed with Aortic Dissection

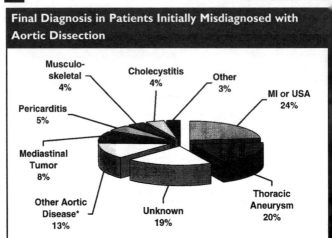

Other aortic disease includes aortic regurgitation (9%), aortic mass (2.5%), and leaking left coronary anastomosis (1.5%).

References: Eagle KA, Quertermous T, Kritzer GA, et al. Spectrum of conditions initially suggesting acute aortic dissection but with negative aortograms. *Am J Cardiol* 1986;57:322-326; Chan KL. Usefulness of transesophageal echocardiography in the diagnosis of conditions mimicking aortic dissection. *Am Heart J* 1991;122:495-504.

GASTROINTESTINAL EMERGENCIES

LOWER GASTROINTESTINAL BLEEDING

Diagnostic Pitfalls in Lower Gastrointestinal Bleeding

- Don't rely on the color of stool to determine the bleeding site. Colors change as transit times vary and blood products break down.

- All that bleeds bright red is not a hemorrhoid. Unless it's bleeding before your eyes, look for another diagnosis.

- Elderly patients may not manifest orthostatic changes from blood loss as readily as their younger counterparts.

- The initial hemoglobin may not be a reliable indicator of the volume of blood lost, as the volume may be contracted.

- Look for other systemic causes if your investigation of the abdominal structures turns up negative and the patient still has abnormal vitals, especially if the rectal bleeding has ceased.

- Drop a nasogastric tube (NGT) in the presence of bright red rectal bleeding.

- Resuscitate the patient aggressively with fluids for abnormal vitals and hypovolemia.

- Order typed blood products.

- Peritoneal signs may take up to 20 hours to manifest.

- Perform a digital exam and anoscopy on a patient with anorectal bleeding.

Most Common Causes of Major Lower GI Bleeding*

Diagnosis	Percentage (%)
Diverticulosis	23
Angiodysplasia	11
Undetermined	6
Radiation proctitis	3
Cancer	3
Polyps	2
Ischemic colitis	1
Anticoagulants	1

* Reference: Boley SJ, et al. Lower intestinal bleeding in the elderly. Am J Surg 1979;137:57-64.

Most Common Causes of Minor Lower GI Bleeding*

Diagnosis	Percentage (%)
Diverticulosis	16
Undetermined	5
Polyps	5
Cancer	4
Hemorrhoids	3
Fecal impaction	2
Anal stricture	2
Stercoral ulcer	2
Ischemic colitis	2
Fistula-in-ano	1
Inflammatory bowel disease	1
Radiation colitis	1

* Reference: Boley SJ, et al. Lower intestinal bleeding in the elderly. *Am J Surg* 1979;137:57-64.

Bleeding and Pain Associated with Sources of GI Bleeding

Presentation	Large amounts of bleeding/ Pain	Minimal bleeding/ No pain	Minimal bleeding/ Pain	Large amounts of bleeding/ No pain
Diverticulitis		✔		
Angiodysplasia				✔
Radiation proctitis			✔	
Colorectal carcinoma		✔		
Colonic polyps		✔		
Ischemic colitis	✔			
Inflammatory bowel disease	✔			
Acute mesenteric ischemia				✔
Hemorrhoids		✔		
Infectious diarrhea			✔	
Vasculitis		✔		

Stratification of Patients Presenting with Acute Upper or Lower GI Bleeding*

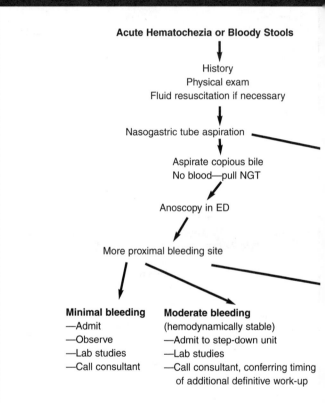

Acute Hematochezia or Bloody Stools

↓

History
Physical exam
Fluid resuscitation if necessary

↓

Nasogastric tube aspiration

↓

Aspirate copious bile
No blood—pull NGT

↓

Anoscopy in ED

↓

More proximal bleeding site

Minimal bleeding
—Admit
—Observe
—Lab studies
—Call consultant

Moderate bleeding
(hemodynamically stable)
—Admit to step-down unit
—Lab studies
—Call consultant, conferring timing
  of additional definitive work-up

* References: Zuccaro G. Management of the adult patient with acute
  lower gastrointestinal bleeding. *Am J Gastroenterol* 1998;93:1202-1208;
  Shoji BT, Becker JM. Colorectal disease in the elderly. *Surg Clin North
  Am* 1994;74:293-316.

All other

↓

Treat as upper GI bleed

↓

Anorectal source identified and patient is stabilized—
patient home

Massive bleeding
—Call GI specialist and surgeon
—ICU bed
—Type and cross/transfuse

Final Diagnosis in Patients Hospitalized for Acute Lower GI Bleed*

Diagnosis	N
Colonic diverticulosis	42%
Colorectal malignancy	9%
Ischemic colitis	9%
Acute colitis	5%
Hemorrhoids	5%
Angiodysplasia	3%
Crohn's disease	2%
Stercoral ulcer	3 patients
Vasculitis	2 patients
Infectious colitis	2 patients
Radiation proctitis	2 patients
Polyp	1 patient
Diverticulitis	1 patient
Meckels' diverticulum	1 patient
Unknown	1 patient

* Reference: Longstreth GF. Epidemiology and outcome of patients hospitalized with acute lower gstrointestinal hemorrhage: A population-based study. *Am J Gastroenterol* 1997;92:419-424

GYNECOLOGIC EMERGENCIES

MEDICAL DISORDERS IN PREGNANCY

Drugs to Avoid in Pregnancy

DRUG	UNTOWARD EFFECTS
Asprin	Increases bleeding risk at delivery, decreased uterine contractility, no teratogenic effects
NSAIDs	Chronic use may lead to oligohydramnios or neonatal pulmonary hypertension, best to avoid use

SELECTED CEPHALOSPORINS:

Cefaclor, Cephalexin, Cephradine	Associated with possible teratogenic effects
Tetracyclines	Discolor teeth
Aminoglycosides	Ototoxicity when taken in first trimester
Quinolones	Bind to cartilage and bone, consequences are debated
Metronidazole (Flagyl)	Effects in humans at normal doses are debated
Lindane	A neurotoxin with toxicity noted primarily in overexposure

Antiseizure Drugs:

Phenytoin, valproic acid Carbamazepine	All associated with defined malformation syndromes—do not prescribe without OB or neurologist recommendation
ACE inhibitors	Renal failure, oligohydramnios, limb and craniofacial deformities
Lithium	Congenital heart disease (Ebstein anomaly)
Warfarin (Coumadin)	Congenital fetal defects

DRUG	UNTOWARD EFFECTS
Antiseizure Drugs: (continued)	
Propranolol (Inderal)	Generally considered safe, may be associated with low birth weight
Terfenadine (Seldane)	Polydactyly
Phenylpropanolamine (Entex LA)	Increased risk of birth defects
Pseudoephedrine (Sudafed)	Increased risk of gastroschisis
Cimetidine (Tagamet)	Possible antiandorgenic effects in fetus
Benzodiazipines	Possible fetal syndrome similar to fetal alcohol syndrome
Oral Contraceptives	Possible cardiac defects in fetus when used in 1st trimester
Isotrentinoin (Accuatane)	Associated with multiple birth defects, spontaneous abortion
Propylthiouracil (PTU)	Induces fetal goiter
Oral hypoglycemics	Cross placenta and induce fetal hypoglycemia
Recreational Drugs:	
Tobacco	Increased prematurity, fetal growth retardation
Alcohol	Fetal alcohol syndrome
Cocaine	Increased spontaneous abortions, placental abruption, preterm labor and microcephaly

Classification of Hypertension During Pregnancy

Chronic Hypertension: Hypertension (BP > 140/90 mmHg) that is present and observable before pregnancy or that is diagnosed before the 20th week of gestation. Hypertension diagnosed for the first time during pregnancy and persisting beyond the 42nd day postpartum.

Preeclampsia-eclampsia: Increased blood pressure accompanied by proteinuria, edema, or both of which usually occur after 20 weeks gestation (or earlier with trophoblastic diseases such as hydatidiform mole or hydrops).

PREECLAMPSIA SUPERIMPOSED

On Chronic Hypertension: Chronic hypertension (defined above) with increase in blood pressure (30 mmHg systolic, 15 mmHg diastolic, or 20 mmHg mean arterial pressure) together with the appearance of proteinuria or generalized edema.

Transient Hypertension: The development of elevated blood pressure during pregnancy or in the first 24 hours postpartum without other signs of preeclampsia or preexisting hypertension (a retrospective diagnosis).

Adapted from: National High Blood Pressure Education Program Working Group Report on High Blood Pressure in Pregnancy. *Am J Obstet Gynecol* 1990:163(5 Pt 1):1691-1712.

Guidelines for Anticoagulation in Pregnancy

PREGNANT:

1. Baseline lab values: CBC, PT, PTT.

2. Heparin loading dose: 60-80 U/kg (or 5000 U) IV bolus.

3. Continuous heparin infusion of 15 U/kg/hr for DVT and 20 U/kg/hr for PE.

4. Check PTT every 6 hours and adjust infusion to maintain PTT between 1.5 and 2.5 times the patient's baseline.

5. Rebolus with 60 U/kg heparin if PTT is not prolonged and increase rate of infusion.

6. Repeat PTT every 6 hours for first 24 hours, then check daily unless outside of therapeutic range.

7. Check platelets every day or every other day for first 10 days of heparin to monitor for heparin-induced thrombocytopenia.

POSTPARTUM:

Heparin therapy as above including:

1. Begin warfarin (Coumadin) therapy on the first day of heparin treatment at 5 mg to 10 mg daily.

2. Check the PT daily and adjust dose to maintain INR between 2.0 and 3.0.

3. Stop heparin after INR of 2.0 to 3.0 is reached for 4 to 7 consecutive days.

4. Continue oral anticoagulation for 3 months to maintain INR of 2.0 to 3.0.

Adapted from: Rutherford SE, Phelan JP. Deep venous thrombosis and pulmonary embolism in pregnancy. *Obstet Gynecol Clin North Am* 1991;18:345-370.

White Classifications of Diabetes in Pregnancy

CLASS	DESCRIPTION
A	Abnormal glucose tolerance test, but asymptomatic or normal glucose achieved with diet control
B	Adult-onset diabetes (> age 20 yr) and short disease duration
C	Youth-onset diabetes (age 1-19 yr) or relatively long disease duration (10 to 19 years)
D	Childhood onset (< age 10 yr), very long disease duration (> 20 yr), or evidence of background retinopathy
E	Any diabetes with evidence of vascular disease in the pelvis (diagnosed by plain films)
F	Any diabetes with the presence of renal disease
R	Any diabetes with the presence of proliferative retinopathy
RF	Any diabetes with both renal disease and proliferative retinopathy
G	Any diabetes with a previous history of multiple pregnancy losses
H	Any diabetes with atherosclerotic heart disease
T	Any diabetes postrenal transplantation

Adapted from: Hare JW. Gestational diabetes and the White Classification. *Diabetes Care* 1980;3:394.

Disorders that May Present as Hyperemesis Gravidarum

CAUSES OF INCREASED VOMITING ASSOCIATED WITH PREGNANCY

■ Hydatidaform mole

■ Multiple gestations

■ Pregnancy-induced hypertension

■ Placental abruption

CAUSES OF VOMITING NOT ASSOCIATED WITH PREGNANCY

■ Appendicitis

■ Cholelithiasis

■ Pancreatitis

■ Hepatitis

■ Thyrotoxicosis

■ Bowel obstruction

■ Peptic ulcers

■ Diabetic ketoacidosis

■ Increased intracranial pressure

■ Pyelonephritis

■ Medications

Adapted from: Hod M, Orvieto R, Kaplan B, et al. Hyperemesis gravidarum: A
review. *J Reprod Med* 1994;39:605-612; Cosmas JM. Nausea and vomiting in early
pregnancy. In: Pearlman MD, Tintinalli JE, (eds). *Emergency Care of the Woman*. New
York: McGraw Hill; 1998:49-56.

Drugs Considered Safe in Pregnancy

PAIN MEDICATIONS

Acetaminophen

Propoxyphene (Darvocet)

Codeine—can lead to addiction and newborn withdrawal if used excessively

ASTHMA MEDICATIONS

Theophylline

Terbutaline

Cromolyn Sodium

Beta-adrenergic agonists (albuterol, isoproterenol, metaproterenol)

Corticosteroids—do cross the placenta, inhaled to a much lesser degree

ANTIBIOTICS

Penicillins

Cephalosporins (except cefaclor, cephalexin and cephradine)[152]

Sulfonamides (except in 3rd trimester)

Sulfamethoxazole/trimethoprim (controversial in 1st trimester)

Nitrofurantoin (Macrodantin—will not treat bacteremia)

Antituberculosis drugs

Erythromycin (except erythromycin estolate Ilosone)

Clindamycin

ANTIVIRALS

Acyclovir

Zidovudine (AZT)

ANTIFUNGALS

Imidazoles (clotrimazole or miconazole—except in 1st trimester)

ANTICOAGULANTS

Heparin (data with low molecular weight heparin is limited)

ANTICONVULSANTS

Phenytoin, valproic acid, and carbamazepine are all associated with
defined malformation syndromes but many physicians feel benefits for
the mother outweigh risks to the fetus. Do not prescribe without OB
or neurologist recommendation.

ANTIEMETICS*

Promethazine (Phenegran)
Proclorperazine (Compazine)
*Stress other remedies first (crackers in a.m., frequent small meals, etc.)
Ginger (shown better than placebo)
Metoclopramide (Reglan)

DECONGESTANTS*

Diphenhydramine (Benadryl)
*Nasal sprays absorbed less than po medications

ANTIHYPERTENSIVES

Methyldopa (Aldomet)
Hydralazine (Apresoline)
Atenolol (Tenormin)

GASTROINTESTINAL DRUGS

H2 blockers:
  Ranitidine (Zantac)
  Famotidine (Pepcid)
Sucralfate (Carafate)

ANTIDEPRESSANTS

Amitriptyline (Elavil)
Fluoxetine (Prozac)

WOUND CARE

Lidocaine

Summary of Laboratory Changes in Pregnancy

LAB TEST	NORMAL RANGE
Sodium	135-145 mEq/L
Potassium	3.5-4.5 mEq/L
Creatinine	0.6-1.1 mg/dL
Creatinine phosphokinase	26-140 U/L
Glucose (fasting)	65-105 mg/dL
Fibrinogen	200-400 mg/dL
Urea nitrogen	12-30 mg/dL
Hematocrit	36-46%
Hemoglobin	12-16 g/dL
Leukocyte count	4000-10,000/mm^3
Platelets	150,000

Adapted from: Barclay ML. Critical physiologic alterations in pregnancy. In: Pearlman MD, Tintinalli JE, eds. *Emergency Care of the Woman*. New York: McGraw Hill; 1998:303-312.

PREGNANCY EFFECT	GESTATIONAL TIMING
lower 2-4 mEq/L	By midpregnancy
lower 0.2-0.3 mEq/L	By midpregnancy
lower 0.3 mg/dL	By midpregnancy
raise 2-4 fold	After labor (mb bands also)
lower 10%	Gradual fall
raise 600 mg/dL	By term
lower 50%	First trimester
lower 4-7%	Nadir at 30-34 weeks
lower 1.4-2.0 g/dL	Nadir at 30-34 weeks
raise 3500/mm^3	Gradual increase to term (up to 25,000/mm^3 in labor)
400,000/mm^3	Slight decrease

Recommended Prophylactic Regimens for Pregnancy in HIV Patients

ALL PATIENTS:

■ Pneumococcal vaccine (0.5 mL IM as a one time dose)

■ Yearly influenza vaccine (0.5 mL IM)

■ Isoniazid for patients with positive TB test, TB history, or chest x-ray evidence of previous TB (300 mg po daily for 12 months)

PATIENTS WITH CD4 COUNT < 200 MM^3:

■ Trimethoprim/sulfamethoxazole for *pneumocystis carinii* pneumonia (1 single strength po daily)

PATIENTS WITH CD4 COUNT < 50 MM^3:

■ Azithromycin for *Mycobacterium avium* complex (1200 mg po weekly)

VAGINAL BLEEDING IN PREGNANCY

Risk Factors for Ectopic Pregnancy

LESSER RISK

Previous pelvic or abdominal surgery

Cigarette smoking

Vaginal douching

Age of 1st intercourse < 18 years

GREATER RISK

Previous genital infections (e.g., pelvic inflammatory disease [PID])

Infertility (In vitro fertilization)

Multiple sexual partners

GREATEST RISK

Previous ectopic pregnancy

Previous tubal surgery or sterilization

Diethystilbestrol exposure in utero

Documented tubal pathology (scarring)

Use of intrauterine contraceptive device

Adapted from Pisa MD, Carson SA. Ectopic pregnancy. In: Scott JR, et al, eds. *Danforth's Obstetrics and Gynecology.* 8th ed. Philadelphia: Lippincott Williams & Wilkins; 1999:155-172; and Mallett VT. Ectopic pregnancy. In: Pearlman MD, Tintinalli JE, eds. *Emergency Care of the Woman.* New York: McGraw Hill; 1998:21-28.

Differential Diagnosis of Ectopic Pregnancy

- Normal intrauterine pregnancy
- Ovarian cysts (rupture, unruptured)
- Acute salpingitis
- Gastroenteritis
- Diverticulitis
- Pyelonephritis

Threatened or incomplete miscarriage

Appendicitis

Tubo-ovarian abscess

Torsion of ovary or fibroid

Renal calculi

Endometriosis

Adapted from: Mallett VT. Ectopic pregnancy. In: Pearlman MD, Tintinalli JE, eds. *Emergency Care of the Woman.* New York: McGraw Hill; 1998:21-28; and Lewis FR, Holcroft JW, Boey J, et al. Appendicitis: A critical review of diagnosis and treatment in 1,000 cases. *Arch Surg* 1975;110:677-684.

Presenting Signs and Symptoms of Ectopic Pregnancy

SYMPTOM	PERCENTAGE OF WOMEN WITH SYMPTOM
Abdominal pain	80-100%
Amenorrhea	75-95%
Vaginal bleeding	50-80%
Dizziness, fainting	20-35%
Urge to defecate	5-15%
Pregnancy symptoms	10-25%
Passage of tissue	5-10%

SIGN	PERCENTAGE OF WOMEN WITH SIGN
Adnexal tenderness	75-90%
Abdominal tenderness	80-95%
Adnexal mass	50%
Uterine enlargement	20-30%
Orthostatic changes	10-15%
Fever	5-10%

Adapted from Weckstein LN. Current perspective on ectopic pregnancy. *Obstet Gynecol Surv* 1985;40:259-272.

Frequency and Sites of Ectopic Pregnancy Implantation

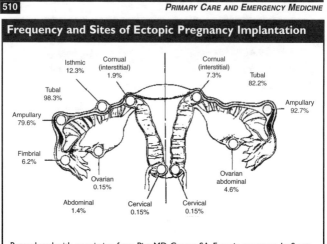

Reproduced with permission from Pisa MD, Carson SA. Ectopic pregnancy. In: Scott JR, et al, eds. *Danforth's Obstetrics and Gynecology*. 8th ed. Philadelphia: Lippincott Williams & Wilkins; 1999:156.

Risk Factors for Placental Abruption

- Maternal hypertension
- Eclampsia and preeclampsia
- History of previous abruption
- Uterine distension (multiple gestations, hydramnios, or tumors)
- Vascular disease (collagen vascular disorders, diabetes)
- Tobacco smoking
- Cocaine use
- Microangiopathic hemolytic anemia
- Premature rupture of membranes
- Uterine blunt trauma (domestic abuse, automobile collisions)
- Short umbilical cord

Algorithm for ED Evaluation of Vaginal Bleeding in First 20 Weeks of Pregnancy

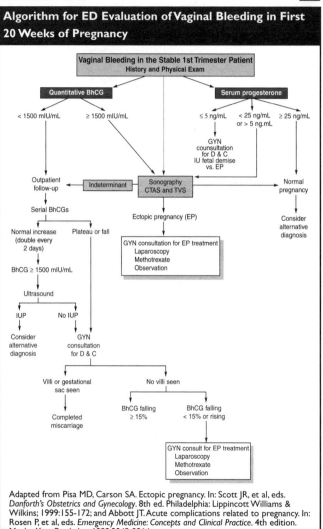

Adapted from Pisa MD, Carson SA. Ectopic pregnancy. In: Scott JR, et al, eds. *Danforth's Obstetrics and Gynecology*. 8th ed. Philadelphia: Lippincott Williams & Wilkins; 1999:155-172; and Abbott JT. Acute complications related to pregnancy. In: Rosen P, et al, eds. *Emergency Medicine: Concepts and Clinical Practice*. 4th edition. Mosby-Year Book, Inc; 1998:2342-2364.

Illustration of the Different Types of Placental Abruption

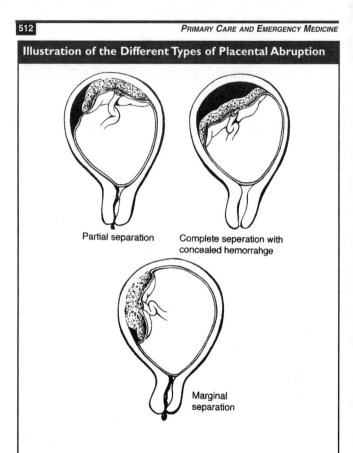

Partial separation

Complete seperation with concealed hemorrahge

Marginal separation

Grade 1 abruption is shown in the bottom diagram as marginal separation. **Grade 2** abruption is shown in the upper left as partial separation. **Grade 3** abruption is shown in the upper right as complete separation with concealed hemorrhage.

Reproduced with permission from: Scott JR. Placenta previa and abruption. In: Scott JR, et al, eds. *Danforth's Obstetrics and Gynecology.* 8th ed. Philadelphia: Lippincott Williams & Wilkins; 1999:412.

Clinical Findings in Placental Abruption: Grade-Dependent Maternal and Fetal Profiles

GRADE 1:

Slight or minimal vaginal bleeding (spotting) and limited uterine irritability (no organized contractions) are typically present. Maternal blood pressure is unchanged, and maternal serum fibrinogen level is normal (normal maternal fibrinogen concentration is 450 mg/percent). Fetal heart rate is normal, between 120 bpm and 160 bpm.

GRADE 2:

External uterine bleeding is mild to moderate, similar to that of a heavy period. Uterine irritability is evident, with tetanic contractions at times. Maternal hypotension is absent in supine position, but orthostatic symptoms may be present. Resting maternal pulse rate may be elevated. Fibrinogen levels are lowered to the range of 150 mg/percent to 250 mg/percent. Fetal distress is evident as manifested by compromised fetal heart rate patterns.

GRADE 3:

Bleeding is moderate to severe but may be underestimated by external losses. Painful uterine contractions are present and they are often tetanic in nature. Hemodynamic instability is evident by maternal hypotension and tachycardia. Fibrinogen levels are often reduced to less than 150 mg/percent, representing a blood loss of approximately 2000 mL. Maternal coagulopathies (thrombocytopenia, clotting factor, and fibrinogen depletion) are often present. Fetal death is common.

RIGHT LOWER QUADRANT PAIN IN WOMEN OF REPRODUCTIVE AGE

Differential Diagnosis of RLQ Pain in Women of Reproductive Age

- Ectopic pregnancy
- Adnexal torsion
- Appendicitis
- Pelvic inflammatory disease
- Urinary tract infection (UTI) and pyelonephritis
- Kidney stones
- Ovarian cysts
- Endometriosis
- Uterine fibroids

Diagnostic Criteria for Pelvic Inflammatory Disease

MAJOR CRITERIA

— Cervical motion tenderness

— Lower abdominal tenderness

— Adnexal tenderness

MINOR CRITERIA

— Temperature > 38°C

— White blood cell count > 10.5

— Erythrocyte sedimentation rate > 15

— Gram stain of vaginal discharge positive for gram-negative diplococci

— Cervical culture positive for gonorrhea or *Chlamydia*

— Purulence on culdocentesis

— Adnexal mass consistent with tubo-ovarian abscess

Complications of Adnexal Torsion

- Infertility
- Infection
- Peritonitis
- Sepsis
- Adhesions
- Chronic pain

ED Management of Cervicitis and Outpatient Treatment of Pelvic Inflammatory Disease

A. CERVICITIS

Gonorrhea treatment:

Ceftriaxone 125 mg IM

or Cefixime 400 mg PO

or Ciprofloxacin 500 mg PO

or Ofloxacin 400 mg PO

Chlamydia treatment

Azithromycin 1 gm PO single dose

or Doxycycline 100 mg PO x 7 d

If pregnant or penicillin allergic:

Azithromycin 2 gm PO single dose

or Erythromycin base 250 mg PO qid x 14 days

or Erythromycin ethylsuccinate 800 mg PO tid x 7 days

B. OUTPATIENT PID:

Choice for gonorrhea treatment from above list

and Doxycycline 100 mg PO bid for 14 days

or Ofloxacin 400 mg PO bid x 14 days plus clindamycin 450 mg PO bid x 14 days

Risk Factors Associated with Delayed or Missed Diagnoses of Ectopic Pregnancy

— Absence of abdominal pain; atypical pain

— Absence of adnexal mass on physical examination

— Negative aspiration on culdocentesis

— Nondiagnostic ultrasound

— Misinterpretation of sonographic image

— Falling hCG level

Algorithm for Differential Diagnosis of RLQ Abdominal Pain in Women of Reproductive Age

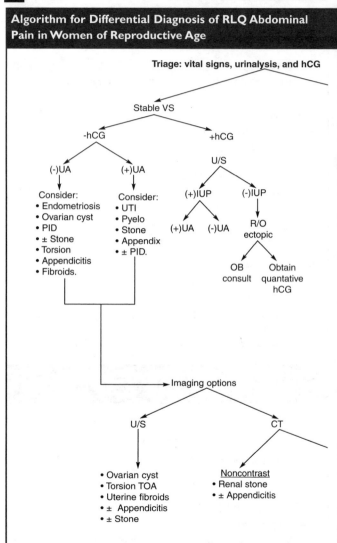

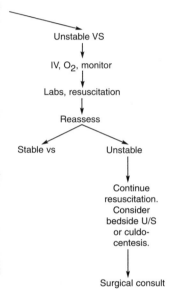

Unstable VS

↓

IV, O$_2$, monitor

↓

Labs, resuscitation

↓

Reassess

Stable vs   Unstable

↓

Continue
resuscitation.
Consider
bedside U/S
or culdo-
centesis.

↓

Surgical consult

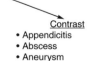

Contrast
• Appendicitis
• Abscess
• Aneurysm
• Malignancy
• Other causes of pain

Key: VS = vital signs; UA = urinalysis; IUP = intrauterine pregnancy; PID = pelvic inflammatory disease; TOA = tubo-ovarian abscess; U/S = ultrasound; R/O = rule out

EYE, EAR, NOSE, AND THROAT EMERGENCIES

"KILLER" SORE THROAT

Conditions Presenting with Sore Throat and Inability to Swallow Saliva

- Epiglottitis
- Peritonsillar abscess
- Retropharyngeal abscess
- Ludwig's angina
- Abscesses in the deep neck space
- Allergic drug reactions
- Lingual tonsillitis
- Ingested foreign body with or without perforation
- Pharyngeal zoster
- Botulism
- Tetanus
- Stevens-Johnson syndrome
- Toxic epidermal necrolysis
- Inhalation or aspiration of toxic chemicals
- Tumors or trauma to the larynx
- Diphtheria

Clinical Findings of Epiglottitis in the Child[*]

- Sudden onset of symptoms
- Rapid progression
- High fever
- Muffled, "hot potato" voice
- Inspiratory stridor
- Sore throat
- Dysphagia
- Drooling
- "Tripod" positioning
- Toxic appearance

* References: Kucera CM, Silverstein MD, Jacobson RM, et al. Epiglottitis in adults and children in Olmstead County, Minnesota, 1976-1990. *Mayo Clin Proc* 1996;71:1155-1161; Murphy P, Colwell C. Prehospital management of epiglottitis. *EMS Magazine* 2000;Jan:41-49.

Predisposing Factors for Retropharyngeal Abscess

- Penetrating trauma: Foreign body such as pencil, Popsicle stick, or fishbone
- Tonsillitis
- Pharyngitis
- Peritonsillar abscess
- Croup
- Otitis media
- Nasal infections
- Dental infections
- Intubation
- Adenoidectomy (recent)

Clinical Findings of Peritonsillar Abscess

- Severe pain
- Fever
- Dysphagia
- Trismus
- Hoarse, "hot potato" voice
- Enlargement of the tonsil
- Uvula deviated to the unaffected side
- Deviation of tonsil toward midline with rotation of anterior tonsillar pillar
- Fluctuance of the soft tissue between the upper pole of the tonsil and the soft palate

Clinical Findings of Epiglottitis in the Adult*

- Gradual onset of symptoms
- Rapid progression
- Severe sore throat (95-100%)
- Dysphagia (76%)
- Pain on swallowing (95%)
- Pain on palpation of the larynx
- High fever (88%)
- Muffled voice (50%)
- Shortness of breath or respiratory difficulty
- Drooling (relatively uncommon)
- "Upright" positioning
- Ear pain
- Toxic appearance

* References: Carey MJ. Epiglottitis in adults. *Am J Emerg Med* 1996;14:421-424; Deeb ZE. Acute supraglottitis in adults: Early indicators of airway obstruction. *Am J Otolaryngol* 1997;18:112-115; Solomon P, Weisbrod M, Irish JC, et al. Adult epiglottitis: The Toronto Hospital experience. *J Otolaryngol* 1998;27:332; Kucera CM, Silverstein MD, Jacobson RM, et al. Epiglottitis in adults and children in Olmstead County, Minnesota, 1976-1990. *Mayo Clin Proc* 1996;71:1155-1161.

Scoring System* for Croup‡

LEVEL OF CONSCIOUSNESS

Normal or sleeping	0
Disoriented	5

CYANOSIS

None	0
With agitation	4
At rest	5

STRIDOR

None	0
With agitation	1
At rest	2

AIR ENTRY

Normal	0
Decreased	1
Markedly decreased	2

RETRACTIONS

None	0
Mild	1
Moderate	2
Severe	3

* Zero represents the normal state or absence of the sign and the highest number represents the most severe distress.

‡ Reference: Westly CR, Cotton EK, Brooks JG. Nebulized racemic epinephrine by IPPB for the treatment of croup. A double blind study. *Am J Dis Child* 1978;132: 484-487.

Complications of Retropharyngeal Abscess

- Rupture of abscess
- Airway rupture
- Asphyxiation
- Aspiration pneumonia
- Spinal rupture
- Lateral pharyngeal space rupture
- Inferior rupture into mediastinum
- Airway compromise

TOXICOLOGIC EMERGENCIES

BIOTERRORISM

Epidemiological Clues of Biologic Warfare

- *Any* single case of an uncommon agent (smallpox, some viral hemorrhagic fevers, anthrax)

- The presence of an unusually large number of patients with similar disease or symptoms

- Many cases of unexplained diseases or deaths

- Dead or dying animals

- More severe disease than is usual for a specific pathogen

- Failure to respond to standard therapy for a specific pathogen

- Disease that is unusual for the geographic area or season

- Disease transmitted by a vector that usually is not present

- Unusual route of exposure for a disease (inhalation anthrax or plague)

- Multiple simultaneous or serial epidemics of different diseases

- A disease that is unusual for an age group or population

- Similar genetic pattern of diseases from distinct sources at different times or locations

- Discrete attack rates among those in a particular building or at a specific event

- Outbreak of disease in non-contiguous areas (not spread by travelers)
- Intelligence of a potential attack

Adapted from: USAMRIID Medical management of biologic casualties handbook. USAMRIID 2001;Fort Detrick, MD.

Samples to Obtain from Representative Patients with Possible Exposure to Biological Warfare Agents

- Nasal swabs for culture and PCR (take several, if possible)

- Blood cultures (take several, if possible)

- Sputum cultures

- Blood and urine for toxin analysis

- Throat cultures and swabs

- Serum for analysis

- Stool samples — particularly if any diarrhea

- Lung washings/suction if any respiratory difficulty

- CBC, clotting studies, chemistries — more important for patient management than for epidemiology

- Clothing for environmental analysis

Availability of Licensed, Pre-exposure Vaccines for Prevention of Bioterrorism-Associated Disease

AGENT	VACCINE
Smallpox	**Yes** (Currently approved on as-needed basis for lab workers)
Anthrax	**Yes** (Vaccine for civilian use must be approved by Dept. of Defense)
Botulism	**No**
Tularemia	**No**
Plague	**Yes** (But not proven effective against pneumonic plague)
Brucellosis	**No**

Ten-Step Approach for Management of Biologic Casualties

1. SUSPECT A PROBLEM

If you don't look for it, you won't find it . . . but it still might find you.

2. PROTECT YOURSELF

Before you approach a potential biological casualty, you need to protect yourself. Gown, gloves, and HEPA-filter mask are essential.

3. ASSESS YOUR PATIENT

The ABCs are addressed before specific management.

4. DETERMINE IF DECONTAMINATION IS NEEDED

Decontamination is possible only for "fresh" exposures.

5. ESTABLISH THE DIAGNOSIS (IF POSSIBLE)

Secondary survey of the patient and in-depth lab examinations.

6. BEGIN EMPIRIC TREATMENT

Treat what you can. Empiric doxycycline and/or fluoroquinolones.

- Respiratory
  —Inhaled anthrax
  —Pneumonic plague
  —Pneumonic tularemia

7. PROTECT OTHERS — INFECTION CONTROL

- Smallpox — all airborne precautions and contact precautions
- Pneumonic plague — droplet precautions
- Viral hemorrhagic fever — contact precautions

8. ALERT THE AUTHORITIES

9. ASSIST IN EPIDEMIOLOGY

Ask questions about potential exposures, immunization history, travel history, occupation, food/water sources, vector exposures, activities over the preceding 3-5 days, potential spray devices; list all of these for each patient. In some of these diseases, you may be the only person able to interview the patient; by the time CDC officials get there, the patient may be intubated and unable to communicate.

10. SPREAD THE WORD

Ensure that you are proficient and that others are aware of the threat.

Online Resources for Bioterrorism Information

- CDC's bioterrorism preparedness and response web site: http://www.bt.cdc.gov
- USAMRIID's Medical Management of Biologic Casualties Handbook: http://www.nbc-med.org
- Anthrax information: http://www.nbc-med.org/SiteContent/MedRef/OnlineRef/GovDocs/Anthrax/index.htm
- Biological Agent Information Papers, U.S. Army Institute of Infectious Diseases: http://www.nbc-med.org/SiteContent/MedRef/OnlineRef/GovDocs/BioAgents.html
- Smallpox information: http://www.nbc-med.org/SiteContent/MedRef/OnlineRef/FieldManuals/medman/SmallPox.htm
- Medical aspects of chemical and biological warfare: http://www.nbc-med.org/SiteContent/HomePage/WhatsNew/MedAspects/contents.html
- USAMRIID web site: www.usamriid.army.mil
- Association of Professionals in Infection Control and Epidemiology (APIC). Site contains bioterrorism response plan: www.apic.org.
- Johns Hopkins University Center for Civilian Biodefense: www.hopkins-biodefense.org.
- Anthrax Vaccine Implementation Program: www.anthrax.osd.mil

Web sites accessed on Jan. 14, 2003.

Biological Agents With Risk for Secondary Transmission of Illness

AGENT	SECONDARY TRANSMISSION RISK
Smallpox	Yes
Anthrax	No
Botulism	No
Tularemia	No
Plague	Yes
Brucellosis	No

Vaccines for Biological Weapons

DISEASE	VACCINE
Anthrax *Bacillus anthracis*	Three versions: Two killed, one live Appear equally effective in prevention (about 90%) Untested (in the United States) in humans for inhalation anthrax Full treatment is six shots plus an annual booster. When combined with administration of antibiotics, probably is effective in prevention of inhalation anthrax.
Argentine hemorrhagic fever	Experimental, live vaccine in IND status. Protects against both Argentine and Bolivian hemorrhagic fevers.
Botulism *Clostridia* species	The CDC provides a pentavalent antitoxin which gives protection from toxin types A, B, C, D, and E. Military heptavalent antitoxin is believed effective against all types of botulism toxin but still is in experimental status. CDC vaccine has been administered to several thousand volunteers and to occupationally at-risk workers (fully licensed). Induces protective levels of antitoxin. A monovalent antitoxin for type A alone is available from the California Health Department for treatment of infant botulism. Pentavalent vaccine in IND status for prophylaxis use only.
Hantaan hemorrhagic fever	Experimental vaccinia-vectored Hantaan vaccine

AVAILABILITY[†]

Only to military personnel and others whose jobs put them at high
   risk.

Approved only for healthy adults age 18-65 years.

....

New drug protocols.

....

Antitoxin not used for prophylaxis.

Toxoid has been recommended only for those at high risk for toxin
   aerosols.

Standard treatment is supportive care.

Post-exposure prophylaxis has been demonstrated in animals.

Horse serum

....

Available only to laboratory workers at USAMRIID

....

Table continued on next page

Vaccines for Biological Weapons *(continued)*

DISEASE	VACCINE
Plague *Yersinia pestis*	Does not prevent pneumonic plague. Somewhat effective against bubonic plague version. Pneumonic plague treated with antibiotics.
Rift Valley fever	Both inactivated and live-attenuated Rift Valley fever vaccines currently are under investigation.
Smallpox *Variola major*	Given prior to exposure, inoculation provides almost 100% protection against the disease. It is mostly effective up to four days after exposure. People who were previously vaccinated will have more protection and faster onset of protection when revaccinated. Some antivirals also may be effective.
Staphylococcal enterotoxin B	Experimental vaccine in development (not at IND status yet)
Tularemia *F. tularensis*	Provides partial protection against infection by inhalation or direct contact. Antibiotics are the treatment of choice for all cases of tularemia
Venezuelan equine encephalitis	Two IND human vaccines: TC-83, a live-attenuated cell, vaccine, produced by the Salk Institute, which has been licensed for horses and used as an IND for humans working in labs with VEE; and C-84, which has been tested but not licensed for use in humans. C-84 is used to boost non-responders to TC-83.
Yellow fever	The only licensed vaccine for any of the hemorrhagic fevers is yellow fever vaccine.

† *Most of these vaccines were developed before bioterrorism emerged as a threat. Only smallpox vaccine was produced in bulk. Few of these vaccines are widely available at this time.*

AVAILABILITY[†]

Recommended only for people who work with the plague pathogen *Yersinia pestis*, or veterinarians who work with animals in plague areas.

....

New drug protocols.

....

Extremely limited. The United States has up to 10 million doses; 40 million more on order.

Contraindicated for immunosuppressed individuals.

Not recommended since 1980

.

....

Animal work appears promising.

....

Only given to those who work routinely with tularemia bacteria.

Not yet approved by the FDA.

....

Available as IND only.

....

Available, required for travel to Africa and South America.

....

The Hemorrhagic Fevers: Location, Vector, and Incubation

DISEASE	LOCATION
Argentine hemorrhagic fever (Junin virus)	South America
Bolivian hemorrhagic fever (Machupo virus)	South America
Brazilian hemorrhagic fever (Guanarito virus)	South America
Congo-Crimean HF	Africa, Asia
Dengue fever	Worldwide
Ebola (Philippines = Reston)	Africa, Philippines
Hantavirus pulmonary syndrome	Americas
Hemorrhagic fever with renal syndrome (HFRS) (Hantaan virus)	Worldwide
Kyanasur Forest disease	India
Lassa fever	Africa
Marburg fever	Africa
Omsk hemorrhagic fever	Siberia
Rift Valley fever	Africa
Venezuelan hemorrhagic fever (Sabia virus)	South America
Yellow fever	Worldwide

Every VHF virus except dengue is infectious by aerosol in the laboratory and therefore requires careful barrier and aerosol quarantine.

VECTOR	INCUBATION	SPECIES
Rodent	3-12 days	Arenavirus
Rodent	3-16 days	Arenavirus
Rodent	3-16 days	Arenavirus
Tick	3-12 days	Bunyavirus
Mosquito		Flavivirus
Unknown	2-21 days	Filovirus
Rodent	3-21	Bunyavirus
Rodent	9-35 days	Bunyavirus (Most common disease of hantaviruses)
Tick		Flavivirus
Mosquito	5-16 days	Arenavirus
Unknown	2-21 days	Filovirus
Tick		Flavivirus
Mosquito	2-5 days	Bunyavirus
Rodent	3-15 days	Arenavirus
Mosquito		Flavivirus

Interim Recommendations for Postexposure Prophylaxis for Prevention of Inhalational Anthrax After Intentional Exposure to *Bacillus anthracis*

CATEGORY	INITIAL THERAPY	DURATION
Adults (including pregnant women and immuno-compromised persons)	Ciprofloxacin 500 mg po BID or Doxycycline 100 mg po BID	60 days
Children	Ciprofloxacin 10-15 mg/kg po Q12 hrs* or Doxycycline:	60 days
> 8 yrs and > 45 kg	100 mg po BID	60 days
> 8 yrs and ≤ 45 kg	2.2 mg/kg po BID	
≤ 8 yrs	2.2 mg/kg po BID	

* Ciprofloxacin dose should not exceed 1 gram per day in children
Source: Oct. 19, 2001. *MMWR Morb Mortal Wkly Rep.*

Characteristics of Effective Biological Weapons

- Potential for massive numbers of casualties
- Ability to produce lengthy illness requiring prolonged and extensive care
- Ability of agents to spread via contagion
- Paucity of adequate detection systems
- Incubation period enables victims (and perpetrators) to widely disperse
- Nonspecific symptoms complicate early diagnosis and mimic endemic infectious diseases

Adapted from: USAMRIID's Medical Management of Biological Casualties Handbook, 4th ed. U.S. Army Medical Research Institute. February 2001.

Clinical Syndromes Suggestive of Bioterrorism-Associated Illness

AGENT	CLINICAL PRESENTATION
Anthrax	Widened mediastinum, not associated with chest trauma
Smallpox	Characteristic vesiculopustular rash, with eruption of palms and soles, involving face sore then chest, and all lesions in same phase of development
Botulism	Prominent neurologic symptoms: descending paralysis beginning with cranial nerve palsies
Plague, Tularemia	Increased incidence of atypical pneumonia in population

Post-Exposure Prophylaxis Against Agents of Bioterrorism

Variola virus	Smallpox vaccine is effective in preventing death if given up to five days after exposure and in preventing illness if given within 72 hours.
Anthrax	Ciprofloxacin 500 mg orally b.i.d. Also initiate anthrax immunization, if available. Antibiotic prophylaxis should continue for at least four weeks and until three doses of vaccine have been given.
Botulism	Trivalent equine antitoxin, available from CDC
Tularemia	Doxycycline 100 mg orally b.i.d. for 14 days
Plague	Doxycycline 100 mg orally b.i.d. for seven days
Brucellosis	Doxycycline 100 mg b.i.d. plus rifampin 600-900 mg/d for three weeks

Postexposure Prophylaxis: Prophylaxis immediately after recognized exposure may be given with doxycycline 100 mg b.i.d. for 14 days. For long-term advanced prophylaxis, a live attenuated vaccine is available in the United States under an investigational new drug protocol.

Potential Biologic Agents Used for Terrorism

CATEGORY A — HIGH-PRIORITY agents include organisms that:

- Can be easily disseminated or transmitted from person to person
- Cause high mortality, with a potential for major public health impact
- Might cause public panic and social disruption
- Require special action for public health preparedness

CATEGORY B — SECOND-PRIORITY agents include agents that:

- Are moderately easy to disseminate
- Cause moderate morbidity and low mortality
- Require specific enhancements of the CDC's diagnostic capacity and disease surveillance

These agents have been used or considered as biological weapons.

DISEASES PROPOSED FOR BIOWARFARE (CATEGORY DESIGNATION [I.E., A, B, C] NOTED WHERE APPLICABLE)*

TOXINS PROPOSED FOR BIOWARFARE

Botulinum toxins[B]
Clostridium perfringens toxins[B]
Mycotoxins (trichothecenes group)
Palytoxin
Ricin[B]
Saxitoxin
Staphylococcal enterotoxin B
Tetrodotoxin

BACTERIA PROPOSED FOR BIOWARFARE

Anthrax[A]
Brucellosis[B]
Cholera[B]
Melioidosis
Plague[A]
Shigella[B]
Tularemia[A]

E. coli O157:H7[B]
Salmonella species[B]
Multidrug-resistant tuberculosis[C]
Burkolderia mallei (glanders)[B]

CHLAMYDIA PROPOSED FOR BIOWARFARE

Psittacosis

RICKETTSIA PROPOSED FOR BIOWARFARE

Q fever[B]
Rocky Mountain spotted fever

VIRUSES PROPOSED FOR BIOWARFARE

Chikun-Gunya fever
Junin Argentine hemorrhagic fever[A]
Bolivian hemorrhagic fever[C]
Crimean-Congo hemorrhagic fever[C]

CATEGORY C — THIRD-PRIORITY agents include organisms that are emerging pathogens that could be genetically engineered for mass dissemination.

■ These agents may be easily available.

■ These agents may be easily produced or disseminated

■ These agents have the potential for high morbidity and mortality and, therefore, may have a major public health impact.

Preparedness for Category-C agents requires ongoing research into disease detection, diagnosis, treatment, and prevention.

Adapted from: Khan AS, Morse S, Lillibridge S. Public health preparedness for biological terrorism in the USA. *Lancet* 2000;356:1179-1182; CDC. Biologic threats http://www.bt.cdc.gov/agent/agentlist.asp accessed on 10/10/2001.

Dengue fever[C]
Eastern equine encephalitis[B]
Ebola fever[A]
Hantavirus[C]
Korean hemorrhagic fever (Hantaan)[C]
Lassa fever[A]
Marburg virus[A]
Omsk hemorrhagic fever[C]
Rift Valley fever
Russian Spring-Summer encephalitis[C]
Smallpox (variola major)[A]
Venezuelan hemorrhagic fever
Western equine encephalitis[B]
Yellow fever[C]
Influenza

Nipah virus[C]
Venezuelan encephalomyelitis[B]
West Nile fever

MISCELLANEOUS PROPOSED FOR BIOWARFARE

Histoplasmosis
Coccidiomycosis
Cryptosporidium parvum[B]

* Note: These Tables are not inclusive. Many other diseases could be adapted to biowarfare.

Prophylaxis and/or Treatment Regimens for Agents of Bioterrorism

AGENT	VACCINE
Variola	Treatment of active smallpox can be attempted with cidofovir, an agent with activity against many pox viruses; three other agents—adefovir dipivoxide, cyclic cidofovir, and ribavirin—may also be candidates for use in this setting.
Anthrax	IV administration of ciprofloxacin 400 mg every 8-12 hrs (post-exposure prophylaxis)
Botulism	Trivalent equine antitoxin if the disease is in a phase of progression. Contact the CDC for release of antitoxin. Skin testing should be done first to avoid the occurrence of anaphylaxis or serum sickness.
Tularemia	Streptomycin given 30 mg/kg/day IM in two divided doses for 10-14 days.
Plague	Streptomycin 30 mg/kg IM per day in two divided doses. (Gentamicin is considered a substitute agent.) IV chloramphenicol may be given for plague meningitis or in sepsis syndrome. IV doxycycline (100 mg every 12 hours for 10-14 days, after an initial loading dose of 200 mg) is also effective.
Brucellosis	Preferred for severe brucellosis (bone, joint, heart, CNS infection) is a combination of doxycycline (100 mg BID) plus rifampin 600-900 mg/day orally for six weeks.

POLYPHARMACY AND ADVERSE DRUG REACTIONS

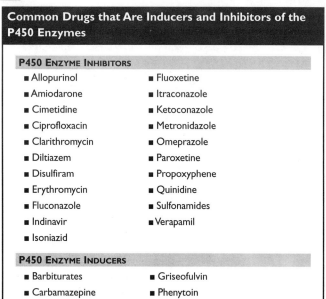

Common Drugs that Are Inducers and Inhibitors of the P450 Enzymes

P450 ENZYME INHIBITORS

- Allopurinol
- Amiodarone
- Cimetidine
- Ciprofloxacin
- Clarithromycin
- Diltiazem
- Disulfiram
- Erythromycin
- Fluconazole
- Indinavir
- Isoniazid
- Fluoxetine
- Itraconazole
- Ketoconazole
- Metronidazole
- Omeprazole
- Paroxetine
- Propoxyphene
- Quinidine
- Sulfonamides
- Verapamil

P450 ENZYME INDUCERS

- Barbiturates
- Carbamazepine
- Chronic ethanol use
- Griseofulvin
- Phenytoin
- Rifampin

Partial List of Medicinal Substances that Have Clinically Significant Interactions with Warfarin

— Acetaminophen

— Amiodarone

— Antibiotics: Ciprofloxacin, clarithromycin, erythromycin, metronidazole, trimethoprim-sulfamethoxazole

— Antifungals: Fluconazole, itraconazole, ketoconazole

— Botanicals: Bromelains, danshen, dong quai, garlic, Ginkgo biloba

— Disulfiram

— Nonsteroidal anti-inflammatory drugs

— Salicylates

Calcium Channel Blockers and Drug Interactions

BETA-BLOCKERS

- Additive effect on chronotropy, inotropy, and conduction
- Hypotension, bradydysrhythmias

CARBAMAZEPINE

- Increased carbamazepine concentration (diltiazem, verapamil)
- Ataxia, altered mental status

DIGOXIN

- Increased digoxin concentration (verapamil)
- Bradydysrhythmias

PRAZOSIN

- Potentiation of effect
- Decreased blood pressure

QUINIDINE

- Increased quinidine concentrations (diltiazem, verapamil)
- Bradydysrhythmias
- Decreased quinidine concentrations (nifedipine)
- Tachydysrhythmias

Factors that Contribute to Adverse Drug Reactions in the Elderly

- Polypharmacy
- Multiple physicians and treatment locales
- Use of over-the-counter medications and herbal products
- Physiologic changes of aging
- Chronic medical illness
- Physical limitations (dementia/hearing impairment/poor vision)
- Look-alike medications
- Sound-alike medication names

Over-The-Counter Agents with Reported Clinical Toxicity

AGENT	OTC APPLICATION	CLINICAL MANIFESTATION
Acetaminophen	Analgesic	
	Antipyretic	Hepatic failure
Antihistamine (H1 receptor) (diphenhydramine, chlorpheniramine, brompheniramine,doxylamine)	Decongestant	Anticholinergic syndrome
		Antipruritic
		Sleep aid
Caffeine	Stimulant	Agitation, seizure
		Nausea, vomiting
		Tachydysrhythmia
		Hypotension, hypertension
Camphor	Rubefacient	Seizures
Dextromethrophan	Antitussive	Altered mental status
		Hypoventilation
Ethanol	Mouthwash/ Germicide	Depressed mental status
		Hypoventilation
		Hypoglycemia
Imidazoline (tetrahydrolozine, naphazoline, oxymetazoline, xylometazoline)	Topical decongestant	Depressed mental status
		Miosis
		Hypoventilation
		Bradycardia
		Alteration of blood pressure
Inorganic salts (magnesium, calcium, aluminum, sodium bicarbonate)	Antacid	Dehydration
	Laxative	Electrolyte abnormalities
Iodine (Povidone-iodine)	Antiseptic/Germicide	Nausea, vomiting
	Vaginal douche	Abdominal pain
		GI tract burns

AGENT	OTC APPLICATION	CLINICAL MANIFESTATION
Iron salts (e.g., ferrous sulfate, ferrous gluconate, etc.)	Mineral supplement	Nausea, vomiting, Abdominal pain GI bleeding Metabolic acidosis Hypotension Decreased mental status
Local anesthetics (benzocaine, dibucaine, dyclonine, lidocaine)	Topical analgesic	Depressed mental status Seizure Bradycardia Methemoglobinemia
Loperamide	Antidiarrheal	Depressed mental status Hypoventilation
Nonsteroidal anti-inflammatory agents (ibuprofen, ketoprofen, naproxen)	Analgesic Anti-inflammatory Antipyretic	GI distress CNS depression
Permethrin	Pediculocide	Hypersensitivity
Pyrethrin	Scabicide	Keratitis
Quartenary ammonium compounds (alkyldimehtylbenzyl-ammonium chlorides)	Antiseptic/ Germicide	Nausea, vomiting Abdominal pain GI tract burns
Salicylate	Analgesic Antipyretic Rubefacient Keratolytic	Nausea, vomiting Tinnitus Altered mental status Mixed acid/base disorder Pulmonary edema
Sympathomimetics (ephedrine, psuedoephedrine, phenylephrine, phenylpropanolamine)	Decongestant Appetite suppressant	Sympathomimetic syndrome

Strategies to Prevent Polypharmacy Adverse Drug Reactions in Elderly Patients

Have a high suspicion of risk
- Always consider the diagnosis
- Complete illness history/medication history

Enhance knowledge
- Study drug information sources
- Understand geriatric prescribing principles

Limit the number of prescriptions

Look for high-risk combinations to avoid potential drug interaction

Follow a low-dose philosophy in prescribing

Avoid prescribing errors
- Use legible handwriting
- Avoid abbreviations
- Take care with decimal points

Consider the use of safer alternative drugs

Adjust dose for organ function impairment

TRAUMA

TRAUMA IN PREGNANCY

Critical Physiologic Changes that Occur During Pregnancy

CARDIOVASCULAR	Cardiac output is increased by 40%; pulse increased by 20-30% to 80-95 beast/min; mild decrease in BP seen in second trimester; blood volume is increased by 40% at term; CVP declines during gestation from 9 mmHg to 4-5 mmHg in third trimester.
ECG	A left axis shift occurs from elevation of the diaphragm.
PULMONARY	Tidal volume and respiratory rate increase; minute ventilation increased by 40-50%; reduced functional residual capacity; increased sensitivity to CO_2 with resulting partially compensated respiratory alkalosis. Oxygen consumption increased 10-20% by term. Diaphragm is elevated by 4 cm at term.
HEMATOLOGIC	Blood volume is increased, more than RBC mass, resulting in dilutional "anemia"; WBC increased (to 18,000); sedimentation rate increased, but CRP remains normal; fibrinogen factors VII, VIII, IX, and X increased.
GASTROINTESTINAL	Hypomotility present; gastric emptying delayed; esophageal reflux more frequent; increased acid production.
GENITOURINARY	Hypomotility of collecting systems; increased GFR. Anterior and superior displacement of bladder with progressing gestation.
CENTRAL NERVOUS	Some decreased coordination in later gestation.

Key: BP = Blood pressure; CVP = central venous pressure; ECG = electrocardiogram; AVF = arteriovenous fistula; RBC = red blood cells; WBC = white blood cells; CRP = C-reactive protein; GFR = glomerular filtration rate; BUN = blood urea nitrogen.

Supine position reduces venous return (treat with left lateral displacement of the uterus); relative tachycardia is normal; blood loss will exceed 30% of total blood volume before hypotension is manifest. Retroperitoneal bleeds may not be readily manifest.

Flattened T waves, possible inversion in lead III, possible Q waves in III and AVF.

Persistent respiratory alkalosis; Mild tachypnea;
Shorter anesthesia induction time.

Thoracostomies performed 1-2 interspaces higher than usual.

False dilutional anemia may be diagnosed;
Potentially false diagnosis of infection based on WBC;
Change in coagulation factors increases risk for thromboembolic problems, especially with immobilization.

Risk of aspiration increased with anesthesia induction or unconsciousness.

Ureteral dilation on radiographic studies (right > left) as early as 10th week; risk of infection increased with stasis and catheterization; BUN and creatinine normally decrease.

Increased emotional lability.

Source: Lavery JP, Staten-McCormick M. Management of moderate to severe trauma in pregnancy. *Obstet Gynecol Clin North Am* 1995;22:69-90.

Use of Studies in Blunt and Penetrating Trauma

	ADVANTAGES	DISADVANTAGES

CT	• Good anatomical detail
	• Identifies retro-
	  peritoneal injury
		• Minimal but present
		  radiation exposure
		• Need a stable patient

Ultrasound	• Can be used in an
	  unstable patient
	• Non-invasive
	• No radiation
	• Good view of fetus
	  as well as abdominal
	  fluid collections
		• Accuracy of results is
		  user dependent
		• Source of fluid not
		  necessarily clear

Deep peritoneal lavage	• Can be done in an
	  unstable patient
	• Sensitivity for hemo-
	  peritoneum is good
		• Invasive
		• Does not identify
		  retroperitoneal or
		  intrauterine injury

Pearls and Pitfalls in Managing the Pregnant Trauma Patient

- The pregnant patient can lose up to 30% of her blood volume before she shows any of the classic vital sign changes of shock.

- Fetal heart rate is an additional vital sign that may be more sensitive than the maternal vital signs for blood loss.

- The majority of injuries during pregnancy are due to blunt trauma.

- The fetus is more sensitive to hypovolemia than the mother.

- Domestic violence increases during pregnancy.

- The suicide rate during pregnancy is lower than that for age-matched women who are not pregnant.

- Perimortem cesarean section should be begun if the mother arrests and does not respond within four minutes.

- Management of the pregnant trauma patient should be directed at maternal survival.

- Fetal outcome is best when the maternal outcome is good.

- Sonogram is a noninvasive way of looking for free fluid in the abdominal cavity.

- A patient at more than 20 weeks gestation can exhibit supine hypotensive syndrome secondary to an enlarged uterus obstructing the inferior vena cava.

- Any diagnostic test that is indicated for the care of the patient should not be modified or delayed because of the pregnancy.

THORACIC TRAUMA

Algorithm for Evaluation of Tracheobronchial Injuries

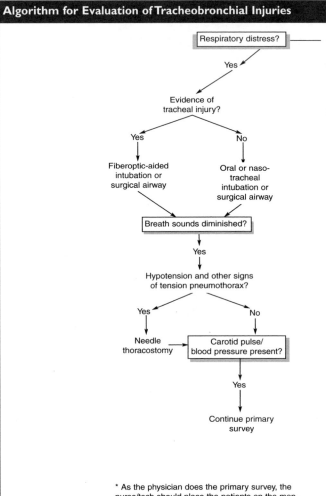

Respiratory distress?

Yes

Evidence of
tracheal injury?

Yes — Fiberoptic-aided intubation or surgical airway

No — Oral or naso-tracheal intubation or surgical airway

Breath sounds diminished?

Yes

Hypotension and other signs of tension pneumothorax?

Yes — Needle thoracostomy

No — Carotid pulse/blood pressure present?

Yes

Continue primary survey

* As the physician does the primary survey, the nurse/tech should place the patients on the monitors, draw blood for type and screen/cross or other labs, and establish large bore peripheral IVs.

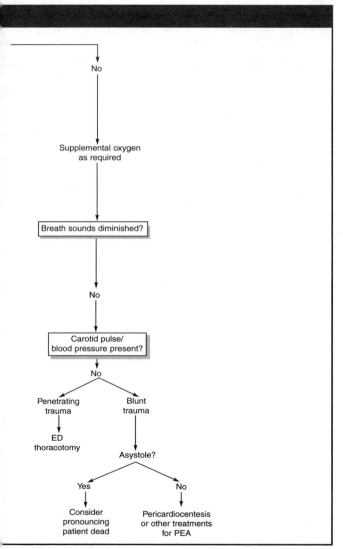

Differential Diagnosis and Radiographic Findings in Chest Trauma

INJURY	SYMPTOMS/SIGNS
ESOPHAGEAL	
	Chest pain, throat pain, fever, crepitus
TRACHEOBRONCHIAL	
	Dyspnea, dysphonia, hoarseness, hemoptysis crepitus, persistent air leak from chest tube
DIAPHRAGM	
	Asymptomatic, chest or abdominal pain, vomiting/signs of obstruction
PULMONARY CONTUSION	
	Dyspnea, tachypnea, hemoptysis, hypoxia, rales on ausculation
FLAIL CHEST	
	Paradoxical chest wall motion, chest pain, dyspnea, tachypnea, hypoxia
PNEUMOTHORAX	
	Diminished breath sounds on affected side, tympanitic to percussion, dyspnea, tachypnea, hypoxia
TENSION PNEUMOTHORAX	
	Signs of pneumothorax + jugular venous distension and/or hypotension, tracheal deviation away from the affected side
HEMOTHORAX	
	Diminished breath sounds on affected side, dullness to percussion, dyspnea, tachypnea, hypotension
TRAUMATIC ASPHYXIA	
	Cervicofacial cyanosis, facial petechiae, subconjunctival hemorrhage, periorbital edema, disorientation

X-RAY FINDINGS

Deep cervical emphysema, pneumomediastinum, pleural effusions

Deep cervical emphysema, pneumomediastinum, persistent pneumothorax after chest tube

Bowel gas or nasogastric tube in the chest, DPL fluid draining from chest tube, elevated or irregular contour of the diaphragm

None or patchy infiltrates on initial film; infiltrates on repeat chest film

3-4 contiguous rib fractures in two or more places

Pneumothorax

Do not wait for a chest x-ray to treat this injury

Hemothorax

None

Indications for Thoracotomy

- Initial chest tube output > 20 mL/kg
- Continued bleeding > 7 mL/kg/hr
- Increasing hemothorax seen on chest x-ray (CXR)
- Continued hypotension despite blood transfusion, after other causes of blood loss have been ruled out
- Decompensation after initial response to resuscitation

Source: Vukich DJ, Morkovchick V. Thoracic trauma. In: Rosen P, Barkin R. *Emergency Medicine: Concepts and Clinical Practice*. Fourth ed. Mosby; 1998.

Resuscitative Thoracotomy Rules

INDICATIONS	CONTRAINDICATIONS
Penetrating thoracic trauma	No qualified surgeon present
Pulseless electrical activity	Blunt injury
	Pulseless, without electrical activity

Source: Subcommittee on Advanced Trauma Life Support of the American College of Surgeons Committee on Trauma, 1993-1997. Thoracic Trauma. In: *Advanced Trauma Life Support*. Chicago: American College of Surgeons; 1997.

Radiographic Findings in Mediastinal Hematoma

FINDING	SENSITIVITY	SPECIFICITY
Mediastinal widening	50-90%	10%
Depression of the left mainstem bronchus	70-80%	80-100%
Deviation of nasogastric tube	23-71%	90-94%
Lateral displacement of trachea	12-100%	80-95%
Left apical pleural cap	20-63%	75-76%
Loss of paravertebral pleural stripe		
Obscured aortic knob		
Widened paratracheal stripe		

HEAD TRAUMA/ SUBDURAL HEMATOMA

Important Historical Facts in Head Injury

MECHANISM OF INJURY

— Condition of car (drivable, windshield, deployment of airbags, steering column)

— Height of fall, landing surface, number of steps

COMORBIDITIES

— Past medical history (coagulopathy, chronic alcoholism, hemophilia)

— Medication history (warfarin)

— Complaints preceding trauma (chest pain, dizziness, headache)

— Drug/alcohol ingestion

CONDITION POST INJURY

— Seizures

— Duration of loss of consciousness

— Repetitive questioning

— Amnesia to event

— Compared to baseline

— Other injuries

Adapted from: Biros MH. Head Trauma. In: Rosen P, Barkin R, eds. *Emergency Medicine: Concepts and Clinical Practice.* 4th ed. Mosby-Year Book; 1998.

Abridged Neurological Examination in the Severe Traumatic Brain Injury (TBI) Patient

- Mental status
- Glasgow Coma Scale
- Pupils (size, responsiveness, asymmetry)
- Motor exam (symmetry, abnormal movements, strength, reflexes)
- Cranial nerves (gag reflex, corneal reflex)
- Brainstem function (respiratory rate and pattern, eye movements)

Adapted from: Biros MH. Head Trauma. In: Rosen P, Barkin R, eds. *Emergency Medicine: Concepts and Clinical Practice.* 4th ed. Mosby-Year Book; 1998.

The Glasgow Coma Scale

EYE OPENING

Spontaneously	4	Reticular activating system is intact; patient may not be aware
To verbal command	3	Opens eyes when told to do so
To pain	2	Opens eyes in response to pain
None	1	Does not open eyes to any stimuli

VERBAL RESPONSE

Oriented—converses	5	Relatively intact CNS. Aware of self and environment
Disoriented—converses	4	Well articulated, organized, but patient is disoriented
Inappropriate words	3	Random, exclamatory words
Incomprehensible	2	Moaning, no recognizable words
No response	1	No response or intubated

MOTOR RESPONSE

Obeys verbal commands	6	Readily moves limbs when told to
Localizes to painful stimuli	5	Moves limb in an effort to remove painful stimuli
Flexion withdrawal	4	Pulls away from pain in flexion
Abnormal flexion	3	Decorticate rigidity
Extension	2	Decerebrate rigidity
No response	1	Hypotonia, flaccid: suggests loss of medullary function or concomitant spinal cord injury

Adapted from: Teasdale G, Jennett B. Assessment of coma and impaired consciousness: A practical scale. *Lancet* 1984;2:81-84.

ABDOMINAL TRAUMA

Algorithm for Managing Blunt Abdominal Trauma

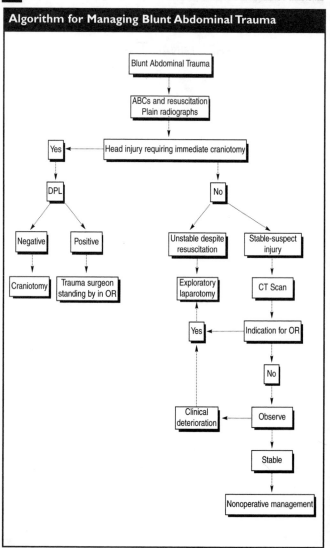

UROLOGIC EMERGENCIES

Differential Diagnosis of the Acute Scrotum

EMERGENT	NON-EMERGENT
Testicular torsion	Appendage torsion
Fournier's gangrene	Acute epididymitis
Abdominal aortic aneurysm	Testicular/scrotal abscess
Traumatic testicular rupture	Testicular cancer with bleeding
Peritonitis with patent processus vaginalis	Renal colic
Incarcerated inguinal hernia	Hydrocele
	Varicocele
	Henoch-Schonlein purpura
	Orchitis

Differentiating Acute Epididymitis from Testicular Torsion

	TESTICULAR TORSION	EPIDIDYMITIS
Average age	14 years (and neonate)	25 years
Pain	Sudden onset (usually)	Gradual onset
	Not affected by position	Worse when standing
Onset	After exercise or sleep	Rarely after sleep
Time to presentation	< 6 hours	> 24 hours
Past episodes	Frequently > 2 weeks past	Only if previous infection
Severity	Peaks in hours	Peaks in days
Vomiting	Common from pain	Unusual
Fever	Up to 20%	Up to 95%
Testicle swelling	Only after about 12 hours	Common
Dysuria or discharge	Rare	Common
Urinalysis	30% have WBCs/ bacteria	50% may be normal
	Voiding complaints rare	Have voiding complaints
Physical exam	Non-tender prostate	Prostate tender
Color Doppler*	Decreased testicular flow	Increased flow

*Imaging studies always are indicated in differentiating between these two disorders.

PSYCHIATRIC EMERGENCIES

ALTERED MENTAL STATUS IN THE ELDERLY

Sedating Drugs to Decrease Agitation in the Elderly

DRUG	DOSE	FREQUENCY
Haloperidol	0.5-2.0 mg IM IV PO	every 30-60 min
Droperidol	5 mg IM IV	every 30 min
Lorazepam	0.5-1.0 mg IM	every 60 min
Phenobarbital	150-100 mg IM IV	every 60 min

Confusion Assessment Method

ACUTE ONSET AND FLUCTUATING COURSE AND INATTENTION

Evidence of an acute change from baseline

Behavior increasing or decreasing in severity

Difficulty focusing attention

Easily distracted

Difficulty keeping track of what was said

OR

DISORGANIZED THINKING AND ALTERED LEVEL OF CONSCIOUSNESS

Rambling or irrelevant conversation

Unclear or illogical flow of ideas

Unpredictable switching from subject to subject

Hyperalertness or lethargy

SIDE EFFECTS

Orthostatic hypotension, decrease in seizure threshold, dystonic reaction, neuroleptic malignant syndrome

Same as haloperidol

Respiratory depression, orthostatic hypotension

Cardiovascular and respiratory depression

Mini Mental Status Exam

		Max. Points
Orientation	date	5
	place	5
Registration	recall three objects	3
Attention	serial 7's, 'world' spelled backwards, backward counting	5
Recall	three objects recalled later	3
Language	name pencil, wristwatch	2
	repeat "no if, ands, or buts"	1
	follow three-part command	3
	read and obey "close your eyes"	1
	write a sentence	1
	copy a design	1

SCORING

A score of 30 is considered normal. Scores are intended to monitor the patient's progress over time.

Assessment Algorithm for Altered Mental Status

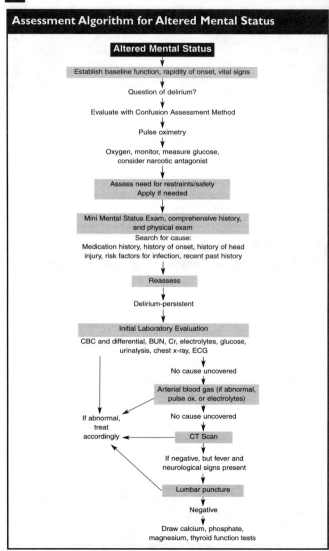

Altered Mental Status

Establish baseline function, rapidity of onset, vital signs

Question of delirium?

Evaluate with Confusion Assessment Method

Pulse oximetry

Oxygen, monitor, measure glucose,
consider narcotic antagonist

Assess need for restraints/safety
Apply if needed

Mini Mental Status Exam, comprehensive history,
and physical exam

Search for cause:
Medication history, history of onset, history of head
injury, risk factors for infection, recent past history

Reassess

Delirium-persistent

Initial Laboratory Evaluation

CBC and differential, BUN, Cr, electrolytes, glucose,
urinalysis, chest x-ray, ECG

No cause uncovered

Arterial blood gas (if abnormal,
pulse ox. or electrolytes)

No cause uncovered

If abnormal,
treat
accordingly   CT Scan

If negative, but fever and
neurological signs present

Lumbar puncture

Negative

Draw calcium, phosphate,
magnesium, thyroid function tests

ONCOLOGIC/HEMATOLOGIC
EMERGENCIES

ONCOLOGIC
EMERGENCIES

Presentation of Superior Vena Cava Syndrome*

- Extreme fatigue (due to poor blood return to the right side of the heart)
- Dyspnea
- Chest pain
- Headache
- Face and neck swelling (e.g., Stokes sign)
- Flushing
- Poor vision
- Syncope
- Confusion

*These symptoms most often are notable upon awakening.

Common Lab Test Results in Patients with Tumor Lysis Syndrome

- Elevated blood urea nitrogen level
- Elevated creatinine level
- Elevated potassium level
- Elevated phosphorus level
- Elevated uric acid level
- Decreased serum calcium level
- Urine (evidence of hematuria and crystals)
- Electrocardiographic abnormalities (depend on degree of electrolyte abnormality, commonly will reflect findings consistent with hyperkalemia)

Common Physical Findings in Patients with Brain Metastasis

- Headache (retro-orbital, associated with nausea and vomiting)
- Blurred and double vision or visual field defects (if cranial nerves involved)
- Alterations in mental status (if the ICP continues to worsen)
- Focal neurologic deficits (e.g., motor or sensory deficits, dysphasia, cerebellar symptoms, changes in personality, and seizures)

Cancers that Commonly Cause Hypercalcemia

SOLID TUMORS:

- Non-small cell lung cancer
- Squamous cell cancers of the head and neck
- Breast cancer
- Renal cell carcinoma
- Cholangiocarcinoma

HEMATOLOGIC CANCERS:

- Multiple myeloma and lymphoma (most common)

Possible Physical Examination Findings in Pericardial Disease Related to Malignancy*

MORE COMMON FINDINGS:

- Tachycardia
- Jugular venous distention
- Hepatic engorgement
- Poor peripheral effusion
- Paradoxical pulse (if the patient is severely dehydrated, the classic features of pericardial tamponade may be absent)
- Pericardial friction rub (though uncommon)

IN SEVERE CASES:

- Hypotension
- Tachycardia
- Cyanosis
- Altered mental status
- Narrowed pulse pressure

* Onset of symptoms may be abrupt or develop slowly over a prolonged period of time.

Criteria for Diagnosis of Hyponatremia Resulting from Syndrome of Inappropriate Antidiuretic Hormone (SIADH)*

- Hyponatremia with hypo-osmolality

- Elevated renal excretion of sodium (> 20 mEq/L)

- Normal volume status

- Inappropriately elevated urine osmolality for the plasma osmolality

* No diuretics and no evidence of pre-existing renal disease, adrenal insufficiency, or hypothyroidism. Recent chemotherapeutic agents should be reviewed, and a search for pulmonary and central nervous system disease.

* SIADH = Syndrome of Inappropriate Antidiuretic Hormone

Physical Examination Findings Common in Epidural Spinal Cord Compression (ESCC)

— Midline bony tenderness (as the compression increases, patient may develop objectively measurable sensory loss distal to the lesion)

— Ataxic gait

— Bilateral weakness

— Autonomic dysfunction (e.g., bowel or bladder dysfunction develops late and parallels the development of weakness)

Diagnosis of Hyperviscosity Syndrome (HVS)

CLASSIC TRIAD:

- Bleeding symptoms (e.g., gingival bleeding, epistaxis, hematuria, and rectal and vaginal bleeding)

- Visual disturbances (e.g., early vision changes: blurring and diplopia that may progress to vision loss. Physical examination may show papilledema, retinal hemorrhage, or retinal detachment.)

- Neurologic symptoms (e.g., headache, vertigo, ataxia, paresthesias, and mental status changes)

Diagnosis of Neutropenic Fever

DEFINITION:

Neutropenia with a single temperature elevation of > 101.3°F, or recurrent temperature elevations of 100.4°F occur over a 24-hour period

PHYSICAL EXAMINATION:

— Evaluate common areas of infection: e.g., sinuses, throat, skin, lungs, urinary tract, prostate, and perirectal area.

— Evaluate any indwelling devices for pain, swelling, redness, and drainage.

HEMATOLOGIC EMERGENCIES

Diseases Related to Abnormal Bleeding Times or Platelet Function/Count

LABORATORY TESTING	DISEASE OR CAUSE
Prolonged aPTT/normal PT	Hemophilias A and B, moderate to severe von Willebrand's disease, heparin therapy
Prolonged PT/normal aPTT	Factor VII deficiency, mild liver disease, initial coumadin therapy, vitamin K deficiency
Prolonged PT and aPTT	Severe liver disease, heparin and coumadin use, DIC, afibrinogenemia
Decreased platelet count	Decreased platelet production, increased platelet destruction, splenic sequestration
Abnormal bleeding time	Thrombocytopenia, von Willebrand's disease, aspirin use, nonsteroidal use, uremia, liver disease, cancer, other drugs

Laboratory Tests and Abnormalities Associated with von Willebrand's Disease

TESTS:

Bleeding time
Activated partial thromboplastin time (aPTT)
Factor VIII coagulant activity
vWF antigen
vWF activity

COMMON ABNORMALITIES:

Prolonged bleeding time
Low or normal vWF antigen
Low vWF activity
Factor VIII activity may be variable
aPTT activity may be variable

Manifestations of Thrombotic Thrombocytopenia Purpura

HEMOLYTIC ANEMIA

Microangiopathic hemolytic anemia manifesting with high lactic dehydrogenase (LDH) and a blood smear with helmet cells and schistoctes.

THROMBOCYTOPENIA

Moderate to severe thrombocytopenia with increased marrow megakaryocytes. Patients may have mucosal bleeding, petechiae, and purpura.

FEVER

Varies in elevation, but may be very high.

CNS SIGNS AND SYMPTOMS

Transient agitation, headache, and disorientation rapidly may progress to: aphasia, seizures, hemiparesis, focal deficits, coma, death.

RENAL DISEASE

Moderate elevation of creatinine and urine protein. Hematuria may be present.

Drugs Causing Immune-Mediated Thrombocytopenia

- Quinine
- Quinidine
- Gold salts
- Sulfonamides
- Digitoxin
- Heparin
- Indomethacin
- Rifampin
- Glycoprotein IIb-IIIa receptor antagonists
- Aspirin
- Furosemide
- Procainamide
- Ranitidine
- Cocaine
- Amidarone
- Valproic acid
- Heroin

Production Deficits Leading to Thrombocytopenia

Type	Acquired/ Congenital	Disorder
	Congenital	Fanconi's syndrome
		Alport's syndrome
		Neonatal rubella/CMV
Platelet		Maternal thiazides
Production	Acquired	Marrow aplasia or hypoplasia
Deficit	Acquired	Marrow infiltration, pancytopenia
	Acquired	Impairment of platelet line production
	Acquired	Inadequate megakaryopoiesis

Acute Chest Syndrome in Sickle Cell Disease

ACUTE CHEST SYNDROME:

Any acute illness with a new pulmonary infiltrate found on radiograph

Onset of chest pain associated with fall in hemoglobin level from normal baseline

PRESENTING SIGNS:

Pleuritic chest pain
Fever
Cough (usually nonproductive)
Tachypnea

TREATMENT:

Closely monitor fluid status
Oxygen
Pain control
Broad-spectrum antibiotics
Transfusion or exchange transfusion (associated with improvement)

CAUSE

Radiation, cytotoxic drugs, idiopathic, renal failure

Leukemia, lymphoma, marrow fibrosis

Multiple medications, infections

Nutritional deficiency (vitamin B_{12}, folic acid), alcohol abuse, myelodysplastic syndrome

Febrile Transfusion Reactions

CLINICAL PRESENTATION:

Mild temperature elevation to fever

Rigors

Headache

Myalgias

Vital sign abnormality

Dyspnea

Chest pain

TREATMENT AND PREVENTION:

Antipyretics (premedication with diphenhydramine and acetaminophen may help prevent)

If recurrent, leukocyte-reduced blood products may be helpful

Causes of Increased Platelet Destruction Leading to Thrombocytopenia

TYPE	DISORDER
Increased platelet destruction or removal	Increased destruction by immune mechanism
	Increased destruction by nonimmune mechanism
	Other causes

ETIOLOGY

Idiopathic thrombocytopenic purpura

Post-transfusion

Systemic lupus erythematosis

Graves' disease

Medication-related antibody production (i.e., heparin, quinine, glycoprotein IIb-IIIa antagonists)

Infections

Sepsis/DIC/infection

Snake envenomation

Extensive burn

Preeclampsia and HELLP syndrome

Vasculitis

Thrombotic thrombocytopenic purpura

Hemolytic-uremic syndrome

Massive transfusion

Aortic valve disease

Fat embolism

von Willebrand's disease (type IIB and platelet T-type)

Giant hemangioma

Hypersplenism, heat stroke, hypothermia, HIV

Factor IX Concentrates Currently Available for the Treatment of Hemophilia B[*]

LOW-PURITY FACTOR IX PROTHROMBIN COMPLEX CONCENTRATES

Bebulin VH *(Immuno)*

Profilnine *(Alpha)*

Proplex T *(Baxter - Hyland)*

Konyne 80 *(Bayer - Miles)*

ACTIVATED FACTOR IX PROTHROMBIN COMPLEX CONCENTRATES

(For use in patients with factor VIII or IX inhibitors)

Autoplex T *(Baxter - Hyland)*

FEIBA VH *(Immuno)*

COAGULATION FACTOR IX PRODUCTS

High-purity factor IX
— AlphaNine SD *(Alpha)*

Monoclonal antibody-purified factor IX
— Mononine *(Centeon)*

RECOMBINANT FACTOR IX—SYNTHETIC

Benefix *(Genetics Institute)*

[*] References: Cohen AJ, Kessler CM. Treatment of inherited coagulation disorders. *Am J Med* 1995;99:675-682; DiMichele D, Neufeld EJ. Hemophilia. *Hematol Oncol Clin North Am* 1998;12:1315-1344; Hemophilia Program Fact Sheet, updated 4/99. Available at http://www.mchb.hrsa.gov.; Lusher JM. Transfusion therapy in congenital coagulopathies. *Hematol Oncol Clin North Am* 1994;8:1167-1180.

Factor VIII Concentrates Currently Available for Treatment of Hemophilia A*

INTERMEDIATE AND HIGH-PURITY FACTOR VIII PRODUCTS

Factor VIII SD *(New York Blood Center)*

Humate-P *(Behringwerke)*

Profilate OSD *(Alpha)*

Melate *(New York Blood Center)*

Koate HP *(Bayer - Miles)*—High purity

Alphanate *(Alpha)*—High purity

Hyate:C *(Speywood/Porton)*—Porcine plasma
(For use in persons with factor VIII inhibitors)

MONOCLONAL ANTIBODY-PURIFIED FACTOR VIII PRODUCTS

Monoclate P *(Armour)*

Hemofil M *(Baxter - Hyland)*

AHF Method M *(Red Cross)*

RECOMBINANT FACTOR VIII PRODUCTS—SYNTHETIC

Recombinate *(Baxter)*

Bioclate *(Centeon)*—Identical to Recombinate

Kogenate *(Bayer - Miles)*

Helixate *(Centeon)*—Identical to Kogenate

---

* References: Cohen AJ, Kessler CM. Treatment of inherited coagulation disorders. *Am J Med* 1995;99:675-682; DiMichele D, Neufeld EJ. Hemophilia. *Hematol Oncol Clin North Am* 1998;12:1315-1344; Hemophilia Program Fact Sheet, updated 4/99. Available at http://www.mchb.hrsa.gov.; Lusher JM. Transfusion therapy in congenital coagulopathies. *Hematol Oncol Clin North Am* 1994;8:1167-1180.

Pathways of Secondary Hemostasis (Coagulation Cascade System)

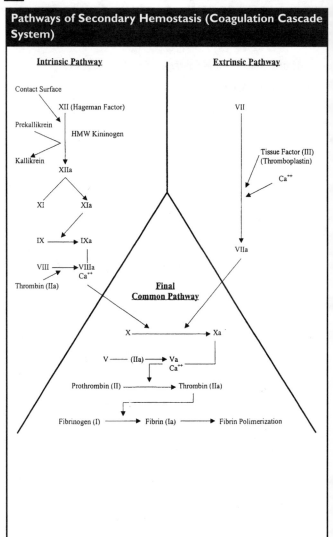

INDEX

Figures and Tables by Title

DIAGNOSTIC AIDS BY DISEASE STATES

ST-ELEVATION MYOCARDIAL INFARCTION (STEMI):
Site-, Specialty-, and Spectrum-of-Care Strategies for Outcome-Effective Management
CATH Panel SOS-ACS Guidelines and Recommendations

ACS CARE LEVEL: A SITE

Interventional cardiology services are available, PCI is the dominant strategy for patients with STEMI, and coronary artery bypass graft (CABG) is available: ACS Care Level A institutions maintain cardiac catheterization facilities and skilled interventional operators capable of performing cardiac angiography and percutaneous coronary intervention (PCI), as well as facilities for performing CABG. As a result, interventional strategies will dominate management of STEMI patients at these sites, and pharmacological antithrombotic therapy should be consistent with this approach.

Level A Site:

EMERGENCY DEPARTMENT

At ACS Care Level A site, STEMI patients should be managed with PCI as the dominant strategy. Pharmacological stabilization and antithrombotic therapy prior to PCI should include:

- **Aspirin 162-325 mg PO**
- **UFH or enoxaparin**

If patient is to be transferred directly from the emergency department to the cardiac catheterization laboratory to undergo coronary angiography and possible PCI, the emergency physician, in consultation with the interventional cardiologist, may initiate antiplatelet therapy with the GP IIb/IIIa inhibitor abciximab in addition to the core regimen above:

- **Abciximab (0.25 mg/kg bolus IV, followed by 0.125 mcg/kg/min [max 10 mcg/min] infusion for 12 hrs).** (Alternative GP IIb/IIIa inhibitor for primary PCI: eptifibatide, 180 mcg/kg IV bolus x 2, 10 min apart, followed by 2.0 mcg/kg/min infusion for 18-24 hrs.)

As dictated by clinical presentation and need to implement appropriate measures for acute medical management of ischemic chest pain, pulmonary edema, hypertension, and other hemodynamic abnormalities in the emergency department, the following agents may be initiated according to clinical protocols:

- Nitroglycerin IV/SC/TC/SL
- Morphine sulfate IV
- Lopressor 5 mg q 5 min x 3 doses

ST-ELEVATION MYOCARDIAL INFARCTION (STEMI):
Site-, Specialty-, and Spectrum-of-Care Strategies for Outcome-
Effective Management *(Continued)*

CATH Panel SOS-ACS Guidelines and Recommendations

ACS CARE LEVEL: A SITE *(continued)*

CARDIAC CATHETERIZATION LABORATORY/PCI

STEMI patients should undergo invasive assessment of their coronary anatomy with the intention for PCI in the cardiac catheterization laboratory. The pharmacological foundation regimen in these patients should include the following:

- **Abciximab (0.25 mg/kg bolus IV, followed by 0.125 mcg/kg/min [max 10 mcg/min] infusion for 12 hrs)** if not already started in the emergency department (alternative GP IIb/IIIa inhibitor for primary PCI: eptifibatide, 180 mcg/kg IV bolus x 2, 10 min apart, followed by 2.0 mcg/kg/min infusion for 18-24 hrs.)[1]

PLUS
- **Clopidogrel 300 mg loading dose**
- **Aspirin 162-325 mg PO**
- **UFH or enoxaparin**[2]

As dictated by clinical presentation and need to implement appropriate measures for acute management of ischemic chest pain, pulmonary edema, hypertension, and/or other hemodynamic abnormalities, adjunctive pharmacology should be employed per standard protocols.

INPATIENT CARE (STEP-DOWN UNIT/CORONARY CARE UNIT/MEDICAL INTENSIVE CARE UNIT)

After coronary angiography/PCI, the following pharmacological agents should be continued or initiated in the CCU or other inpatient setting prior to discharge:

- **Aspirin 162 mg PO QD**
- **Abciximab (continue infusion for 12 hours)** (alternative GP IIb/IIIa inhibitor for primary PCI: eptifibatide, 180 mcg/kg IV bolus x 2, 10 min apart, followed by 2.0 mcg/kg/min infusion for 18-24 hrs.)
- **Clopidogrel 75 mg PO QD**[3]

As dictated by presentation, and based on the presence of ischemic symptoms, abnormal hemodynamic parameters, cardiac risk factors, hypertension, diabetes, and/or left ventricular dysfunction, the following agents, if not contraindicated, should be considered for administration during acute hospitalization; when indicated, these agents should be continued for cardioprotection and/or management of symptoms following discharge:

- Statin therapy (within 96 hours of acute ischemic event)
- Beta-blockers
- ACE inhibitors
- Maintenance nitrate therapy

ACS CARE LEVEL: B SITE

Medical management is the dominant strategy at ACS Care Level B site, although rapid patient transfer is possible. Level B institution or site-of-care has no facilities for performing percutaneous coronary intervention (PCI), although transfer of STEMI patients to an institution capable of PCI is possible or likely.

Level B Site:

EMERGENCY DEPARTMENT

Medical Management (Fibrinolysis is Dominant Strategy at ACS Care Level B Site)[4]

Recommended First-Line Fibrinolytic Regimen*

- **Aspirin 162-325 mg PO**
- **Enoxaparin 30 mg IV bolus[5] followed by 1 mg/kg SC q 12 hrs** (maximum dose 100 mg SC q 12 hrs for first 24 hours)
- **Full-dose tenecteplase (TNK), weight-based dosing per package insert**

* **Alternative first-line fibrinolytic regimens:** tPA in combination with either of the following anticoagulant regimens: enoxaparin 30 mg IV bolus[5] followed by 1 mg/kg SC q 12 hrs, or unfractionated heparin (60 U/kg bolus, followed by 12 U/kg/hr); OR rPA in combination with UFH. As dictated by clinical presentation and need to implement appropriate measures for acute medical management of ischemic chest pain, pulmonary edema, hypertension, and other hemodynamic abnormalities in the emergency department, the following agents may be initiated according to clinical protocols:
- Nitroglycerin IV/SC/TC/SL
- Morphine sulfate IV

ST-ELEVATION MYOCARDIAL INFARCTION (STEMI):
Site-, Specialty-, and Spectrum-of-Care Strategies for Outcome-Effective Management (Continued)
CATH Panel SOS-ACS Guidelines and Recommendations

KEY

1 A GP IIb/IIIa inhibitor (abciximab) should be used for rescue PCI in the STEMI patient. If PCI is performed after successful fibrinolysis, and following initial stabilization, a GP IIb/IIIa inhibitor is indicated but the choice of which agent is less clear.

2 Anticoagulation for STEMI patients undergoing PCI may be accomplished with either enoxaparin or UFH. Results of one study (ENTIRE-TIMI 23B) evaluating outcomes in STEMI patients undergoing fibrinolysis-facilitated mechanical reperfusion suggests anti-coagulation with enoxaparin ± 30 mg IV bolus infusion followed by 1 mg/kg SC q 12 hrs plus full-dose tenecteplase was preferable (less death/MI at 30 days) to full-dose tenecteplase plus UFH. Head-to-head studies comparing enoxaparin vs. UFH in STEMI patients undergoing PCI who are being treated with GP IIb/IIIa inhibitors are not current-ly available. Weight-adjusted heparin dosing can be utilized during PCI. In those not treated with a GP IIb/IIIa inhibitor, 100 IU/kg IV initially should be administered; the target ACT is 300-350 sec when measured by the Hemochron device. In those who are treated with a GP IIb/IIIa inhibitor, 60-70 IU/kg should initially be administered; the target ACT is generally given as 200-300 sec, with some recommending a target ACT of 200-250 sec. If, after sheath removal manual compression is to be utilized, sheaths can be removed when the ACT is < 180 sec. (Popma JJ, Ohman EM, Weitz J, et al. Antithrombotic thera-py in patients undergoing percutaneous coronary intervention. *Chest* 2001;119 (Suppl):321S-336S; Smith SC, Dove JT, Jacobs AK, et al. ACC/AHA guidelines for percu-taneous coronary intervention. *J Am Coll Cardiol* 2001;37:1-66.)

3 Although studies evaluating outcomes in STEMI patients placed on chronic clopidogrel therapy (plus aspirin) following PCI are not currently available, the CATH Panel recom-mends consideration of clopidogrel-based antiplatelet therapy in patients with document-ed coronary heart disease whether or not PCI is performed.

4 Patient transfer for cardiac catheterization/PCI is strongly recommended in STEMI patients who are unstable so they can receive definitive, interventional and/or cardiology-directed specialty care at appropriate sites of care.

5 Results from the ASSENT-3 PLUS study indicate that STEMI patients > 75 years of age who were treated in the prehospital setting with 30 mg IV enoxaparin followed by 1 mg/kg enoxaparin SC had a higher risk of intracranial hemorrhage than patients treated with UFH plus TNK. Consequently, until further data are forthcoming, it is recommended that in STEMI patients > 75 years of age who are managed using fibrinolysis, the 30 mg enoxaparin IV bolus dose be withheld, and that the subcutaneous dose of enoxaparin be reduced to 0.75 mg/kg SC q 12 hrs. In the ASSENT-3 trial, a maximum dose of 100 mg of enoxaparin was used for the first two doses of enoxaparin in the first 24 hours, after which full 1 mg/kg SC q 12 h dosing is resumed.

ACUTE CORONARY SYNDROME (NSTE-ACS)
Site-, Specialty-, and Spectrum-of-Care Strategies for Outcome-Effective Management
CATH Clinical Consensus Panel Guidelines and Recommendations

ACS CARE LEVEL: A SITE

Interventional cardiology services are available at ACS Care Level A sites; revascularization (PCI or CABG) is doimant strategy for appropriately selected ACS patients. ACS Care Level A institutions maintain cardiac catheterization facilities and skilled interventional operators capable of performing cardiac catheterization and percutaneous coronary intervention (PCI), as well as facilities for performing CABG. As a result, interventional strategies will dominate management of NSTE-ACS patients, and pharmacological antithrombotic therapy should be consistent with this approach.

Level A Site:

EMERGENCY DEPARTMENT

Initiate Risk Stratification and Pharmacological Antithrombotic Management

HIGH-RISK FEATURES PRESENT: NSTE-ACS patient with high-risk features and/or treatment trigger criteria will benefit from an interventional strategy, which is the evidence-based management option of choice for this subgroup of ACS patients. The antithrombotic regimen for NSTE-ACS patients for whom coronary angiography is planned should include:

- **Aspirin 162-325 mg PO** (immediately)
- **Clopidogrel 300 mg loading dose** (only if it is confirmed that patient is not a CABG candidate. If CABG is possible, clopidogrel should be withheld until coronary anatomy is defined at time of catheterization)
- **Enoxaparin 30 mg IV bolus** (optional[1]) **followed by 1 mg/kg SC q 12 hrs** (alternative: UFH)[2]

As dictated by clinical presentation and need to implement appropriate measures for acute medical management of ischemic chest pain, pulmonary edema, hypertension, and other hemodynamic abnormalities in the emergency department, the following agents may be initiated according to clinical protocols:

- Nitroglycerin IV/SC/TC/SL
- Morphine sulfate IV

PLUS *(GP IIb/IIIa inhibitor)*

ACS CARE LEVEL: A SITE *(continued)*

EMERGENCY DEPARTMENT *(CONTINUED)*

If patient is admitted from the emergency department to the hospital and it is anticipated that cardiac catheterization will be performed during the hospitalization, the emergency physician, in consultation with the interventional cardiologist, may initiate antiplatelet therapy with the GP IIb/IIIa receptor antagonist, eptifibatide, which should be added to the core regimen above:

- **Eptifibatide 180 mcg/kg IV bolus, followed by 2.0 mcg/kg/min infusion for 18-72 hrs** (alternative: tirofiban 0.4 mcg/kg loading dose, followed by 0.1 mcg/kg/min infusion for 48 hrs)

-------------------------------- *OR* --------------------------------

If patient is to be transferred directly from the emergency department to the cardiac catheterization laboratory to undergo cardiac catheterization for evaluation of coronary architecture and possible PCI, abciximab may be administered in the cardiac catheterization laboratory.

- **Abciximab (0.25 mg/kg bolus IV, followed by 0.125 mcg/kg/min [max 10 mcg/min] infusion for 12 hrs).** (Alternative GP IIb/IIIa inhibitor for primary PCI: eptifibatide 180 mcg/kg IV bolus x 2, 10 min apart, followed by 2.0 mcg/kg/min infusion for 18-72 hrs)

NO HIGH-RISK FEATURES: For the NSTE-ACS patient who does not have high-risk features or treatment trigger criteria[3] supporting inclusion of small molecule GP IIb/IIIa receptor antagonist, and in whom cardiac catheterization is not planned, initial management would include:

- **Aspirin 162-325 mg PO**
- **Clopidogrel 300 mg loading dose[4]**
- **Enoxaparin 30 mg IV bolus (optional[1]) followed by 1 mg/kg SC q 12 hrs** (alternative: UFH)[2]

As dictated by clinical presentation and need to implement appropriate measures for acute medical management of ischemic chest pain, pulmonary edema, hypertension, and other hemodynamic abnormalities in the emergency department, the following agents may be initiated according to clinical protocols:

- Nitroglycerin IV/SC/TC/SL
- Morphine sulfate IV

ACS CARE LEVEL: A SITE *(continued)*

CARDIAC CATHETERIZATION LABORATORY/PCI

NSTE-ACS patients with moderate- to high-risk features and/or aggressive treatment trigger points should undergo invasive assessment of their coronary anatomy. The pharmacological foundation regimen in those patients should include the following:

- **Aspirin 162-325 mg PO** (immediately, or in the emergency department)
- **Clopidogrel 300 mg loading dose** (to be initiated upstream only if it is confirmed that patient is not a CABG candidate; if CABG remains a therapeutic option, clopidogrel should be held until coronary anatomy is defined by cardiac catheterization)

PLUS *(LMWH)*[2]

- **Enoxaparin 30 mg IV bolus** (optional[1]) **followed by 1 mg/kg SC q 12 hrs** (for cardiac catheterization/PCI considerations, see dosing algorithm on next page),[5,6,7] initiated prior to catheterization upon initial presentation

PLUS *(GP IIb/IIIa Antagonist)*[8]

At PCI:
- **Abciximab (0.25 mg/kg bolus IV, followed by 0.125 mcg/kg/min [max 10 mcg/min] infusion for 12 hrs)**

---------- *OR* ----------

- **Eptifibatide 180 mcg/kg IV bolus x 2, 10 min apart, followed by 2.0 mcg/kg/min infusion for 18 hrs** (alternative: tirofiban 0.4 mcg/kg loading dose, followed by 0.1 mcg/kg/min infusion for 48 hrs)

IN-PATIENT CARE (STEP-DOWN, CORONARY CARE/MEDICAL INTENSIVE CARE UNIT)

POST-CARDIAC CATHETERIZATION
Subsequent inpatient pharmacological management will depend upon coronary anatomy findings at time of catheterization, whether or not stent insertion has been successfully completed, and/or if the patient has coronary anatomy that is conducive to and is scheduled for CABG.

In a patient who has undergone cardiac catheterization and is found to have normal coronary anatomy:
- **Aspirin 162 mg PO QD** (for insignificant CAD or for cardioprotection in patients with significant CAD risk factors)

ACS CARE LEVEL: A SITE *(continued)*

Enoxaparin Dosing Algorithm[5,6,7] for PCI

Therapeutic Anti-Xa Levels. To ensure that ACS patients promptly achieve therapeutic anti-Xa levels, a 30 mg IV loadng dose of enoxaparin is recommended, followed immediately by administration of 1 mg/kg SC q 12 hrs. Therapeutic anti-Xa levels also are achieved after ≥ **2 doses** of enoxaparin 1 mg/kg SC q 12 hrs have been administered, even in the absence of an initial loading dose.

If an initial 30 mg IV loading dose of enoxaparin has been administered, or ≥ 2 doses of SC enoxaparin have been administered (without IV loading dose):
  — If procedure is performed within 8 hours of the last SC dose, no additional enoxaparin needs to be administered.
  — If procedure is performed at a point within 8-12 hours of the last SC dose, 0.3 mg/kg enoxaparin IV should be administered in the catheterization laboratory.

If an initial 30 mg IV dose of enoxaparin has not been administered and if only one dose of SC enoxaparin has been administered (in a patient without an IV loading dose):
  — At time of procedure, patient should receive a booster dose of 0.3 mg/kg prior to catheterization/PCI. The ENOX clotting time may be measured in such patients; if it is found to be > 260 seconds, the booster dose may be withheld.

If no enoxaparin has been previously administered:
  — At time of procedure, 1.0 mg/kg enoxaparin IV should be administered in the catheterization laboratory if a GP IIb/IIIa inhibitor is not given; 0.75 mg/kg enoxaparin IV should be administered when a GP IIb/IIIa will be used.

Sheath Removal. Timing of sheath removal depends on a number of factors, among them, whether or not a closure device is employed and time and route of last enoxaparin dose:
  — Sheath can be removed 6-8 hours after the last SC dose of enoxaparin without a closure device, or immediately if a closure device has been employed.
  — Sheath can be removed 4 hours after the 0.3 mg/kg IV supplemental dose for the 8-12 hour group, as well as after the 1.0 mg/kg IV (0.75 mg/kg with a GP IIb/IIIa inhibitor) for the group undergoing PCI > 12 hours after their last SC dose or who have not received any pretreatment.

ACS CARE LEVEL: A SITE *(continued)*

IN-PATIENT CARE (STEP-DOWN, CORONARY CARE/MEDICAL INTENSIVE CARE UNIT) *(continued)*

POST-CARDIAC CATHETERIZATION *(continued)*

In a patient who has undergone cardiac catheterization, has had stent insertion, and is not going to CABG:
- **Aspirin 162 mg PO QD**
- **Clopidogrel 75 mg PO QD for 1 year** (assumes that 300 mg loading dose already given)
- **GP IIb/IIIa inhibitor:** (Continue 12 hours for abciximab; 18 hours for eptifibatide or tirofiban)

As dictated by the presence of ischemic symptoms, abnormal hemodynamic parameters, cardiac risk factors, hypertension, diabetes, and/or left ventricular dysfunction, the following agents, if not contraindicated, should be considered for administration during the acute hospitalization, and when indicated, should be continued for cardioprotection and/or management of symptoms following discharge:
- Statin therapy (within 96 hours of acute ischemic event)
- Beta-blockers
- ACE inhibitors
- Nitrate therapy

In a patient with anatomy appropriate for surgical revascularization, who is scheduled for and awaiting CABG:
- **Aspirin 325 mg PO QD**
- **Clopidogrel** (should be discontinued, with a plan to restart clopidogrel at 75 mg PO QD the day following surgery, provided there is no bleeding)
- **GP IIb/IIIa** (eptifibatide or tirofiban continued up to 4-6 hours before induction)
- **Enoxaparin** (discontinue 24 hours before surgery) OR
- **UFH** (continue up to the time of surgery)

As dictated by the presence of ischemic symptoms, abnormal hemodynamic parameters, cardiac risk factors, hypertension, diabetes, and/or left ventricular dysfunction, the following agents, if not contraindicated, should be considered for administration during the acute hospitalization, and when indicated, should be continued for cardioprotection and/or management of symptoms following discharge:
- Statin therapy (within 96 hours of acute ischemic event)
- Beta-blockers
- ACE inhibitors
- Nitrate therapy

ACS CARE LEVEL: A SITE *(continued)*

IN-PATIENT CARE (STEP-DOWN, CORONARY CARE/MEDICAL INTENSIVE CARE UNIT) *(continued)*

NO INITIAL CARDIAC CATHETERIZATION ··

Low-risk feature patients with NSTE-ACS who are are not undergoing cardiac catheterization and who are being managed medically in the hospital:

- Aspirin 162 mg PO QD
- Clopidogrel 75 mg PO QD
- Enoxaparin 1 mg/kg SC q 12 hrs (or UFH) x 3-8 days

As dictated by the presence of ischemic symptoms, abnormal hemodynamic parameters, cardiac risk factors, hypertension, diabetes, and/or left ventricular dysfunction, the following agents, if not contraindicated, should be considered for administration during the acute hospitalization, and when indicated, should be continued for cardioprotection and/or management of symptoms following discharge:

- Statin therapy (within 96 hours of acute ischemic event) • ACE inhibitors
- Beta-blockers   • Nitrate therapy

High-risk feature patients with NSTE-ACS who did not undergo cardiac catheterization initially, who are being managed medically in the hospital, but in whom cardiac catheterization prior to discharge is planned:

- Aspirin 162 mg PO QD
- Enoxaparin 30 mg IV (optional), **followed by 1 mg/kg SC q 12 hrs (or UFH) x 3-8 days**
- Eptifibatide 180 mcg/kg IV bolus, **followed by 2.0 mcg/kg/min infusion for 18-72 hours** (alternative: tirofiban)

As dictated by the presence of ischemic symptoms, abnormal hemodynamic parameters, cardiac risk factors, hypertension, diabetes, and/or left ventricular dysfunction, the following agents, if not contraindicated, should be considered for administration during the acute hospitalization, and when indicated, should be continued for cardioprotection and/or management of symptoms following discharge:

- Statin therapy (within 96 hours of acute ischemic event) • ACE inhibitors
- Beta-blockers   • Nitrate therapy

ACUTE CORONARY SYNDROME (NSTE-ACS)
Site-, Specialty-, and Spectrum-of-Care Strategies for Outcome-Effective Management *(Continued)*
CATH Clinical Consensus Panel Guidelines and Recommendations

ACS CARE LEVEL: B SITE

Level B Site:

Medical management is the dominant strategy at ACS Care Level B site, although patient transfer is possible and routinely can be facilitated for individuals with high-risk features requiring invasive care. Level B institution or site-of-care has no facilities for performing percutaneous cardiac catheterization, PCI, or CABG, but inter-institutional communication, physician-to-physician referrals, and transfer networks permit transfer of NSTE-ACS patient to a Level A institution.

EMERGENCY DEPARTMENT

Medical Management[9]
> *Initiate Risk Stratification*

> **NO HIGH-RISK FEATURES:** For the NSTE-ACS patient who does not have high-risk features or treatment trigger criteria,[3] initial medical management would include:

>> • **Aspirin 162-325 mg PO**
>> • **Enoxaparin 30 mg IV bolus (optional)[1] followed by 1 mg/kg SC q 12 hrs** (alternative: UFH)[2]
>> • **Clopidogrel 300 mg loading dose[4]** (assuming low likelihood of surgical revascularization)

> As dictated by clinical presentation and need to implement appropriate measures for acute medical management of ischemic chest pain, pulmonary edema, hypertension, and other hemodynamic abnormalities in the emergency department, the following agents may be initiated according to clinical protocols:

>> • Nitroglycerin IV/SC/TC/SL
>> • Morphine sulfate IV

> **HIGH-RISK FEATURES PRESENT:** For the NSTE-ACS patient who has high-risk features or treatment trigger criteria[3] supporting maximal medical therapy, addition of a small molecule GP IIb/IIIa receptor antagonist is recommended:

>> • To above regimen, add small molecule GP IIb/IIIa receptor antagonist, **eptifibatide**, 180 mcg/kg IV bolus, followed by 2.0 mcg/kg/min infusion for 18-72 hrs (alternative GP IIb/IIIa antagonist: tirofiban).[10]

ACUTE CORONARY SYNDROME (NSTE-ACS)
Site-, Specialty-, and Spectrum-of-Care Strategies for Outcome-Effective Management *(Continued)*
CATH Clinical Consensus Panel Guidelines and Recommendations

ACS CARE LEVEL: B SITE *(continued)*

INPATIENT CARE (STEP-DOWN, CORONARY CARE/MEDICAL INTENSIVE CARE UNIT)

Continue Medical Management and Ongoing Risk Feature Evaluation and Stratification:

NO HIGH-RISK FEATURES: During ongoing risk level stratification, in the NSTE-ACS patient who does not manifest highrisk features or treatment trigger criteria[1] that would support addition of small molecule GP IIb/IIIa receptor antagonist, continuing antithrombotic management should include:

- **Aspirin 162 mg PO QD**
- **Clopidogrel 75 mg PO QD[4]**
- **Enoxaparin 1 mg/kg SC q 12 hrs x 3-8 days** (alternative: UFH)[2]

As dictated by the presence of ischemic symptoms, abnormal hemodynamic parameters, cardiac risk factors, hypertension, diabetes, and/or left ventricular dysfunction, the following agents, if not contraindicated, should be considered for administration during the acute hospitalization, and when indicated, should be continued for cardioprotection and/or management of symptoms following discharge:

- Nitroglycerin IV/SC/TC/SL
- Morphine sulfate IV
- Statin therapy (within 96 hours of acute ischemic event)
- Beta-blockers
- ACE inhibitors

....

HIGH-RISK FEATURES PRESENT:[1] For the NSTE-ACS patient who has—or during ongoing risk stratification and evaluation develops—high-risk features or treatment trigger criteria[3] indicating need for maximal medical therapy, addition of a small molecule GP IIb/IIIa receptor antagonist is recommended. It also should be stressed that transfer to ACS Care Level A site is strongly recommended for NSTE-ACS patients with high-risk features.

- **Aspirin 162 mg PO QD**
- **Clopidogrel 75 mg PO QD[4]** (only if not CABG candidate)
- **Enoxaparin 1 mg/kg SC q 12 hrs x 3-8 days**
- **Eptifibatide 180 mcg/kg IV bolus, followed by required 2.0 mcg/kg/min infusion for 18-72 hrs** (alternative: tirofiban 0.4 mcg/kg loading dose, followed by 0.1 mcg/kg/min infusion for 48 hrs)

As dictated by the presence of ischemic symptoms, abnormal hemodynamic parameters, cardiac risk factors, hypertension, diabetes, and/or left ventricular dysfunction, the following agents, if not contraindicated, should be considered for administration during the acute hospitalization, and when indicated, should be continued for cardioprotection and/or management of symptoms following discharge:

- Nitroglycerin IV/SC/TC/SL
- Morphine sulfate IV
- Statin therapy (within 96 hours of acute ischemic event)
- Beta-blockers
- ACE inhibitors

ACS CARE LEVEL: B SITE *(continued)*

TRANSFER TO CARDIAC CATHETERIZATION LABORATORY/PCI (LEVEL A SITE)

Because ACS Care Level B sites-of-care do not maintain interventional cardiology capabilities, transfer to an ACS Care Level A site (interventional cardiology, PCI, and CABG services available) is strongly recommended for NSTE-ACS patients who present with or, during ongoing risk feature evaluation, manifest high-risk features and/or aggressive treatment trigger criteria. Patient outcomes in these high-risk patient subgroups are optimized using an invasive strategy.

KEY:

1 From a pharmacodynamic perspective, administration of a 30 mg IV bolus immediately prior to the first 1 mg/kg SC dose of enoxaparin permits the patient to promptly achieve therapeutic factor anti-Xa levels; therefore, when prompt/immediate PCI is possible, administration of 30 mg IV enoxaparin bolus (followed by 1 mg/kg SC q 12 hrs) is recommended by the CATH Consensus Panel. When PCI is likely to be delayed, the possible advantages of a 30 mg IV bolus of enoxaparin is less well defined. It should be noted that the risk of bleeding associated with administration of an IV enoxaparin (30 mg) bolus dose plus a GP IIb/IIIa inhibitor is not known; however, the risk of bleeding associated with combined use of enoxaparin 1 mg/kg SC 12 hrs (i.e., no IV bolus) plus GP IIb/IIIa inhibitors has been shown to be comparable to, and in some studies lower than, bleeding resulting from combined use of unfractionated heparin (UFH) plus GP IIb/IIIa receptor antagonists. Use of an initial enoxaparin 30 mg IV bolus is not recommended in patients > age 75 who are concomitantly being treated with thrombolytics or GP IIb/IIIa inhibitors.

2 Unfractionated heparin (UFH) can be used as an alternative to enoxaparin. If UFH is used in the setting of PCI, activated clotting time (ACT) should be followed to achieve an appropriate level of anticoagulation. Use weight-based dosing according to guidelines. Weight-adjusted heparin dosing can be utilized during PCI. In those not treated with a GP IIb/IIIa inhibitor, 100 IU/kg IV should initially be administered; the target ACT is 300-350 sec when measured by the Hemochron device. In those who are treated with a GP IIb/IIIa inhibitor, 60-70 IU/kg should initially be administered; the target ACT is generally given as 200-300 sec, with some recommending a target ACT of 200-250 sec. If, after sheath removal manual compression is to be utilized, sheaths can be removed when the ACT is < 150-180 sec. (Popma JJ, Ohman EM, Weitz J, et al. Antithrombotic therapy in patients undergoing percutaneous coronary intervention. *Chest* 2001;119(Suppl):321S-336S; Smith SC, Dove JT, Jacobs AK, et al. ACC/AHA guidelines for percutaneous coronary intervention. *J Am Coll Cardiol* 2001;37:1-66.)

3 High-risk criteria that support more aggressive medical therapy (i.e., addition of small molecule GP IIb/IIIa inhibitor to aspirin, enoxaparin, and in most cases, clopidogrel) *and/or support invasive (mechanical or surgical) revascularization* include, but are not limited to the presence of one or more of the following: (1) elevated troponin level (or elevated CK-MB); (2) elevated C-reactive protein (CRP); (3) age > 65 years; (4) ST-T wave segment changes; (5) TIMI Risk Score greater than or equal to 5; and/or (6) failure to respond to maximal medical therapy. Additional factors that may suggest the need for more intensive medical therapy or support PCI as the dominant approach include the presence of heart failure, and other co-existing risk factors, which, at the clinician's discretion, suggest that maximally intensive pharmacotherapeutic approaches combined with interventional modalities will yield optimal patient outcomes.

KEY *(continued):*

4 Because clopidogrel increases the risk of bleeding in patients undergoing CABG, the decision to initiate clopidogrel therapy in the emergency department (prior to PCI) or in the peri-PCI period should be based primarily on whether the patient is likely to undergo CABG surgery. Unless contraindications exist, all patients with documented coronary heart disease should be discharged from the hospital on clopidogrel therapy for a minimum of 12 months. Clopidogrel is administered as a 300 mg loading dose, and 75 mg QD thereafter. It is the panel's recommendation that when clopidogrel therapy is initiated in patients who are not candidates for surgical revascularization, it should be initiated in the cath lab.

5 Enoxaparin-mediated anticoagulation for PCI is supported by pharmacokinetic modeling data showing that patients who have been receiving subcutaneously-administered enoxaparin for NSTE-ACS and who undergo PCI within 8 hours, will have anti-Xa levels in the range of 0.6-1.8 IU/mL. Those who have received an IV loading dose or two (2) or more doses of subcutaneous enoxaparin and undergo PCI 8-12 hours after the last SC dose achieve these levels with an additional "booster" dose of 0.3 mg/kg administered intravenously. Investigators have demonstrated that anti-Xa levels were generally within 10% of the predicted values, and in the targeted range in 96% of patients. If an initial 30 mg IV dose of enoxaparin has not been administered and if only one dose of SC enoxaparin has been administered (in a patient with out an IV loading dose), then at the time of procedure, patient should receive a booster dose of 0.3 mg/kg prior to catheterization/ PCI. The ENOX clotting time may be measured in such patients, and if it is found to be > 260 seconds, the booster dose may be withheld.

6 In conjunction with the dosing algorithm for enoxaparin presented above, interventional cardiologists may employ a point-of-care device approved for assessment of anticoagulation in patients receiving enoxaparin while undergoing PCI. Use of this tool should be considered in patients receiving subcutaneous doses, and/or in those in whom steady state levels may not have been achieved. Guidelines for its use and target values in the setting of PCI are presented (see table of enoxaparin dosing guidelines). Note: The activated clotting time (ACT) is not useful for assessing therapeutic levels or anticoagulation effects of enoxaparin and should not be monitored in patients receiving enoxaparin in the setting of PCI.

7 In patients with severe renal failure (Cr clearance < 30 mL/min) receiving enoxaparin, dose adjustment may be required. Consult the package insert for detailed dosing information.

8 If patient is not on GP IIb/IIIa inhibitor prior to PCI, use abciximab (0.25 mg/kg bolus IV, followed by 0.125 mcg/kg/min [max 10 mcg/min] infusion for 12 hrs) or eptifibatide (180 mcg/kg IV bolus x 2, 10 min apart, followed by 2.0 mcg/kg/min infusion for 18 hrs).

9 Patient transfer for cardiac catheterization/PCI is strongly recommended.

10 Tirofiban dosing (PRISM-PLUS, TIMI-18): 0.4 mcg/kg loading dose, followed by 0.1 mcg/kg/min infusion for 18 hours post PCI.

ENOXAPARIN DOSING GUIDELINES AND ALGORITHM FOR NSTE-ACS PATIENTS UNDERGOING PCI

DOSING GUIDELINES FOR INITIAL ENOXAPARIN-BASED ANTICOAGULATION THERAPY IN PATIENTS WITH NSTE-ACS:

General Recommendations. Enoxaparin 30 mg IV bolus (optional[1]) followed immediately by 1 mg/kg SC q 12 hrs (until diagnostic cardiac catheterization or for 72-96 hrs.). An IV bolus dose should be given when cardiac catheterization is to be performed before therapeutic factor anti-Xa levels are achieved, or shortly after presentation.

ENOXAPARIN DOSING GUIDELINES AND ALGORITHM[1-5] FOR PCI:

Therapeutic Anti-Xa Levels. To ensure that ACS patients promptly achieve therapeutic anti-Xa levels, a 30 mg IV loading dose of enoxaparin is recommended, followed immediately by administration of 1 mg/kg SC q 12 hrs. Therapeutic anti-Xa levels also are achieved after ≥ 2 doses of enoxaparin 1 mg/kg SC q 12 hrs have been administered, even in the absence of an initial loading dose.[6]

If an initial 30 mg IV loading dose of enoxaparin has been administered, or ≥ 2 doses of SC enoxaparin have been administered (with or without IV loading dose):

- If procedure is performed within 8 hours of the last SC dose, no additional enoxaparin needs to be administered.

- If procedure is performed at a point within 8-12 hours of the last SC dose, 0.3 mg/kg enoxaparin IV should be administered in the catheterization laboratory.

If an initial 30 mg IV dose of enoxaparin has not been administered and if only one dose of SC enoxaparin has been administered (in a patient without an IV loading dose):

- At time of procedure, patient should receive a booster dose of 0.3 mg/kg prior to catheterization/PCI. The ENOX clotting time may be measured in such patients, and if it is found to be > 260 seconds, the booster dose may be withheld.

If no enoxaparin has been previously administered:

- At time of procedure, 1.0 mg/kg enoxaparin IV should be administered in the catheterization laboratory if GP IIb/IIIa inhibitor is not given; 0.75 mg/kg enoxaparin IV should be administered when a GP IIb/IIIa will be used.

ENOXAPARIN DOSING GUIDELINES AND ALGORITHM[1-5] FOR PCI *(continued)*:

Sheath Removal. Timing of sheath removal depends on a number of factors, among them, whether or not a closure device is employed and time and route of last enoxaparin dose:

– Sheath can be removed 6-8 hours after the last SC dose of enoxaparin without a closure device, or immediately if a closure device has been employed.

– Sheath can be removed 4 hours after the 0.3 mg/kg IV supplemental dose for the 8-12 hour group, as well as after the 1.0 mg/kg IV (0.75 mg/kg with a GP IIb/IIIa inhibitor) for the group undergoing PCI > 12 hours after their last SC dose or who have not received any pretreatment.

ENOX CLOTTING TIME:[3] AN ALTERNATIVE AND ADJUNCTIVE STRATEGY USING A POINT OF CARE DEVICE

Times cited for the Pharmanetics® ENOX coag assay should be used only as guidelines for efficacy, based on clinical judgment and other factors. These parameters are based on corresponding anti-Xa activity and the results of the ELECT trial. It also should be emphasized that because of the predictable pharmacokinetic properties of enoxaparin, such monitoring is generally unnecessary, provided the time from last administration is known accurately. Clinicians should consult the ENOX® package insert for additional, detailed information.[7]

KEY

1 From a pharmacodynamic perspective, administration of a 30 mg IV bolus immediately prior to the first 1 mg/kg SC dose of enoxaparin permits the patient to promptly achieve therapeutic factor anti-Xa levels; therefore, when prompt/immediate PCI is possible, administration of 30 mg IV enoxaparin bolus (followed by 1 mg/kg SC q 12 hrs) is recommended by the CATH Consensus Panel. When PCI is likely to be delayed, the possible advantages of a 30 mg IV bolus of enoxaparin is less well defined. It should be noted that the risk of bleeding associated with administration of an IV enoxaparin (30 mg) bolus dose plus a GP IIb/IIIa inhibitor is not known; however, the risk of bleeding associated with combined use of enoxaparin 1 mg/kg SC 12 hrs (i.e., no IV bolus) plus GP IIb/IIIa inhibitors has been shown to be comparable, and in some studies lower than, bleeding resulting from combined use of unfractionated heparin (UFH) plus GP IIb/IIIa receptor antagonists. Use of an initial enoxaparin 30 mg IV bolus is not recommended in patients > 75 years of age who are concomitantly being treated with thrombolytic drugs.

KEY *(CONTINUED)*

2 This dosing regimen for enoxaparin-mediated anticoagulation for PCI is supported by pharmacokinetic modeling data showing that patients who have been receiving subcutaneously-administered enoxaparin for ACS for $\geq$ 24 hours and who undergo PCI within 8 hours will have anti-Xa levels in the currently recommended range of 0.6-1.8 IU/mL. Those who undergo PCI 8-12 hours after the last SC dose achieve these levels with an additional "booster" dose of 0.3 mg/kg administered intravenously. Investigators have demonstrated that anti-Xa levels were generally within 10% of the predicted values, and in the targeted range in 96% of patients. (Martin JL, Fry ETA, Serano A, et al. Pharmacokinetic study of enoxaparin in patients undergoing coronary intervention after treatment with subcutaneous enoxaparin in acute coronary syndromes. The PEPCI study. *Eur Heart J* 2001;22 (suppl):14.)

3 In conjunction with the dosing algorithm for enoxaparin, interventional cardiologists may employ a point-of-care device approved for assessment of anticoagulation in patients receiving enoxaparin while undergoing PCI. Use of this tool is may be considered in patients receiving SC doses, in whom steady state levels and/or therapeutic anti-Xa levels may not have been achieved. The device generates an ENOX clotting time. Guidelines for its use are presented in the table. Clinicians should consult the ENOX® package insert for additional, detailed information. The activated clotting time (ACT) is not useful for assessing therapeutic levels or anticoagulation effects of enoxaparin and should not be monitored in patients receiving enoxaparin in the setting of PCI.

4 In patients with severe renal failure (Cr clearance < 30 mL/min) receiving enoxaparin, dose adjustment may be required. Consult the package insert for detailed dosing information.

5 Precautions regarding enoxaparin use in "special patient groups" such as renal insufficiency (Cr > 2.5 g/dL, creatinine clearance < 30 cc/min), morbid obesity (arbitrarily > 150 kg), and the elderly (> 75 yrs) must be considered and dosage modifications should be made accordingly. As a rule, patients with renal dysfunction receiving < 4 doses are at low risk for drug accumulation and bleeding. However, when > 4 doses are required in patients with severe renal impairment, additional dosing should be guided by anti-Xa levels or patients should be switched to UFH. Similarly, levels of activity in morbidly obese patients may be unreliable. Elderly patients treated with an initial loading dose of enoxaparin and another class of antithrombotic agent (i.e., fibrinolytics or GP IIb/IIIa inhibitors) may be at increased risk for bleeding, including ICH, and may need to be managed with alternative agents or combinations.

KEY (CONTINUED)

6 Collet JP, Montalescot G, Golmard JL, et al. Safety and efficacy of subcutaneous enoxaparin in early invasive strategy of unstable angina. American College of Cardiology Poster Presentation, Apr. 1, 2003; presentation 1176-199.

7 ENOX® package insert. ENOX® is a trademark of Pharmanetics, Inc., Rapidpoint is a trademark of Bayer Corporation. Lovenox and Clexane are registered trademarks of Aventis Pharmaceuticals Products, Inc. © 2002 Pharmanetics, Inc. 9401Globe Center Drive, Morrisville, NC 27560 US Pats 4,849,340; 5,110,727; 5,350,676.

CME INSTRUCTIONS

Physicians participate in this CME program by reading the monographs, using the provided references for further research, and studying the questions. Participants should select what they believe to be the correct answers, then refer to the answer key (see below) to test their knowledge.

To clarify confusion surrounding any questions answered incorrectly, please consult the source material. **After completing this CME activity, you must complete the evaluation form included with this Quick Consult and return it to Thomson American Health Consultants to receive a certificate of completion.** When your evaluation is received, a certificate will be mailed to you. ■

Answer key:

Community-Acquired Pneumonia, pages 1-98
1. E; 2. E; 3. A; 4. E; 5. D; 6. B; 7. D; 8. A

Urinary Tract Infection, pages 99-154
9. B; 10. D; 11. A; 12. B; 13. A; 14. B; 15. E

OMBIRT, pages 155-224
16. D; 17. D; 18. C; 19. D; 20. D; 21. A; 22. D

Acute Coronary Syndromes, pages 225-270
23. E; 24. E; 25. C; 26. E; 27. A; 28. C; 29. A; 30. B

Evidence-Based, Outcome-Effective Management of Acute Coronary Syndromes: Management of Non ST-Elevation Myocardial Infarction

CEVAT (Centers of Excellence in Venous and Arterial Thrombosis) Leadership Council Guidelines and Protocols

PATIENT PRESENTS WITH CHEST PAIN OR POTENTIAL CHEST PAIN EQUIVALENT
(Jaw, shoulder, arm, back, or epigastric pain; unexplained dyspnea; syncope; palpitations, etc)

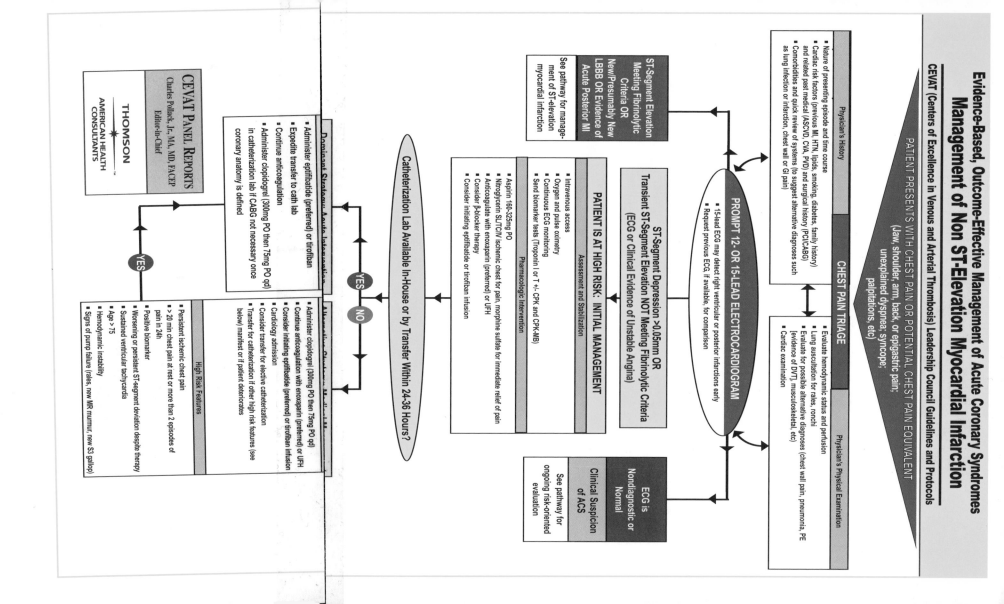

Physician's History

- Nature of presenting episode and time course
- Cardiac risk factors (previous MI, HTN, lipids, smoking diabetes, family history) and related past medical (ASCVD, CVA, PVD) and surgical history (PCI/CABG)
- Comorbidities and quick review of systems (to suggest alternative diagnoses such as lung infection or infarction, chest wall or GI pain)

CHEST PAIN TRIAGE

Physician's Physical Examination

- Evaluate hemodynamic status and perfusion
- Lung auscultation for rales, ronchi
- Evaluate for possible alternative diagnoses (chest wall pain, pneumonia, PE [evidence of DVT], musculoskeletal, etc)
- Cardiac examination

PROMPT 12- OR 15-LEAD ELECTROCARDIOGRAM

- 15-lead ECG may detect right ventricular or posterior infarctions early
- Request previous ECG, if available, for comparison

ST-Segment Elevation Meeting Fibrinolytic Criteria OR New/Presumably New LBBB OR Evidence of Acute Posterior MI

See pathway for management of ST-elevation myocardial infarction

ST-Segment Depression >0.05mm OR Transient ST-Segment Elevation NOT Meeting Fibrinolytic Criteria (ECG or Clinical Evidence of Unstable Angina)

PATIENT IS AT HIGH RISK: INITIAL MANAGEMENT

Assessment and Stabilization
- Intravenous access
- Oxygen and pulse oximetry
- Continuous ECG monitoring
- Send biomarker tests (Troponin I or T +/- CPK and CPK-MB)

Pharmacologic Intervention
- Aspirin 160-325mg PO
- Nitroglycerin SL/TC/IV ischemic chest for pain, morphine sulfate for immediate relief of pain
- Anticoagulate with enoxaparin (preferred) or UFH
- Consider β-blocker therapy
- Consider initiating eptifibatide or tirofiban infusion

ECG is Nondiagnostic or Normal

Clinical Suspicion of ACS

See pathway for ongoing risk-oriented evaluation

Catheterization Lab Available In-House or by Transfer Within 24-36 Hours?

YES

NO

Dominant Strategy: Acute Intervention

- Administer eptifibatide (preferred) or tirofiban
- Expedite transfer to cath lab
- Continue anticoagulation
- Administer clopidogrel (300mg PO then 75mg PO qd) in catheterization lab if CABG not necessary once coronary anatomy is defined

YES

Alternative Strategy: Medical Management

- Administer clopidogrel (300mg PO then 75mg PO qd)
- Continue anticoagulation with enoxaparin (preferred) or UFH
- Consider initiating eptifibatide (preferred) or tirofiban infusion
- Cardiology admission
- Consider transfer for elective catheterization
- Transfer for catheterization if other high risk features (see below) manifest or if patient deteriorates

NO

High Risk Features

- Persistent ischemic chest pain
- > 20 min chest pain at rest or more than 2 episodes of pain in 24h
- Positive biomarker
- Worsening or persistent ST-segment deviation despite therapy
- Sustained ventricular tachycardia
- Age > 75
- Hemodynamic instability
- Signs of pump failure (rales, new MR murmur, new S3 gallop)

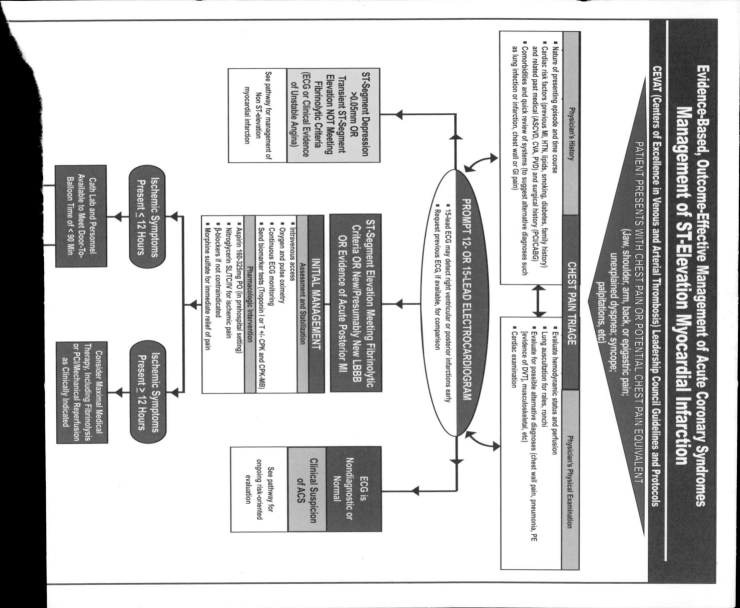

Evidence-Based, Outcome-Effective Management of Acute Coronary Syndromes
Management of ST-Elevation Myocardial Infarction

CEVAT (Centers of Excellence in Venous and Arterial Thrombosis) Leadership Council Guidelines and Protocols

PATIENT PRESENTS WITH CHEST PAIN OR POTENTIAL CHEST PAIN EQUIVALENT
(Jaw, shoulder, arm, back, or epigastric pain; unexplained dyspnea; syncope; palpitations, etc)

Physician's History
- Nature of presenting episode and time course
- Cardiac risk factors (previous MI, HTN, lipids, smoking, diabetes, family history) and related past medical (ASCVD, CVA, PVD) and surgical history (PCI/CABG)
- Comorbidities and quick review of systems (to suggest alternative diagnoses such as lung infection or infarction, chest wall or GI pain)

CHEST PAIN TRIAGE

Physician's Physical Examination
- Evaluate hemodynamic status and perfusion
- Lung auscultation for rales, ronchi
- Evaluate for possible alternative diagnoses (chest wall pain, pneumonia, PE [evidence of DVT], musculoskeletal, etc)
- Cardiac examination

PROMPT 12- OR 15-LEAD ELECTROCARDIOGRAM
- 15-lead ECG may detect right ventricular or posterior infarctions early
- Request previous ECG, if available, for comparison

ST-Segment Depression >0.05mm OR Transient ST-Segment Elevation NOT Meeting Fibrinolytic Criteria (ECG or Clinical Evidence of Unstable Angina)

See pathway for management of Non ST-elevation myocardial infarction

ST-Segment Elevation Meeting Fibrinolytic Criteria OR New/Presumably New LBBB OR Evidence of Acute Posterior MI

INITIAL MANAGEMENT

Assessment and Stabilization
- Intravenous access
- Oxygen and pulse oximetry
- Continuous ECG monitoring
- Send biomarker tests (Troponin I or T +/- CPK and CPK-MB)

Pharmacologic Intervention
- Aspirin 160-325mg PO (in prehospital setting)
- Nitroglycerin SL/TC/IV for ischemic pain
- β-blockers if not contraindicated
- Morphine sulfate for immediate relief of pain

Ischemic Symptoms Present ≤ 12 Hours

Cath Lab and Personnel Available to Meet Door-To-Balloon Time of < 90 Min

Ischemic Symptoms Present ≥ 12 Hours

Consider Maximal Medical Therapy, Including Fibrinolysis or PCI/Mechanical Reperfusion as Clinically Indicated

ECG is Nondiagnostic or Normal

Clinical Suspicion of ACS

See pathway for ongoing risk-oriented evaluation

YES →

Dominant Strategy — PCI/Mechanical Reperfusion
▪ Enoxaparin or UFH
▪ Consider IIb/IIIa receptor blockade in cath lab
▪ Administer clopidogrel as indicated in catheterization lab

NO →

Primary Alternative Strategy — Fibrinolysis Via ASSENT-3 Protocol
▪ Enoxaparin 30mg IV then 1mg/kg SQ q 12h
plus
▪ TNKase 30-50mg based on weight

Secondary Alternative Strategy* — Fibrinolysis Via Conventional Protocol
▪ Enoxaparin or UFH
plus
▪ tPA or rPA

* GUSTO-V supports the use of 1/2 dose rPA plus abciximab in STEMI patient < 75 years of age and non-diabetic. Risk of hemorrhage increased.

CEVAT PANEL REPORTS
Charles Pollack, Jr., MA, MD, FACEP
Editor-in-Chief

THOMSON
AMERICAN HEALTH CONSULTANTS

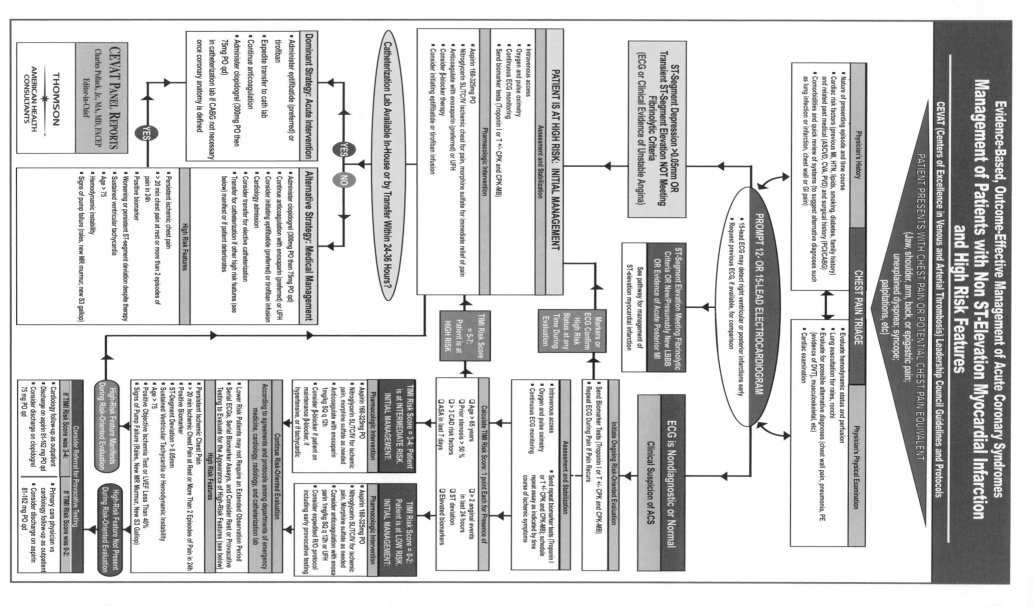

Evidence-Based, Outcome-Effective Management of Acute Coronary Syndromes
Management of Patients with Non ST-Elevation Myocardial Infarction and High Risk Features

CEVAT (Centers of Excellence in Venous and Arterial Thrombosis) Leadership Council Guidelines and Protocols

PATIENT PRESENTS WITH CHEST PAIN OR POTENTIAL CHEST PAIN EQUIVALENT
(Jaw, shoulder, arm, back, or epigastric pain; unexplained dyspnea; syncope; palpitations, etc)

CHEST PAIN TRIAGE

Physician's History
- Nature of presenting episode and time course
- Cardiac risk factors (previous MI, HTN, lipids, smoking, diabetes, family history) and related past medical (ASCVD, CVA, PVD) and surgical history (PCI/CABG)
- Comorbidities and quick review of systems (to suggest alternative diagnoses such as lung infection or infarction, chest wall or GI pain)

Physician's Physical Examination
- Evaluate hemodynamic status and perfusion
- Lung auscultation for rales, ronchi
- Evaluate for possible alternative diagnoses (chest wall pain, pneumonia, PE (evidence of DVT), musculoskeletal, etc)
- Cardiac examination

PROMPT 12- OR 15-LEAD ELECTROCARDIOGRAM
- 15-lead ECG may detect right ventricular or posterior infarctions early
- Request previous ECG, if available, for comparison

ST-Segment Elevation Meeting Fibrinolytic Criteria OR New/Presumably New LBBB OR Evidence of Acute Posterior MI
See pathway for management of ST-elevation myocardial infarction

ST-Segment Depression >0.05mm OR Transient ST-Segment Elevation NOT Meeting Fibrinolytic Criteria (ECG or Clinical Evidence of Unstable Angina)

ECG is Nondiagnostic or Normal
Clinical Suspicion of ACS

PATIENT IS AT HIGH RISK: INITIAL MANAGEMENT
Assessment and Stabilization
- Intravenous access
- Oxygen and pulse oximetry
- Continuous ECG monitoring
- Send biomarker tests (Troponin I or T +/- CPK and CPK-MB)

Pharmacologic Intervention
- Aspirin 160-325mg PO
- Nitroglycerin SL/TC/IV ischemic chest for pain, morphine sulfate for immediate relief of pain
- Anticoagulate with enoxaparin (preferred) or UFH
- Consider β-blocker therapy
- Consider initiating eptifibatide or tirofiban infusion

Markers or ECG Confirm High Risk Status at any Time During Evaluation

Catheterization Lab Available In-House or by Transfer Within 24-36 Hours?

YES → **NO**

Dominant Strategy: Acute Intervention
- Administer eptifibatide (preferred) or tirofiban
- Expedite transfer to cath lab
- Continue anticoagulation
- Administer clopidogrel (300mg PO then 75mg PO qd) in catheterization lab if CABG not necessary once coronary anatomy is defined

Alternative Strategy: Medical Management
- Administer clopidogrel (300mg PO then 75mg PO qd)
- Continue anticoagulation with enoxaparin (preferred) or UFH
- Consider initiating eptifibatide (preferred) or tirofiban infusion
- Cardiology admission
- Consider transfer for elective catheterization
- Transfer for catheterization if other high risk features (see below); manifest or if patient deteriorates

YES → **High Risk Features?**
High Risk Features
- Persistent ischemic chest pain
- > 20 min chest pain at rest or more than 2 episodes of pain in 24h
- Positive biomarker
- Worsening or persistent ST-segment deviation despite therapy
- Sustained ventricular tachycardia
- Age > 75
- Hemodynamic instability
- Signs of pump failure (rales, new MR murmur, new S3 gallop)

TIMI Risk Score = 5-7; Patient is at HIGH RISK

TIMI Risk Score = 3-4: Patient is at INTERMEDIATE RISK. INITIAL MANAGEMENT.

Pharmacologic Intervention
- Aspirin 160-325mg PO
- Nitroglycerin SL/TC/IV for ischemic pain, morphine sulfate as needed
- Anticoagulate with enoxaparin 1mg/kg SQ q 12h
- Consider β-blocker if patient on maintenance β-blocker, if hypertensive, or if tachycardic

Continue Risk-Oriented Evaluation
According to agreements and protocols among departments of emergency medicine, cardiology, radiology, and catheterization lab
- Lower Risk Patients may not Require an Extended Observation Period
- Serial ECGs, Serial Biomarker Assays, and Consider Rest or Provacative Testing to Evaluate for the Appearance of High-Risk Features (see below)

High Risk Features
- Persistent Ischemic Chest Pain
- > 20 min Ischemic Chest Pain at Rest or More Than 2 Episodes of Pain in 24h
- Positive Biomarker
- ST-Segment Deviation > 0.05mm
- Sustained Ventricular Tachycardia or Hemodynamic Instability
- Age > 75
- Positive Objective Ischemia Test or LVEF Less Than 40%
- Signs of Pump Failure (Rales, New MR Murmur, New S3 Gallop)

Calculate TIMI Risk Score; 1 point Each for Presence of
- ☐ Age > 65 years
- ☐ Prior stenosis > 50 %
- ☐ ≥ 3 CAD risk factors
- ☐ ASA in last 7 days
- ☐ > 2 anginal events in last 24 hours
- ☐ ST deviation
- ☐ Elevated biomarkers

Assessment and Stabilization
- Intravenous access
- Oxygen and pulse oximetry
- Continuous ECG monitoring
- Send repeat biomarker tests (Troponin I or T +/- CPK and CPK-MB); schedule repeat assay as indicated by time course of ischemic symptoms

Initiate Ongoing Risk-Oriented Evaluation
- Send repeat biomarker tests (Troponin I or T +/- CPK and CPK-MB)
- Repeat ECG During Pain if Pain Recurs

TIMI Risk Score = 0-2: Patient is at LOW RISK. INITIAL MANAGEMENT.

Pharmacologic Intervention
- Aspirin 160-325mg PO
- Nitroglycerin SL/TC/IV for ischemic pain, Morphine sulfate as needed
- Consider anticoagulation with enoxaparin 1mg/kg SQ q 12h or UFH
- Consider expedited R/O protocol including early provocative testing

---

High-Risk Feature Manifest During Risk-Oriented Evaluation

High-Risk Feature Not Present During Risk-Oriented Evaluation

Consider Referral for Provocative Testing

If TIMI Risk Score was 3-4:
- Cardiology follow-up as outpatient
- Discharge on aspirin 81-162 mg PO qd
- Consider discharge on clopidogrel 75 mg PO qd

If TIMI Risk Score was 0-2:
- Primary care physician vs cardiology follow-up as outpatient
- Consider discharge on aspirin 81-162 mg PO qd

CEVAT PANEL REPORTS
Charles Pollack, Jr., MA, MD, FACEP
Editor-in-Chief

THOMSON™
AMERICAN HEALTH CONSULTANTS